Global Women's Health

Editors

JEAN R. ANDERSON
CHI CHIUNG GRACE CHEN

OBSTETRICS AND GYNECOLOGY CLINICS OF NORTH AMERICA

www.obgyn.theclinics.com

Consulting Editor
WILLIAM F. RAYBURN

December 2022 • Volume 49 • Number 4

ELSEVIER

1600 John F. Kennedy Boulevard • Suite 1800 • Philadelphia, Pennsylvania, 19103-2899

http://www.theclinics.com

OBSTETRICS AND GYNECOLOGY CLINICS OF NORTH AMERICA Volume 49 Number 4
December 2022 ISSN 0889-8545, ISBN-13: 978-0-323-98713-4

Editor: Kerry Holland
Developmental Editor: Hannah Almira Lopez

Obstetrics and Gynecology Clinics (ISSN 0889-8545) is published quarterly by Elsevier Inc., 360 Park Avenue South, New York, NY 10010-1710. Months of issue are March, June, September, and December. Periodicals postage paid at New York, NY, and additional mailing offices. Subscription price per year is $345.00 (US individuals), $963.00 (US institutions), $100.00 (US students), $416.00 (Canadian individuals), $982.00 (Canadian institutions), $100.00 (Canadian students), $473.00 (international individuals), $982.00 (international institutions), and $225.00 (international students). To receive student/resident rate, orders must be accompanied by name of affiliated institution, date of term, and the signature of program/residency coordinator on institution letterhead. Orders will be billed at individual rate until proof of status is received. Foreign air speed delivery is included in all *Clinics* subscription prices. All prices are subject to change without notice. POSTMASTER: Send address changes to *Obstetrics and Gynecology Clinics*, Elsevier Health Sciences Division, Subscription Customer Service, 3251 Riverport Lane, Maryland Heights, MO 63043. **Customer Service: Telephone: 1-800-654-2452 (U.S. and Canada); 314-447-8871 (outside U.S. and Canada). Fax: 314-447-8029. E-mail: journalscustomerservice-usa@elsevier.com (for print support); journalsonlinesupport-usa@elsevier. com (for online support).**

Reprints. For copies of 100 or more of articles in this publication, please contact the Commercial Reprints Department, Elsevier Inc., 360 Park Avenue South, New York, New York 10010-1710. Tel.: 212-633-3874; Fax: 212-633-3820; E-mail: reprints@elsevier.com.

Obstetrics and Gynecology Clinics of North America is also published in Spanish by McGraw-Hill Interamericana Editores S.A., P.O. Box 5-237, 06500, Mexico; in Portuguese by Reichmann and Affonso Editores, Rio de Janeiro, Brazil; and in Greek by Paschalidis Medical Publications, Athens, Greece.

Obstetrics and Gynecology Clinics of North America is covered in MEDLINE/PubMed (Index Medicus), Excerpta Medica, Current Concepts/Clinical Medicine, Science Citation Index, BIOSIS, CINAHL, and ISI/BIOMED.

Contributors

CONSULTING EDITOR

WILLIAM F. RAYBURN, MD, MBA
Affiliate Professor, Department of Obstetrics and Gynecology and College of Graduate Studies, Medical University of South Carolina, Charleston, South Carolina, USA; Emeritus Distinguished Professor, Department of Obstetrics and Gynecology, University of New Mexico, School of Medicine, Albuquerque, New Mexico, USA

EDITORS

JEAN R. ANDERSON, MD
Professor Emerita, Gynecology and Obstetrics and Medicine; Past Director, Johns Hopkins HIV Women's Health Program and Johns Hopkins Global Women's Health Fellowship, Department of Gynecology and Obstetrics, Johns Hopkins Unviersity School of Medicine; Senior Technical Advisor, Jhpiego, Baltimore, Maryland, USA

CHI CHIUNG GRACE CHEN, MD, MHS
Associate Professor, Female Pelvic Medicine and Reconstructive Surgery, Director, Johns Hopkins Global Women's Health Fellowship, Department of Gynecology and Obstetrics, Johns Hopkins University School of Medicine, Baltimore, Maryland, USA

AUTHORS

ADENIYI KOLADE ADEROBA, MBBS, FWACS (OBGYN), FMCOG, MSc
Centre for Population Health and Interdisciplinary Research, HealthMATE 360, Ondo Town, Ondo State, Nigeria; National Perinatal Epidemiology Unit, Nuffield Department of Population Health, University of Oxford, Oxford, United Kingdom

KWAME ADU-BONSAFFOH, MBCHB, FWACS (OBGYN), MPhil (Physiology), MSc (Epidemiology)
Department of Obstetrics and Gynecology, University of Ghana Medical School, Department of Obstetrics and Gynecology, Korle-Bu Teaching Hospital, Accra, Ghana

TITUS K. BEYUO, BSC, MBCHB, MPHIL, MGCS, FWACS
Department of Obstetrics and Gynaecology, University of Ghana Medical School, Accra, Ghana

MOHAN CHANDRA REGMI, MBBS, MD
Professor of Obstetrics and Gynecology, BP Koirala Institute of Health Sciences, Dharan, Nepal

BENJAMIN H. CHI, MD, MSC
Department of Obstetrics and Gynecology, The University of North Carolina at Chapel Hill, Chapel Hill, North Carolina, USA

CARLA J. CHIBWESHA, MD, MSc
Clinical HIV Research Unit, Wits Health Consortium, Themba Lethu Clinic, Helen Joseph Hospital, Johannesburg, South Africa; Division of Global Women's Health, Department of Obstetrics and Gynecology, The University of North Carolina at Chapel Hill, Chapel Hill, North Carolina, USA

MEGAN A. COHEN, MD, MPH
Adjunct Faculty, Department of Obstetrics and Gynecology, Oregon Health & Science University, Portland, Oregon, USA; Assistant Professor, Division of Complex Family Planning, Department of Gynecology and Obstetrics, Emory University, Atlanta, Georgia, USA

JODIE A. DIONNE, MD, MSPH
Associate Professor, Department of Medicine, Division of Infectious Diseases, The University of Alabama at Birmingham, Birmingham, Alabama, USA

ALISON M. EL AYADI, ScD, MPH
Department of Obstetrics, Gynecology and Reproductive Sciences, University of California, San Francisco, San Francisco, California, USA

REINOU SYBRECHT GROEN, MD, MIH, PhD
OBGYN at Alaska Native Medical Center, Anchorage, Alaska, USA

MARK HATHAWAY, MD, MPH
Adjunct Assistant Professor, Johns Hopkins University, Technical Advisor for SRH/FP, Jhpiego, Baltimore, Maryland, USA; Medical Director, Carafem, Technical Advisor for Family Planning and Title X, Unity Health Care, Inc, Washington, DC, USA

LAURA KEYSER, PT, DPT, MPH
Department of Physical Therapy and Rehabilitation Science, University of California, San Francisco, San Francisco, California, USA

THOMAS J. KLEIN, MD, MPH
Department of Obstetrics and Gynecology, University of Michigan, Ann Arbor, Michigan, USA

SOMESH KUMAR, MBBS, MSc, PhD
Country Director, Jhpiego India, New Delhi, India; Senior Director, Technical Leadership and Innovations, Jhpiego, Associate Faculty, Johns Hopkins Bloomberg School of Public Health, Baltimore, Maryland, USA

EMMA R. LAWRENCE, MD, MS
Department of Obstetrics and Gynecology, University of Michigan, Ann Arbor, Michigan, USA

SAIFUDDIN T. MAMA, MD, MPH, FACOG, FACS
Associate Professor, Obstetrics and Gynecology, Division Head, FPMRS & MIGS, Cooper Medical School of Rowan University, Cooper University Health Care, Camden, New Jersey, USA

RAHA MAROYI, MD
Department of Urogynecology, Panzi General Reference Hospital, Faculty of Medicine, Evangelical University in Africa (U.E.A.), Bukavu, Democratic Republic of Congo

MWANGELWA MUBIANA-MBEWE, BSc, MBChB, MMed, MBA
Centre for Infectious Diseases Research, Lusaka, Zambia

DENIS MUKWEGE, MD, PHD
Department of Urogynecology, Panzi General Reference Hospital, Faculty of Medicine, Evangelical University in Africa (U.E.A.), Bukavu, Democratic Republic of Congo

MASANGU MULONGO, MBBCh
Clinical HIV Research Unit, Wits Health Consortium, Themba Lethu Clinic, Helen Joseph Hospital, Johannesburg, South Africa

NEIL JOSEPH MURPHY, MD
OBGYN at Alaska Native Medical Center, Anchorage, Alaska, USA

VICTOR MIVUMBI NDICUNGUYE, MD, MMed, MSc
Department of Reproductive, Maternal, Newborn, and Child Health, Jhpiego, Kigali, Rwanda

ALPHONSE N. NGALAME, MD, DES O&G, MPH
Department of Obstetrics and Gynecology, Faculty of Health Sciences, University of Buea, Buea, Cameroon

ANMOL PATTED, MBBS
MPH Graduate Student: Focus on Global Reproductive Health Systems and Policies, Johns Hopkins Bloomberg School of Public Health, Baltimore, Maryland, USA

KRISTA S. PFAENDLER, MD, MPH
Division of Gynecologic Oncology, WVU Cancer Institute Mary Babb Randolph Cancer Center, West Virginia University, Morgantown, West Virginia, USA

DAISY RUTO, MMED
Senior Technical Advisor, MNH and Safe Surgery, Jhpiego Kenya, Nairobi, Kenya

FRIDAY SAIDI, MBBS, MMED
UNC Project Malawi, Lilongwe, Malawi

ACHILLE VAN CHRIST MANIRAKIZA, MD
Oncology Service, Department of Medicine, King Faisal Hospital, Kigali, Rwanda

JOHN E. VARALLO, MD, MPH, FACOG
Global Director, Safe Surgery, Jhpiego, Washington, DC, USA

Contents

A life-course approach incorporating appropriate preconception and contraception care is key to achieving optimal maternal, neonatal, and child health outcomes. In low- and middle-income countries (LMIC), there is a large unmet need for contraception and an estimated 49% of pregnancies are unintended. In this article, we discuss preconception and contraception care in LMIC settings including key recommendations for content and service delivery. We discuss barriers and facilitators to contraceptive provision, discuss considerations for providers who may practice in LMIC settings, and highlight strategies for achieving increased contraceptive uptake including several examples of successful programs.

Optimal care during the antenatal and postnatal phases of the life cycle is a potentially positive determinant of health elsewhere in the continuum. A successful transition from the antenatal to the postnatal period requires early detection, optimal management, and prevention of disease; health promotion; birth preparedness; and complication readiness. Women, their babies, and families need appropriate evidence-based care based on their dignity and human rights before, during, and after birth. In this review, we present an overview of the components of antenatal and postnatal care needed to provide women a culturally sensitive and positive pregnancy and postnatal experience. The challenge of antenatal and postnatal care is determining their core components and underpinning them with evidence without overmedicalizing their practice.

Efforts to prevent mother-to-child transmission of human immunodeficiency virus (HIV) have led to dramatic reductions in pediatric HIV worldwide. New advances in HIV treatment and prevention, focused on pregnant and breastfeeding women living with HIV, have improved maternal health while decreasing vertical and horizontal HIV transmission.

In this article, we describe how such interventions—including antiretroviral therapy and HIV pre-exposure prophylaxis—can be incorporated into antepartum and postpartum care in global settings.

Despite a 38% decrease in global maternal mortality during the last decade, rates remain unacceptably high with greater than 800 maternal deaths occurring each day. There exists significant regional variation among rates and causes of maternal mortality, and the vast majority occurs in low-income and middle-income countries. The leading causes of direct maternal mortality are hemorrhage, hypertensive disorders of pregnancy, sepsis, complications of abortion, and thromboembolism. Eliminating preventable maternal mortality hinges on improving clinical management of these life-threatening obstetric conditions, as well as addressing the complex social and economic barriers that pregnant women face to access quality care.

Pelvic floor disorders (PFDs) and obstetric fistula (OF) are common across the globe. PFDs include stress and urge urinary incontinence, overactive bladder, pelvic organ prolapse, fecal incontinence, sexual dysfunction, and pelvic pain. Although PFD and OF are common in low- and middle-income countries (LMIC) there is a lack of awareness and constraints in health care resources. This article focuses on epidemiology, risk factors, assessment, and treatment of PFD and OF in resource-poor settings. Adherence to basic medical ethics principles has to be maintained at all times, coupled with knowledge of and respect for local cultures, traditions, and perceptions of health norms.

Treatable genital tract infections in women are common and most are transmitted via sexual contact with the potential for vertical transmission during pregnancy. Adverse infection outcomes include pelvic inflammatory disease, infertility, ectopic pregnancy, preterm delivery, and congenital or neonatal infection. Highly sensitive molecular diagnostic testing for genital tract infections is now recommended in many countries. Unfortunately, this testing is not yet widely available in low- and middle-income countries because of cost. Improved access to early diagnosis and treatment for curable genital tract infections is critical to improving women's health and reaching global STI elimination targets by 2030.

Cervical cancer is a leading cause of cancer among women. Approximately 350,000 women die from cervical needlessly from cancer each year, and 85% of the global burden occurs in low- and middle-income countries (LMICs). Disparities in the incidence and mortality between

LMICs and industrialized countries can be attributed to differences in access to human papillomavirus (HPV) vaccination and cervical cancer screening and treatment. The World Health Organization (WHO) is leading a renewed international effort to reduce the global burden of cervical cancer. In this article, we discuss recommendations for HPV vaccination, primary HPV screening, and treatment of precancerous lesions.

Breast, ovarian, uterine, vaginal, and vulvar cancers pose a significant risk to women's lives in low- and middle-income countries due to increasing incidence and presentation with advanced stage disease. There are challenges to screening and early detection and limitations in access to treatment and palliative care, and the current global health care workforce is insufficient. However, there is promise in development of telehealth strategies, task shifting, and increasing number of physician training programs to help address currently unmet needs.

Globally, an inequitable surgical burden exists. Greater than 90% of people in low- and middle-income countries (LMICs) lack access to safe, affordable surgical care. Also, patients undergoing surgery in LMICs suffer much higher rates of perioperative complications and death. In many LMICs, cesarean section is both underused and overused, and frequently performed unsafely. Obstetric fistula and women's cancers contribute to the surgical burden of women in LMICs. Surgical team nontechnical skills (eg, teamwork and communication) and use of tools such as the WHO Surgical Safety Checklist and Enhanced Recovery after Surgery program have the potential to greatly improve surgical outcomes.

Gender-based violence (GBV) affects more than 700 million women and girls, worldwide, manifesting systemically (eg, human trafficking) and at the interpersonal level (eg, rape, intimate partner violence) and conveying significant negative economic, social, mental, and physical health impacts. It is important for the clinician to be prepared for providing emergency, urgent, and longer-term care to women who are survivors of GBV. Panzi Hospital in the Democratic Republic of the Congo provides an example of person-centered, holistic care for survivors of GBV, including conflict-related and nonconflict-related sexual violence.

Optimizing maternal health in lower-resource settings requires a joint focus to simultaneously increase skilled delivery care access and improve the quality of preventive and emergency maternal health care provided. Evidence-based interventions are largely established, yet despite increasing access, poor quality is limiting health gains. Assessing quality and implementing quality improvement approaches across varied health system levels is imperative to address health priorities. Evaluations of maternal care quality improvement suggest the need for enhancing standardized monitoring strategies and identifying optimal implementation strategies for translating findings into practice within different lower-resource settings to increase adoption and sustainability.

Interprofessional care relates to providing care to an individual in an integrated system of professionals who share and shift the care given, depending on the individual and population need. By broadening the scope of care given by health-care workers (HCWs) or shifting tasks through interprofessional care in Obstetrics and Gynecology, more women and their newborns can benefit from safe deliveries, decreased perinatal morbidity and mortality and through screening and early treatment prevent morbidity and mortality secondary to gynecologic diseases.

OBSTETRICS AND GYNECOLOGY CLINICS

SERIES OF RELATED INTEREST

Clinics in Perinatology
www.perinatology.theclinics.com
Pediatric Clinics of North America
https://www.pediatrics.theclinics.com

THE CLINICS ARE AVAILABLE ONLINE!
Access your subscription at:
www.theclinics.com

SERIES OF RELATED INTEREST

Foreword

Global Women's Health: Not Merely Focusing on Disease

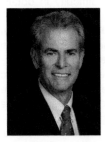

William F. Rayburn, MD, MBA
Consulting Editor

We live in a world where global travel is more easily attainable, and global communications and information technology have improved access to health care expertise. The World Health Organization defines health as a state of complete physical, mental, and social well-being and not merely the absence of disease. Women's health is an example of a specifically defined population.

This issue is our first to deal with global women's health. Edited with the expertise of Dr Jean Anderson and Dr Grace Chen from Johns Hopkins University, this issue covers timely women's health topics, such as contraception and preconception care, gynecologic cancers, maternal health and mortality, HIV, genital tract infections, violence against women, and pelvic floor disorders. While developed countries have lower mortalities overall, there are still major inequalities in outcomes within these countries.

Women's experiences of health and disease can differ from those of men due to unique biological and surrounding environmental conditions. Gender differences in susceptibility and symptoms of disease and response to treatment are particularly evident when viewed from a global perspective. Women's and men's experiences of the same illnesses can differ, especially for cardiovascular disease, cancer, depression, dementia, and urinary tract infections. The gender gap in health is even more acute in developing countries, where women are more disadvantaged.

A large focus of global women's health is on reproduction and pregnancy. Women who are socially marginalized are more likely to die at younger ages. Underappreciated health conditions faced by women and girls in resource-poor regions include female genital cutting, violence, abortion, and lack of access to the appropriate diagnostic and clinical resources, reflecting unique political and cultural considerations relating to the status of women in these societies. Adolescent pregnancy often stems from a person's lack of choice or abuse. Maternal mortality remains

Obstet Gynecol Clin N Am 49 (2022) xiii–xiv
https://doi.org/10.1016/j.ogc.2022.08.007
0889-8545/22/© 2022 Published by Elsevier Inc.

a major problem in global health and is considered a sentinel event in judging the quality of health care systems.

Providing quality and interprofessional medical and surgical care can be a challenge in both developing and developed countries. In the absence of adequate health insurance, women are likely to avoid self-care steps, such as routine physical examination, screening and prevention testing, and prenatal and postpartum care. Added to the financial burden are other barriers in accessing health care: poor educational achievement, lack of transportation, inflexible work schedules, and difficulty in obtaining childcare.

To improve global women's health care, more data are crucial about the burden of disease and evidence of intervention effectiveness. Much of the available information comes from developed countries, yet there are marked differences between low-income and higher-income countries. Research needs of women should include diseases that either are unique or add more risk than to men. Gender differences need to be considered when interpreting what is "normal" for laboratory values, criteria for growth and development, and drug metabolism and dosing.

Written by experts in the field, this issue is easy to read for practitioners pursuing careers in global health. Looking ahead, it should be helpful as a starting point for policymakers and anyone with a general interest in the subjects. With practical comparisons between developing and developed countries, this issue should be a valuable resource for those involved in women's health everywhere.

William F. Rayburn, MD, MBA
Department of Obstetrics and Gynecology
Medical University of South Carolina
Charleston, SC 29425, USA

E-mail address:
wrayburnmd@gmail.com

Preface

Global Women's Health: Health Equity for Women

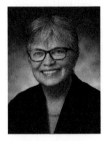 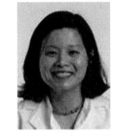

Jean R. Anderson, MD   Chi Chiung Grace Chen, MD, MHS
Editors

Today we live in a globalized world. International travel is easier than ever, and advances in communications and information technology have resulted in increasing access to cellular communications and the Internet in low- and middle-income countries (LMIC). This has resulted in improved education, training, and learning opportunities through work, in public spaces such as Internet cafes, in schools, and in the home. We also live in times of rapid advances in medical care, but these have not had the same reach into lower-resource areas, which continue to suffer from significant health disparities due to an inadequate number of health care workers and lack of economic resources devoted to health, poverty, and conflict.

In LMIC, as in high-income countries, women are the linchpin of the family and the community. Their health reflects the broader health of society, but in too many instances, health indicators for women, such as maternal mortality, rates of obstetric fistula, and unmet need for contraception, demonstrate the burden of health disparities on women and also reflect the low status of women in many societies. While we have focused the discussion of these women's health topics to LMIC, it is imperative that we keep in mind that these conditions and related health disparities experienced by many women are also present in high-income countries. The COVID-19 pandemic has further underscored the interconnectedness of all people around the world and the globalization of all aspects of life, including health.

The authors in this special issue are experts in the specific topic areas they address and include distinguished colleagues from several LMIC. Notably, we were fortunate to include Nobel Peace Prize winner Dr Denis Mukwege and his colleagues at Panzi Hospital (Bukavu Congo) to present their experience working with women survivors of gender-based violence. Although it is impossible to comprehensively cover all relevant topics, the topics chosen represent a broad survey of critical current health issues and innovations in women's health. We hope that these articles will be thought

Obstet Gynecol Clin N Am 49 (2022) xv–xvi
https://doi.org/10.1016/j.ogc.2022.08.005
0889-8545/22/© 2022 Published by Elsevier Inc.

obgyn.theclinics.com

provoking and enlightening, demonstrating both how far we have come and how far we still have to go.

Jean R. Anderson, MD
Gynecologic Specialties
Department of Gynecology and Obstetrics
Johns Hopkins University School of Medicine
Baltimore, MD 21224, USA

Chi Chiung Grace Chen, MD, MHS
Female Pelvic Medicine and Reconstructive Surgery
Department of Gynecology and Obstetrics
Johns Hopkins University School of Medicine
Baltimore, MD 21224, USA

E-mail addresses:
janders@jhmi.edu (J.R. Anderson)
cchen127@jhmi.edu (C.C. Grace Chen)

Global Preconception and Contraception Care

Using a Life-Course Approach to Improve Health Outcomes in Lower-Resource Settings

Megan A. Cohen, MD, MPH[a,b,]*,
Somesh Kumar, MBBS, MSc, PhD[c,d,e,1],
Mark Hathaway, MD, MPH[f,g,h,i,1]

KEYWORDS

- Preconception care • Contraception • Low- and middle-income countries
- Task-shifting • Postabortion care • Contraceptive method mix • Family planning
- Postpartum family planning

KEY POINTS

- A life-course approach including access to appropriate preconception and contraception care is key to achieving optimal maternal, neonatal, and child health outcomes.
- Preconception care should be tailored to local settings, but includes optimizing maternal nutrition and screening for and treating infections, noncommunicable diseases, mental health conditions, and intimate partner violence.
- Determinants of unmet need for family planning are complex, but are influenced by local cultural factors, patient preferences, government and donor environments, supply issues, and access barriers.
- Engaging community members, key stakeholders, and male partners can improve culturally competent care and health outcomes.
- Integrating family planning services with other services such as childhood immunizations, HIV care, postabortion care, and postpartum care can increase contraceptive intake. Specifically, immediate postpartum contraceptive provision is a proven high-impact practice.

[a] Department of Obstetrics and Gynecology, Oregon Health & Science University, Portland, Oregon, USA; [b] Division of Complex Family Planning, Department of Gynecology and Obstetrics, Emory University School of Medicine, 49 Jesse Hill Jr. Drive, SE - Faculty Office Building. Atlanta, GA 30303, USA; [c] Jhpiego India, New Delhi, India; [d] Technical Leadership and Innovations, Jhpiego, Baltimore, MD, USA; [e] Johns Hopkins Bloomberg School of Public Health, Baltimore, MD, USA; [f] Johns Hopkins University, Baltimore, MD, USA; [g] Carafem, Washington, DC, USA; [h] Jhpiego, Baltimore, MD, USA; [i] Unity Health Care, Inc, Washington, DC, USA
[1] Present address: 1776 Massachusetts Avenue, Northwest (Suite 300), Washington, DC 20036.
* Corresponding author.
E-mail address: megan.a.cohen@emory.edu

Obstet Gynecol Clin N Am 49 (2022) 647–663
https://doi.org/10.1016/j.ogc.2022.07.003
0889-8545/22/© 2022 Elsevier Inc. All rights reserved.

INTRODUCTION

In 2015, United Nations member states adopted the Sustainable Development Goals (SDGs), composed of 17 goals to help achieve global improvements in health, peace, and prosperity for all. The SDGs assert the importance of sexual and reproductive health, as evidenced by SDG target 3.7: "By 2030, ensure universal access to sexual and reproductive health-care services, including for family planning (FP), information and education, and the integration of reproductive health into national strategies and programs."[1] Under the banner of FP2030, the world united to promote rights-based FP through global partnerships with government and nongovernmental organization commitments, clear targets, goal-tracking, and a platform for accountability through collection and dissemination of key FP indicators from 82 countries.[2]

Reproductive health care can best be understood through a life-course approach, where childhood and adolescent nutritional and health status can have large impacts on later reproductive and maternal health, while pregnancy morbidities such as pre-eclampsia and gestational diabetes or delivery via cesarean section can have lifelong health consequences and implications for future pregnancies.[3] The life-course approach, therefore, emphasizes improved health and well-being starting in the childhood and adolescent periods, and delaying first pregnancy or subsequent pregnancies until optimal health is achieved. Key to this is access to preconception care and FP services. This helps ensure healthy pregnancies and appropriate birth spacing, which enhances maternal and neonatal health and can have intergenerational effects.[4,5]

Though there have been great strides made in improving sexual and reproductive health care in low- and middle-income countries (LMIC), significant gaps remain. Approximately 111 million pregnancies each year are unintended, or 49% of annual pregnancies in LMIC.[6] An estimated 218 million reproductive-aged women (15–49 years) have an unmet need for modern contraception, meaning that they desire to prevent pregnancy but are not using a modern method.[6] This lack of services has significant ramifications for the health of women and children, and specifically for maternal mortality. It is estimated that provision of adequate contraceptive needs with modern methods would decrease unintended pregnancy by 68%, unsafe abortions by 72%, and avert 70,000 maternal deaths annually.[6] Therefore, simple, safe, and universal access to contraceptive methods should be included in any maternal mortality reduction strategy.

In this article, we explore preconception and contraceptive care within LMIC, situating these reproductive health services within a life-course and rights-based approach. We review specific challenges in contraceptive provision in LMIC, explore differences by region, and discuss considerations for providers who may go practice in LMIC settings. We also highlight ways of achieving increased contraceptive uptake including several success stories from LMIC settings. See **Box 1** for pertinent resources.

PRECONCEPTION

Preconception care is any health care that helps improve women's health before pregnancy, aiming to ensure optimal maternal, neonatal, and child health outcomes. In 2012, a global consensus meeting convened by the World Health Organization (WHO) emphasized that preconception care should be tailored to local environments and individual health needs, but suggested several key components to incorporate. These include addressing any underlying chronic health conditions such as diabetes or hypertension, ensuring optimal maternal nutrition, addressing adverse health

---

Box 1
Resources

World Health Organization Medical Eligibility Criteria for Contraceptive Use https://www.who.int/publications/i/item/9789241549158)

World Health Organization Selected Practice Recommendations for Contraceptive Use (https://www.who.int/publications/i/item/9789241565400)

Family Planning: A Global Handbook for Providers (https://apps.who.int/iris/handle/10665/260156)

Contraceptive eligibility for women at high risk of HIV (https://apps.who.int/iris/bitstream/handle/10665/326653/9789241550574-eng.pdf?ua=1)

Training Resource for Family Planning (https://www.fptraining.org/)

Family Planning High Impact Practices (HIP) Briefs (https://www.fphighimpactpractices.org/briefs/)

Family Planning Program Models (https://toolkits.knowledgesuccess.org/toolkit-topics/family-planningreproductive-health-programs-and-services)

FP2030 (https://fp2030.org/)

Minimum Initial Service Package for Sexual and Reproductive Health in Crisis Situations (https://www.unfpa.org/resources/minimum-initial-service-package-misp-srh-crisis-situations)

---

exposures, screening for genetic conditions, discussing vaccine-preventable illnesses and providing catch-up vaccinations, encouraging avoidance or offering treatment for substance use including tobacco, screening for mental health issues and intimate partner violence, and screening for and treating STIs such as HIV, syphilis, gonorrhea, and chlamydia.[7] Strategies for providing preconception care include community-based preconception counseling, which has been shown to increase likelihood of preconception smoking cessation, folic acid and iron-folic acid supplementation, breast-feeding, safe delivery kit use, and antenatal care (ANC) attendance.[8] As health care utilization in LMIC may be low, all contacts with the health care system should be used to address preconception issues.[9]

Both maternal over and undernutrition can lead to maternal and neonatal adverse effects. Maternal undernutrition contributes to 20% of maternal deaths, and increases risk for poor neonatal outcomes such as preterm birth and small for gestational age neonates.[10] Maternal obesity increases risk for developing gestational diabetes and pregnancy-induced hypertension. In addition, maternal malnutrition may affect fetal developmental programming leading to future cardiovascular and metabolic risks such as increasing childhood obesity rates.[9,11] Evidence-based strategies for improving preconception nutrition include iron and folic acid supplementation, consuming fortified foods, and encouraging a diversified diet.[10]

Anemia is also a modifiable condition in the preconception period and treatment can avert adverse health outcomes, as anemia during pregnancy is associated with pre-term birth, low birth weight, and perinatal and neonatal mortality.[12] Anemia can have multifactorial etiologies: it may be a consequence of iron or other micronutrient deficiencies; due to infectious etiologies such as malaria, HIV, TB, helminths, or schistosomiasis; a result of a hemoglobinopathy; or a result of chronic inflammation.[13] These conditions should be screened for and appropriately treated. For example, all patients in areas at risk for malaria transmission should be encouraged to sleep under insecticide-treated nets and provided a WHO-prequalified insecticide-treated net if not in an area that performs indoor residual spraying.[14] In addition, WHO recommends twice yearly antihelminth treatment for nonpregnant adolescents and women of reproductive age in areas with baseline prevalence >50% and once yearly treatment for those in areas with baseline prevalence >20% to help address non-nutritional causes of anemia.[13] Prevention of infection is also important in preconception care; for example, providing tetanus vaccination in the preconception period has been shown to significantly avert neonatal deaths.[15]

Preconception care is an important time to address sexually transmitted infections, which may be more commonly seen in LMIC settings. HIV counseling and testing can help identify women who have HIV infection and ensure they are started on antiretroviral therapy, optimizing their health and reducing risk of vertical transmission in a subsequent pregnancy. Patients who are HIV negative in serodiscordant relationships can be prescribed HIV preexposure prophylaxis (PrEP), which has been shown to decrease risk of HIV acquisition. Providers should recommend that patients in serodiscordant relationships engage in condom use or dual contraception use to help prevent transmission of HIV.[7] Patients can also be screened and treated for syphilis, gonorrhea, and chlamydia.

CONTRACEPTION

Unmet need for contraception varies widely both within and between regions, countries, and specific populations, given the many complex determinants of contraceptive use. Just as in higher-income countries, in LMIC settings, additional barriers remain for certain populations such as those of low income, those living in rural areas, and adolescents.[16] For example, approximately 43% of adolescents aged 15-19 years have an unmet need for contraception in LMICs compared to 24% for women over age 19 years.[6] Other issues like lack of awareness of contraceptive methods; misperceptions and persistent myths; religious preferences; and lack of commodities, trained providers, or instruments also influence the ability to obtain contraception.[16,17] Access to contraception is especially difficult in humanitarian emergencies, where instability has led to only 16% of programs offering FP services in such settings in sub-Saharan Africa.[18]

Even within similar geographical regions, there is substantial variation in contraceptive prevalence between countries. A systematic review conducted in 2019 analyzing postpartum contraceptive prevalence found an overall pooled modern contraceptive prevalence rate (mCPR) of 41.2%. The mCPR was highest in South Asia/South East Asia region (42.4%), but this ranged from 4.0% in Pakistan to 65.6% in India. Overall mCPR for East Africa was 39.5%, ranging from 10.3% in Ethiopia to 73.7% in Uganda.[19] Another study found overall mCPR for sub-Saharan countries was 22% using DHS data up to 2020, ranging from 3.5% in the Central African Republic to 49.7% in Namibia.[16] For adolescents and young women ages 15-24 years, estimates of modern contraceptive prevalence in sub-Saharan Africa ranged from 5.1% in Chad to 59.2% in Lesotho, with an overall prevalence of 24.7%.[17]

Importance of Method Mix

The contraceptive method mix, or percentage of specific methods used by contraceptive users, also varies greatly between countries and is influenced by both supply and demand factors. Supply factors include methods or contraceptive formulations in country formularies, stock-outs, cost or access barriers. Donor influence is also important, as in the case of increasing contraceptive implant use in sub-Saharan Africa. In 2012, multiple donors negotiated with pharmaceutical firms to lower implant costs and increase supply by providing a "volume guarantee"—an agreement to buy increased implant quantities for focused in-country programs designed to increase demand for implant use.[20] Indeed, approximately 45% of total expenditures for FP in LMIC settings come from international donors.[2] User demand factors include individual, religious, and sociocultural factors that influence method preferences, for example, the cultural favoring of withdrawal in North Africa. In Muslim countries, religious barriers limit the use of female and male sterilization,[21] and may impact the use of other modern contraceptive methods.[22]

The most common contraceptive method used worldwide according to 2019 estimates is female sterilization, followed by male condoms, intrauterine device (IUD), and contraceptive pills.[23] Globally, approximately 45% of individuals on contraception use permanent or long-acting reversible contraception (LARC); 46% use short-acting methods such as barrier methods, the pill, patch, or ring; and 9% use traditional methods such as withdrawal and the rhythm method.

Currently, most IUDs in use are copper IUDs; hormone-releasing IUDs are becoming more available with newer lower cost options but at this time are still predominantly only available in the private sector. Introducing any new method is a long-term process that includes cost, education and training, and public marketing/promotion, including correction of misconceptions. There has recently been a concerted global effort to improve introduction and access to hormone-releasing IUDs (https://www.usaid.gov/global-health/health-areas/family-planning/news-and-updates/introduction-long-acting-family-planning and https://www.hormonaliud.org/contact).

The advent of subcutaneous injectable depot medroxyprogesterone (DMPA-SC) has proven particularly successful as a self-administered, discreet, intermediate-acting contraception with high continuation rates.[24,25] Lactational amenorrhea (LAM) is a common method of contraception globally, but mandates 3 conditions to be met in order to be effective:

1. Woman is less than 6 months postpartum
2. Menses have not resumed (patient is amenorrheic)
3. Full or nearly full breastfeeding (no interval of >4–6 hours between feeds)

Though vasectomy rates are decreasing,[21] successful global programs have been developed to increase vasectomy provision, including promotion through the World Vasectomy Day (WVD) Project, launched in 2013.[26] See **Box 2** for a success story from WVD in Mexico.

Regional method mix also varies. For example, in Asia, the IUD is the dominant method, comprising 22% of the method mix.[21] In Latin America, female sterilization (31%) is predominant.[21] In Northern Africa and Western Asia, 32% of contraceptive users choose the pill,[21] but this is also the region with the largest percentage of women that rely on withdrawal for cultural reasons.[27] In sub-Saharan Africa, injectable contraception (36%) remains the most common method, but use of the implant (14%) has also been increasing and is more common there than in other regions.[21] Of 113 LMIC countries, 34 countries (30%) have a skewed method mix, meaning that one method predominates with >50% of the contraceptive method share.[21] For example, injectables (64%) dominate in Malawi, female sterilization (68%) in India, and IUDs (88%) in Turkmenistan.[21]

Having a varied method mix within a country is important to support method choice based on contraceptive user preferences. To that end, the WHO recommends that country FP programs include a range of modern contraceptive methods including at least one of the following four contraception types: short-acting reversible, long-

> **Box 2**
> **Vasectomy in Mexico**
>
> When World Vasectomy Day (WVD) first arrived in Mexico in 2016, our objective was to support their Ministry's commitment to increase male engagement in FP. Vasectomy was then, and remains today, a free service available to all men, but the number of procedures done, in a country of over 123 million, was only 16,000.
>
> During the following 5 years, WVD worked hand in hand with the Ministry to train doctors, produce public education campaigns, and build a sense of shared purpose among its over 350 doctors and certified vasectomy providers.
>
> This included innovative ideas such as a staged 'battle' before 10,000 spectators between 2 wrestlers (one who had a vasectomy and one who did not) https://youtu.be/_VwP-C-iWTc and competitions for best video between more than 100 clinics scattered throughout the country. The 2017 winner alone had over 1 million views in under a week https://www.facebook.com/WorldVasDay/posts/1732563763485720.
>
> Creating a shared purpose, supporting providers with technical assistance and acknowledging the critical contributions of young physicians has gone a long way to building a much more robust vasectomy program. In 2021, during WVD alone over 9,000 men got a vasectomy and the numbers surpassed 40,000 for the year (**Fig. 1**)

acting reversible, permanent, and emergency.[28] There is controversy surrounding what an "ideal" method mix constitutes, but this may be achieved if every woman of reproductive age who desires to prevent pregnancy is using their method of choice.[21] As such, to help ensure contraception is provided within a human rights framework, FP programs should provide culturally-appropriate counseling and access to and provision of available contraceptives of the patient's choice, without discrimination or coercion.[28]

Providers should familiarize themselves with methods readily available within a country's health system and the ability to provide at specific health facilities. In addition, it is helpful to understand the common contraceptive method choices within a specific context and the sociocultural dynamics driving or constraining patient decision-making. There also may be methods that are unfamiliar and require extra training to provide, such as two-rod levonorgestrel implants that are not typically available in North America. Specific helpful resources for providers are provided in **Box 1**.

Contraceptive care for women at high risk of Human Immunodeficiency Virus acquisition or living with Human Immunodeficiency Virus

For women and adolescents who are at high risk of HIV acquisition, there are certain special contraceptive considerations. In 2010, there was concern that the use of DMPA may increase the risk of HIV acquisition based on observational studies. However, a well-designed recent study dispelled this notion,[29] and the WHO now suggests that DMPA and IUDs may be used without restriction in individuals at high risk of HIV acquisition.[30] Furthermore, use of oral contraceptives, norethisterone enanthate injectable contraception, or other progestin implants is not associated with increased risk of HIV acquisition.[31] However, high-risk individuals should avoid nonoxynol-9 spermicide use as spermicide can abrade the vaginal mucosa leading to a higher risk of genital lesions and increased risk of HIV transmission.[32,33] Dual contraceptive use with male and female condoms should be discussed as these are the only contraceptive methods that can decrease the risk of HIV transmission. However, condom use for HIV prevention has recently been de-emphasized, given the data that effective

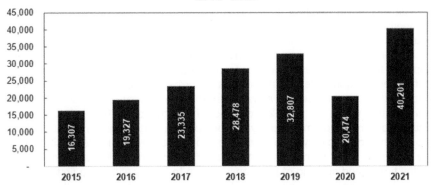

Fig. 1. Number of vasectomies performed per year in Mexico, 2015-2021. (*Courtesy of* Jonathan Stack, World Vasectomy Day Program.)

antiretroviral treatment (ART) with maximal viral suppression is associated with essentially no chance of HIV transmission (U=U, undetectable = untransmissible)[34]; nevertheless, condoms are still an important tool to prevent transmission of other sexually transmitted infections and transmission of HIV when adequate ART of an HIV-infected partner cannot be assured or partner status is unknown.

Women who are living with HIV, as well as women being treated for Mycobacterium tuberculosis or avium complex, may be on certain antiretrovirals or other medications that can interact with hormonal contraception. Providers should consult the WHO Medical Eligibility Criteria for Contraceptive Use (MEC) or another resource such as the HIV Drug Interactions Web site (https://www.hiv-druginteractions.org/checker) to check for pertinent drug interactions if in doubt.

Reasons for Nonuse of Contraception

Reasons for nonuse of contraception are multifactorial and include individual, household, and sociocultural factors. For young women or women not in a union, there are often pervasive cultural sexual mores promoting abstinence for these groups, so women using contraceptive methods may face stigma. In some areas, such as reported in rural Kenya, irregular bleeding associated with progestin-only methods may impact women's ability to complete daily activities, as women are viewed as "unclean" when bleeding.[22] Women also report avoiding modern methods of contraception due to fears of future infertility or illness.[22] Pervasive myths and misconceptions regarding contraceptive methods abound.

Fear of side effects, abstinence, lack of preferred contraceptive method, and husband's disapproval are also common reasons for contraceptive nonuse.[35–38] In West Africa, studies have indicated that male partners frequently make decisions regarding contraception and other reproductive health.[39] Though women may express a desire to space or limit births, partners may disapprove of contraceptive use, given desire for having more children, perceptions of virility, concern over loss of female libido, and myths that contraceptive use leads promiscuity.[22] Given this, women may opt for discreet methods that can be used without partner knowledge, such as injectables.[22]

Postpartum family planning

The postpartum period has been identified as a common crucial missed opportunity for FP uptake, leading to short interpregnancy intervals that are detrimental to maternal and child health.[35] Postpartum FP (PPFP), or use of FP within the first 12 months of childbirth, can improve maternal and neonatal health outcomes by reducing 10% of child deaths[40] and 32% of maternal deaths.[41] Postnatal care utilization is often low, particularly in sub-Saharan Africa.[42] Unmet need for PPFP in LMIC is estimated to be as high as 61%.[35] Reasons stated for nonuse of postpartum contraception frequently include breastfeeding, amenorrhea, and low perceived risk of pregnancy.[35–37] Return to sexual activity, return to ovulatory cycle, and nonuse of contraception within the first 12 months of childbirth lead to 61% of all births that occur before the recommended 3 years postpartum birth to birth interval.[43] Women who are amenorrheic may have unrealistic expectations regarding fecundity, particularly if greater than 6 months postpartum;[19] hence, improving awareness about healthy timing and spacing of pregnancy, return to fertility within the first few weeks after childbirth, and improving access to contraception for women in their first year postpartum requires a policy and program approach.

Studies show that high-intensity antenatal counseling for women may be needed to produce an improvement in contraceptive uptake. Combined antenatal and postnatal interventions have shown a substantial impact on contraceptive use at various points in the first year postpartum.[36,44] Joint counseling of patient and partners at ANC appointments or in the delivery ward led to significant increases in contraceptive use postpartum.[45] Group ANC, where women develop peer support in longitudinal small groups over the course of several sessions, has also facilitated increased PPFP uptake. In Ghana, women in group ANC had 8 times adjusted odds of using a modern PPFP method, despite receiving similar counseling messages as women receiving individual ANC.[46] Other facilitators for postpartum contraception use include delivery at a birthing facility; access to contraception; perceived ease of use; personal characteristics such as previous favorable experience with contraception; desire to space/limit pregnancy; or monogamous partnership or having a partner supportive of contraception; and demographic factors such as higher education, higher socioeconomic status, urban residence, and young age at first birth.[19]

Ways to Improve Contraceptive Uptake

Integration with immunization services

Immunization is one of the highest services used in LMIC as evidenced by high vaccination coverage which affords multiple contacts with families to complete the recommended vaccination schedule, thus increasing the chances for counseling and possible service FP provision. Multiple studies show high acceptability by providers and users and increased contraceptive uptake.[47–50] Models can include integrated service provision where both immunization and FP services are available on site, integrated service provision plus referrals to trained providers for more complex FP needs such as IUD insertions, and screening for FP needs and referral at immunization service provision sites.

Integration of FP and child immunization services in one study allowed for improved counseling and dispelling of misinformation related to modern contraceptive use.[22] Having FP services available in the same location as child immunization services allowed women to increase uptake by removing the need to seek their husband's permission, and by bringing FP services closer to remote communities through outreach clinics or community health workers at local health posts.[22]

Integration with HIV services

Integrating FP counseling and services with HIV testing/care has been shown to increase modern contraceptive uptake and dual method use and decrease unmet need for contraception.[51,52] Dual method use, meaning use of a condom or other barrier method to protect against HIV transmission plus use of more effective contraception method, may be particularly important for key populations like female sex workers who experience higher rates of condom failure, inconsistent condom use, or nonconsensual sex.[53] Similar to integration with immunization services, integration in HIV services can take on several different models including counseling plus referral to either onsite or offsite services, or direct provision of FP services in an integrated clinic. FP for women living with HIV can also allow patients to prevent unintended or mistimed pregnancies, ensure they are well-controlled and virally suppressed if they do desire fertility, and help prevent perinatal HIV transmission. Thus, some clinics perform FP counseling and screening regarding fertility intentions at each visit. Key challenges include staff turnover or budget constraints particularly limiting clinic ability to maintain trained clinicians in long-acting reversible contraceptive provision.[52] FP clinics can also incorporate HIV counseling and testing with provision of pre-exposure prophylaxis for seronegative patients at risk or referrals for treatment for seropositive patients.[54]

Immediate postpartum family planning

Providing immediate PPFP (IPPFP) is a proven high-impact practice that increases contraception uptake and continuation, thereby mitigating aforementioned barriers to postpartum contraception use and serving to decrease unmet need.[55] Strategies include performing postpartum bilateral tubal ligation, insertion of postpartum copper or levonorgestrel intrauterine devices (PPIUDs) within 48 hours of delivery, insertion of contraceptive implants before facility discharge, and provision of injectable contraception for nonbreastfeeding parturients.[55-57] Data from 6 LMIC countries in the FIGO initiative showed the safety and success of PPIUD insertion by a range of trained health staff.[58] Immediate postpartum long-acting reversible contraception provision may be especially useful in humanitarian settings (**Box 3**).[59] Safety of postpartum contraceptive use varies between breastfeeding and nonbreastfeeding patients, but any nonhormonal or progestin-only contraception (except injectables) can be initiated immediately postpartum without any adverse health effects or interference with breastfeeding.[33] Often, demand generation is required to increase IPPFP acceptance. For example, in Nepal, discussing immediate postpartum FP during ANC visits increased uptake of immediate postpartum IUD insertion.[60] Another example from India of a highly successful program to increase immediate postpartum copper IUD use is featured in **Box 4**. For further implementation strategies, such as engaging key community influencers through home visits or community group outreach, see the Family Planning High Impact Practices brief (Web site listed in **Box 1**).[55]

Postabortion care family planning

Postabortion care (PAC) FP is a crucial component of PAC and is also a proven high-impact practice for increasing FP uptake.[61] Interventions designed to improve FP counseling and access in postabortion settings greatly increase uptake of postabortion contraception before facility discharge. Investing in provider training on counseling skills, provider job aids, patient educational materials, and free contraceptive provision increase program success.[62] Including male partners in PAC FP counseling and decision-making also leads to increased contraceptive uptake. Best practice is to offer PAC contraception to all individuals who are seeking PAC, whether they had a

---

Box 3
Contraception in humanitarian settings

As of 2022, over 270 million people around the globe live in humanitarian settings,[68] a quarter of which are women and adolescent girls of reproductive age. Structural instability and limited resources in these settings cause service gaps which can result in high rates of unplanned pregnancies, unsafe abortions, and even higher maternal and neonatal mortality rates.

The Minimum Initial Service Package (MISP) for reproductive health is a set of priority activities that are implemented at the onset of every humanitarian emergency to prevent mortality, morbidity, and disability among crisis-affected populations. Objective 5 of the MISP is to reduce unintended pregnancies by improving availability of contraceptive services. This includes providing contraceptive counseling; provision of a wide range of contraceptive methods, inclusive of LARC; and promoting community awareness of contraceptives.[69]

To address the issue of FP access, Save the Children implemented a program focused on providing a broad range of voluntary contraceptive services in a diversity of humanitarian settings beginning in 2012. Working in collaboration with the Ministries of Health, governments, local partners, and other relevant stakeholders, Save the Children applied a 4-pronged approach to ensure voluntary, high-quality FP and PAC services in humanitarian settings; this included capacity building, assurance of supplies and infrastructure, community collaboration and mobilization, and consistent data management for ongoing monitoring, evaluation, and data use. Since 2011, over 500 providers were trained to provide long-acting reversible contraception and over 850,000 clients initiated FP or switched methods of whom more than 36% chose a long-acting reversible or permanent contraceptive method.

(*Courtesy of* Meghan Gallagher, PhD, MPH, Save the Children.)

---

spontaneous incomplete abortion or induced abortion, as this helps reduce stigma surrounding induced abortion. Individuals who do not opt for PAC contraception should be advised of rapid return to fertility within 2-3 weeks.[62]

IUDs can be inserted immediately after surgical abortions; there is little to no increased risk of expulsion, particularly after first trimester abortion. If medical management is used, IUDs are typically inserted at 1-2 week follow-up. Implants may be inserted immediately at the time of surgical or medical management of abortion. Prompt LARC insertion is associated with increased uptake and decreased subsequent unintended pregnancy compared to a delay of 3-6 weeks.[62] However, in rare cases of septic abortion, IUD insertion should be delayed by at least several weeks until the infection is resolved.

Task-shifting/task-sharing and community health workers

Task-shifting decreases the burden on highly trained medical specialists by shifting certain tasks to midwives, nurses, and lay health workers; it has been recommended by the WHO as a strategy to increase access to maternal and neonatal health care, including expanding long-acting reversible and permanent contraceptive services. A useful WHO guide (available at http://apps.who.int/iris/bitstream/10665/259633/1/WHO-RHR-17.20-eng.pdf) for FP programs provides guidelines regarding which health care worker types can safely provide which services with or without additional training, monitoring, and supervision.[63]

Community health workers can safely administer injectable contraceptives and contraceptive implants. In Nigeria, trained community health extension workers demonstrated safe and proficient implant insertion, appropriate patient counseling, and increased demand generation.[64] Overall, evidence shows that community health workers can competently screen clients for DMPA, administer DMPA injections, and

---

Box 4
Postpartum IUD in India

Jhpiego partnered with the Ministry of Health and Family Welfare, Government of India (GoI) to introduce post-partum copper IUD (PPIUCD) services to the method mix of PPFP services by adopting a 'Health Systems Approach Building Blocks' model. The 6 building blocks include leadership and governance, service delivery, human resources, medicine and technology, financing, and information. Key factors included establishing PPIUCD as a government priority; developing systematic monitoring mechanisms; focusing on task shifting through training a core group of master trainers competent in PPIUCD provision including auxiliary nurse midwives; increasing client follow-up and generating demand; secure significant financial investments from GoI for establishment of training sites, counselors, and commodity procurement; and ensuring quality through standardization of processes including creating checklists and performance standards.

Work that began in 2009 with one facility at Queen Mary Hospital in Lucknow, Uttar Pradesh (UP), spread to more than 2,000 facilities across 320 Districts in 19 States, establishing 83 training sites training more than 20,000 providers undertaking more than 2.08 million PPIUCD insertions during 2010-2018 (**Fig. 2**). Over 6 years, the program helped save the lives of an estimated 86,000 children and 10,000 women through improved contraceptive services. Averting an estimated 16.9 million unintended pregnancies and 10 million abortions saved an estimated US$ 579 million in direct health care spending.

Program Implications and Lessons
- System-based approach with focused interventions during rapid scale-up led to a significant number of PPIUCD acceptors, low expulsion and premature removals; and low adverse infection events
- Postinsertion follow-up, data analysis, and findings are important for constructive feedback on the quality of PPIUCD services

---

counsel clients on side effects with high satisfaction for community-based provision, thereby increasing access and uptake.[65] A technical consultation held in 2009 concluded that CHWs can indeed safely provide progestin-only injectable contraception with appropriate training, monitoring, and supervision.[66] It is anticipated this expansion would specifically help reach traditionally marginalized populations including indigenous women, unmarried women, and those with unsupportive partners, given their ability to navigate community dynamics.[67]

SUMMARY

Preconception and contraception care are key components of providing care within a life-course approach. Access to culturally competent, accessible, and acceptable sexual and reproductive health care is essential to ensuring optimal maternal, neonatal, and child outcomes and crucial to achieving SDG 3. To best achieve this, it is important to have a thorough understanding of local determinants of health, important health risks, cultural forces influencing reproductive health care, knowledge and training on provision of available contraceptive methods, and an understanding of health care system influences. Although there remains a significant unmet need for contraception globally, improvements continue and many evidence-based strategies exist to improve availability and meet the needs of patients. Given low overall health care utilization in many LMIC settings, integrating preconception and FP services into other services like child immunization, HIV care, and PAC can improve uptake. Community-based counseling using CHWs and engaging important decision-makers including male partners can help provide important health messages, dispel

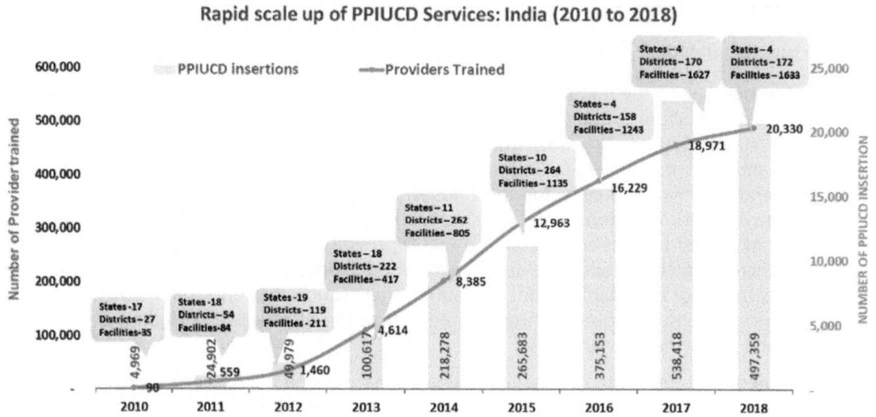

Rapid scale up of PPIUCD Services: India (2010 to 2018)

Fig. 2. Number of providers trained and number of PPIUCD performed in India, 2010 to 2018. (*Courtesy of* Somesh Kumar, Jhpiego India.)

myths and misconceptions surrounding contraception, and can expand access to service provision for some of the most vulnerable populations. Using a rights-based approach, providers can help women best attain their reproductive goals if, when, and however they desire to conceive.

CLINICS CARE POINTS

- Discuss preconception, contraception, and reproductive planning at each contact with the health care system as many people do not seek regular care.
- Know the availability of service, contraceptive options, and provider scope of care within various facility settings in your area. Adhere to local guidelines.
- Be aware of the multiple complex social and cultural contexts that influence contraceptive choices; encourage couples contraceptive counseling whenever possible.
- Use the WHO Medical Eligibility Criteria for Contraceptive Use to break down non–evidence-based restrictions in contraceptive provision and increase options for patients.
- Consider integration of FP services with other care such as immunizations/well-baby care and HIV services
- Provide postpartum and postabortion FP counseling and immediate service provision wherever possible
- Use midlevel providers and community health workers to task-shift and improve access to services

ACKNOWLEDGMENTS

The authors wish to acknowledge the following individuals who provided input in creation of this article: Meghan Gallagher, PhD, MPH, Save the Children; Jonathan Stack, World Vasectomy Day; and Rhoda Njeru, Jhpiego Kenya.

DISCLOSURE

Megan Cohen has been a trainer for AccessMatters. Mark Hathaway is a Nexplanon trainer for Organon and clinical advisory board member for Afaxys. He was previously on speakers' bureaus for Medicines360 and Bayer, but these affiliations ended in December 2021. Somesh Kumar has no conflicts to disclose.

REFERENCES

1. Transforming our world: the 2030 Agenda for Sustainable Development | Department of Economic and Social Affairs. Available at: https://sdgs.un.org/2030agenda. Accessed March 21, 2022.
2. FP2030. The Transition to FP2030: Measurement Report 2021. FP2030. 2021. Available at: https://fp2030.org/sites/default/files/Data-Hub/FP2030_DataReport_v5.pdf. Accessed March 19, 2022.
3. Firoz T, McCaw-Binns A, Filippi V, et al. A framework for healthcare interventions to address maternal morbidity. Int J Gynaecol Obstet 2018;141(Suppl Suppl 1):61–8.
4. Filippi V, Chou D, Barreix M, et al. A new conceptual framework for maternal morbidity. Int J Gynecol Obstet 2018;141(S1):4–9. https://doi.org/10.1002/ijgo.12463.
5. Conde-Agudelo A, Rosas-Bermúdez A, Kafury-Goeta AC. Birth spacing and risk of adverse perinatal outcomes: a meta-analysis. JAMA 2006;295(15):1809–23.
6. Sully E.A., Biddlecom A., Darroch J.E., et al. Adding it up: investing in sexual and reproductive health 2019. Guttmacher Institute, 2020, Available at: https://www.guttmacher.org/report/adding-it-upinvesting-in-sexual-reproductive-health-2019. Accessed March 15, 2022.
7. World Health Organization. Meeting to Develop a Global Consensus on Preconception Care to Reduce Maternal and Childhood Mortality and Morbidity: World Health Organization Headquarters, Geneva, 6–7 February 2012: Meeting Report. World Health Organization; 2013. Accessed March 19, 2022. https://apps.who.int/iris/handle/10665/78067
8. Dean SV, Lassi ZS, Imam AM, et al. Preconception care: closing the gap in the continuum of care to accelerate improvements in maternal, newborn and child health. Reprod Health 2014;11(Suppl 3):S1.
9. Jacob CM, Killeen SL, McAuliffe FM, et al. Prevention of noncommunicable diseases by interventions in the preconception period: a FIGO position paper for action by healthcare practitioners. Int J Gynaecol Obstet 2020;151(Suppl 1):6–15.
10. Dean SV, Lassi ZS, Imam AM, et al. Preconception care: nutritional risks and interventions. Reprod Health 2014;11(Suppl 3):S3.
11. Fleming TP, Watkins AJ, Velazquez MA, et al. Origins of lifetime health around the time of conception: causes and consequences. Lancet 2018;391(10132):1842–52.
12. Rahman MM, Abe SK, Rahman MS, et al. Maternal anemia and risk of adverse birth and health outcomes in low- and middle-income countries: systematic review and meta-analysis. Am J Clin Nutr 2016;103(2):495–504.
13. World Health Organization. Global anaemia reduction efforts among women of reproductive age: impact, achievement of targets and the way forward for optimizing efforts. World Health Organization; 2020. Available at: https://apps.who.int/iris/handle/10665/336559. Accessed March 29, 2022.
14. World Health Organization. WHO guidelines for malaria, 18 february 2022. World Health Organization; 2022. Available at: https://apps.who.int/iris/handle/10665/351995. Accessed March 29, 2022.
15. Lassi ZS, Imam AM, Dean SV, et al. Preconception care: preventing and treating infections. Reprod Health 2014;11(Suppl 3):S4.

16. Boadu I. Coverage and determinants of modern contraceptive use in sub-Saharan Africa: further analysis of demographic and health surveys. Reprod Health 2022;19(1):18.

17. Ahinkorah BO. Predictors of modern contraceptive use among adolescent girls and young women in sub-Saharan Africa: a mixed effects multilevel analysis of data from 29 demographic and health surveys. Contracept Reprod Med 2020; 5(1):32.

18. Casey SE, Chynoweth SK, Cornier N, et al. Progress and gaps in reproductive health services in three humanitarian settings: mixed-methods case studies. Confl Health 2015;9(Suppl 1):S3.

19. Dev R, Kohler P, Feder M, et al. A systematic review and meta-analysis of post-partum contraceptive use among women in low- and middle-income countries. Reprod Health 2019;16(1):154.

20. Bank D. Guaranteed Impact: Increasing supplies and cutting prices for contraceptives without spending a dime. Stanf Soc Innov Rev 2016;14(3):A16–8.

21. Bertrand JT, Ross J, Sullivan TM, et al. Contraceptive method mix: updates and implications. Glob Health Sci Pract 2020;8(4):666–79.

22. Hoyt J, Krishnaratne S, Hamon JK, et al. "As a woman who watches how my family is… I take the difficult decisions": a qualitative study on integrated family planning and childhood immunisation services in five African countries. Reprod Health 2021;18(1):41.

23. United Nations. Contraceptive use by method 2019: data booklet. UN; 2019. https://doi.org/10.18356/1bd58a10-en.

24. World Health Organization. WHO guideline on self-care interventions for health and well-being. World Health Organization; 2021. Available at: https://apps.who.int/iris/handle/10665/342741. Accessed March 22, 2022.

25. Lerma K, Goldthwaite LM. Injectable contraception: emerging evidence on subcutaneous self-administration. Curr Opin Obstet Gynecol 2019;31(6):464–70.

26. World vasectomy day – an act of love – vasectomy. Available at: https://wvd.org/. Accessed April 3, 2022.

27. Senderowicz L, Maloney N. Supply-side versus demand-side unmet need: implications for family planning programs. Popul Dev Rev. n/a(n/a). doi:10.1111/padr.12478

28. World Health Organization. Ensuring human rights in the provision of contraceptive information and services: guidance and recommendations. World Health Organization; 2014. Available at: http://www.who.int/reproductivehealth/publications/family_planning/human-rights-contraception/en/. Accessed March 22, 2022.

29. Ahmed K, Baeten JM, Beksinska M, et al. HIV incidence among women using intramuscular depot medroxyprogesterone acetate, a copper intrauterine device, or a levonorgestrel implant for contraception: a randomised, multicentre, open-label trial. Lancet 2019;394(10195):303–13.

30. World Health Organization. Contraceptive eligibility for women at high risk of HIV. Guidance statement: recommendations on contraceptive methods used by women at high risk of HIV. World Health Organization; 2019. Available at: https://apps.who.int/iris/handle/10665/346345. Accessed March 22, 2022.

31. Curtis KM, Hannaford PC, Rodriguez MI, et al. Hormonal contraception and HIV acquisition among women: an updated systematic review. BMJ Sex Reprod Health 2020;46(1):8–16.

32. World Health Organization Department of Reproductive Health and Research (WHO/RHR), Johns Hopkins Bloomberg School of Public Health/Center for Communication Programs (CCP), Knowledge for Health Project. Family Planning:

A Global Handbook for Providers. 2018 Update. Baltimore and Geneva: CCP and WHO; 2018.

33. World Health Organization, Medical Eligibility Criteria for Contraceptive Use, 5th Edition, 2015, World Health Organization; Geneva. Available at: https://www.who.int/publications-detail-redirect/9789241549158. Accessed March 22, 2022.

34. Eisinger RW, Dieffenbach CW, Fauci AS. HIV viral load and transmissibility of hiv infection: undetectable equals untransmittable. JAMA 2019;321(5):451–2.

35. Moore Z, Pfitzer A, Gubin R, et al. Missed opportunities for family planning: an analysis of pregnancy risk and contraceptive method use among postpartum women in 21 low- and middle-income countries. Contraception 2015;92(1):31–9.

36. Gahungu J, Vahdaninia M, Regmi PR. The unmet needs for modern family planning methods among postpartum women in Sub-Saharan Africa: a systematic review of the literature. Reprod Health 2021;18(1):35.

37. Gebeyehu NA, Lake EA, Gelaw KA, et al. The intention on modern contraceptive use and associated factors among postpartum women in public health institutions of sodo town, southern ethiopia 2019: an institutional-based cross-sectional study. Biomed Res Int 2020;2020:9815465.

38. Wulifan JK, Brenner S, Jahn A, et al. A scoping review on determinants of unmet need for family planning among women of reproductive age in low and middle income countries. BMC Womens Health 2016;16:2.

39. Ayanore MA, Pavlova M, Groot W. Unmet reproductive health needs among women in some West African countries: a systematic review of outcome measures and determinants. Reprod Health 2016;13(1):5.

40. Conde-Agudelo A, Belizán JM. Maternal morbidity and mortality associated with interpregnancy interval: cross sectional study. BMJ 2000;321(7271):1255–9.

41. Cleland J, Bernstein S, Ezeh A, et al. Family planning: the unfinished agenda. Lancet Lond Engl 2006;368(9549):1810–27.

42. Geremew AB, Boke MM, Yismaw AE. The effect of antenatal care service utilization on postnatal care service utilization: a systematic review and meta-analysis study. J Pregnancy 2020;2020:7363242.

43. Ross JA, Winfrey WL. Contraceptive use, intention to use and unmet need during the extended postpartum period. Int Fam Plann Persp 2001;27(1):20.

44. Cleland J, Shah IH, Daniele M. Interventions to improve postpartum family planning in low- and middle-income countries: program implications and research priorities. Studies in Family Planning 2015;46(4):423–41.

45. Blazer C, Prata N. Postpartum family planning: current evidence on successful interventions. Open Access J Contracept 2016;7:53–67.

46. Lori JR, Chuey M, Munro-Kramer ML, et al. Increasing postpartum family planning uptake through group antenatal care: a longitudinal prospective cohort design. Reprod Health 2018;15(1):208.

47. Family Planning and Immunization Integration Services Postpartum. HIPs. Available at: https://www.fphighimpactpractices.org/briefs/family-planning-and-immunization-integration/. Accessed March 19, 2022.

48. Balasubramaniam S, Kumar S, Sethi R, et al. Quasi-experimental Study of Systematic Screening for Family Planning Services among Postpartum Women Attending Village Health and Nutrition Days in Jharkhand, India. Int J Integr Care 2018;18(1). https://doi.org/10.5334/ijic.3078.

49. Cooper CM, Fields R, Mazzeo CI, et al. Successful proof of concept of family planning and immunization integration in Liberia. Glob Health Sci Pract 2015;3(1):71–84.

50. Dulli LS, Eichleay M, Rademacher K, et al. Meeting Postpartum women's family planning needs through integrated family planning and immunization services: results of a cluster-randomized controlled trial in rwanda. Glob Health Sci Pract 2016;4(1):73–86.

51. Grant-Maidment T, Kranzer K, Ferrand RA. The effect of integration of family planning into HIV services on contraceptive use among women accessing HIV services in low and middle-income countries: a systematic review. Front Glob Womens Health 2022;3. Available at: https://www.frontiersin.org/article/10.3389/fgwh.2022.837358. Accessed March 21, 2022.

52. Haberlen SA, Narasimhan M, Beres LK, et al. Integration of family planning services into HIV care and treatment services: a systematic review. Stud Fam Plann 2017;48(2):153–77.

53. Ippoliti NB, Nanda G, Wilcher R. Meeting the reproductive health needs of female key populations affected by HIV in low- and middle-income countries: a review of the evidence. Stud Fam Plann 2017;48(2):121–51.

54. World Health Organisation (Geneva). Integration of HIV Testing and Linkage in Family Planning and Contraception Services: Implementation Brief. 2021. Available at: https://www.who.int/publications-detail-redirect/9789240035188. Accessed March 22, 2022.

55. Immediate Postpartum Family Planning Counseling and Services. HIPs. Available at: https://www.fphighimpactpractices.org/briefs/immediate-postpartum-family-planning/. Accessed March 19, 2022.

56. Goldthwaite LM, Shaw KA. Immediate postpartum provision of long-acting reversible contraception. Curr Opin Obstet Gynecol 2015;27(6):460–4.

57. Harrison MS, Goldenberg RL. Immediate postpartum use of long-acting reversible contraceptives in low- and middle-income countries. Matern Health Neonatol Perinatol 2017;3. https://doi.org/10.1186/s40748-017-0063-z.

58. Makins A, Taghinejadi N, Sethi M, et al. FIGO postpartum intrauterine device initiative: complication rates across six countries. Int J Gynaecol Obstet Off Organ Int Fed Gynaecol Obstet 2018;143(Suppl 1):20–7.

59. Gallagher MC, Morris CN, Fatima A, et al. Immediate postpartum long-acting reversible contraception: a comparison across six humanitarian country contexts. Front Glob Womens Health 2021;2:613338.

60. Pradhan E, Canning D, Shah IH, et al. Integrating postpartum contraceptive counseling and IUD insertion services into maternity care in Nepal: results from stepped-wedge randomized controlled trial. Reprod Health 2019;16(1):69.

61. Postabortion family planning care and services. HIPs. Available at: https://www.fphighimpactpractices.org/briefs/postabortion-family-planning/. Accessed March 19, 2022.

62. Huber D, Curtis C, Irani L, et al. Postabortion care: 20 years of strong evidence on emergency treatment, family planning, and other programming components. Glob Health Sci Pract 2016;4(3):481–94. https://doi.org/10.9745/GHSP-D-16-00052.

63. World health organization & UNDP/UNFPA/WHO/world bank special programme of research, development and research training in human reproduction H. Task Shifting to improve Access to contraceptive methods: improve Access to key Maternal and newborn health interventions. World Health Organization; 4. Available at: https://apps.who.int/iris/handle/10665/94831. Accessed March 27, 2022.

64. Charyeva Z, Oguntunde O, Orobaton N, et al. Task shifting provision of contraceptive implants to community health extension workers: results of operations research in northern nigeria. Glob Health Sci Pract 2015;3(3):382–94.

65. Malarcher S, Meirik O, Lebetkin E, et al. Provision of DMPA by community health workers: what the evidence shows. Contraception 2011;83(6):495–503.
66. Stanback J, Spieler J, Shah I, et al. Expanding Access to Injectable Contraceptives Technical Consultation Participants. Community-based health workers can safely and effectively administer injectable contraceptives: conclusions from a technical consultation. Contraception 2010;81(3):181–4.
67. High-impact practices in family planning (HIPs). *Community health workers: bringing family planning Services to where people Live and work.* USAID; 2015. Available at: https://www.fphighimpactpractices.org/briefs/community-health-workers/. Accessed March 19, 2022.
68. Global Humanitarian Overview 2022 | Global Humanitarian Overview. Available at: https://gho.unocha.org/. Accessed April 4, 2022.
69. IAWG | inter-agency working group on reproduction health in crises. Available at: https://iawgfieldmanual.com/. Accessed April 4, 2022.

Antenatal and Postnatal Care

Adeniyi Kolade Aderoba, MBBS, FWACS (OBGYN), FMCOG, MSc[a,b,*],
Kwame Adu-Bonsaffoh, MBChB, FWACS (OBGYN), MPhil (Physiology), MSc (Epidemiology)[c,d]

KEYWORDS

- Antenatal care • Postnatal care • Maternal health • Newborn health
- Evidence-based care • Obstetric care

KEY POINTS

- Antenatal care (ANC) and postnatal care (PNC) should be of sufficient scope and quality to help women and their families explore care options and make shared decisions with their caregivers that are relevant to their context without over medicalizing its practices.
- In many areas, the care of women during pregnancy and after childbirth have shifted from relying on caregivers' opinions to underpinning ANC and PNC with high-quality evidence.
- Despite increasing evidence that supports the components of the care needed to promote a positive pregnancy and postnatal experience, research gaps, and other health systems challenges, including limited resources, exist. Therefore, the content and quality of ANC and PNC vary across settings.

INTRODUCTION

Since Archibald Leman Cochrane flagged obstetric care as a discipline that lacked evidence in many of its practices approximately 4 decades ago, evidence-based obstetric care has evolved.[1] Many aspects of the care of women during pregnancy, delivery, and the period after childbirth have shifted from reliance on caregivers' opinions to underpinning obstetric practices with high-quality evidence. Despite the increase in obstetric evidence, global or context-specific gaps exist. Additionally, the resources available for obstetric care are not identical in all settings. Therefore, the content, quality, and implementation of evidence-based obstetrics vary across countries and contexts.

[a] Centre for Population Health and Interdisciplinary Research, HealthMATE 360, Ondo Town, Ondo State, Nigeria; [b] National Perinatal Epidemiology Unit, Nuffield Department of Population Health, University of Oxford, Oxford, United Kingdom; [c] Department of Obstetrics and Gynecology, University of Ghana Medical School, Accra, Ghana; [d] Department of Obstetrics and Gynecology, Korle-Bu Teaching Hospital, Accra, Ghana
* Corresponding author. Centre for Population Health and Interdisciplinary Research, Health-MATE 360, Box 603, Ondo Town, Ondo State, Nigeria
E-mail address: adeniyi.aderoba@gmail.com

Obstet Gynecol Clin N Am 49 (2022) 665–692
https://doi.org/10.1016/j.ogc.2022.07.005

The World Health Organization (WHO) Quality of Care framework for maternal health describes two interlinked dimensions that underpin good-quality care.[2] This includes the health care provided and how the pregnant woman experiences it. Despite the complex nature of the definition of health with dimensions of physical, mental, and social well-being,[3] the current emphasis is on preventing death and severe morbidity. Health equally prioritizes person-centered health and well-being as a human right. This review is focused on an overview of the components of antenatal care (ANC) and postnatal care (PNC) needed to promote a culturally sensitive and positive pregnancy experience.

The terms "antenatal," "antepartum," and "prenatal" are usually used interchangeably to refer to events regarding obstetric care before birth; likewise, "postnatal" and "postpartum" are used to refer to events after birth.[4] Occasionally, postpartum suggests more maternal issues, while postnatal concerns the baby.[4] Although some professional guidelines describe the period after birth as postpartum,[5] for clarity, the WHO technical panel advised using postnatal for all maternal and child issues after birth.[4] Therefore, this review will use the terms antenatal and postnatal to refer to the period before and after birth, respectively.

ANTENATAL CARE

ANC refers to the "care provided by skilled health care professionals (HCPs) to pregnant women and adolescent girls to ensure the best health conditions for both mother and baby during pregnancy."[6] Antenatal care visits offer an opportunity for risk identification, health education, health promotion, disease prevention, early identification and management of pregnancy-related or concurrent disorders, birth preparedness and complication readiness. Maternal mortality and complications during pregnancy, childbirth, and puerperium are important contributors to the global disease burden.[7] Compared with less than half of the pregnant women in resource-limited regions, more than 80% attend ANC in well-resourced areas.[8] Women who register early for ANC and receive regular care tend to have better pregnancy outcomes.[9,10]

Women are more empowered to engage in shared decision-making with their caregivers when they feel respected, safe, and supported.[11,12] Thus, respectful maternity care is a human right while implementing programs to reduce preventable maternal morbidity and mortality[13] and a critical consideration in providing quality maternity care.[14] Maternity care should be of sufficient quality and scope to help women and their families explore treatment options and preferences and make shared decisions with their providers. Shared decision-making requires a trusting woman–provider relationship. Occasionally, a consensus is reached over more than one clinic visit. Alternative consultations or multidisciplinary reviews, including ethics professionals, may be needed when a woman's preference contrasts with professional recommendations and ethical codes.

Organization of Antenatal Care

ANC may be provided by a team of providers or a single professional such as a midwife, medical officer, obstetrician-gynecologist, family medicine physician, or maternal-fetal medicine (MFM) specialist. Typically, ANC is midwifery-led or offered by a multidisciplinary team with midwives caring for pregnancies that are not expected to be associated with complications. In contrast, obstetrician-gynecologists and MFM specialists manage pregnancies with increasing complications.

Continuity of care with the same HCP or team is recommended when possible.[15] Midwife-led continuity of care offer some benefitl to low-risk women and their babies.[16] A Cochrane review shows that midwife-led continuity of care appears associated with fewer interventions such as regional analgesia and instrumental births but no difference in cesarean births in low-risk pregnancies.[16] With the need for higher-level care, transfer of care between HCPs or teams is critical,[15] and with effective communication, women generally accept transfers between HCPs.[17] However, cross-cutting guidelines on HCPs' professional scope of practice and contracts on remuneration and liabilities are essential.[18]

Efficient medical record systems with clear documentation have the potential to improve care and enhance effective communication between multiple providers.[15] Medical records are often in case notes stored in Health Management Information Systems or held by women. Beyond their clinical use, case notes can have quality assurance, audit, or medico-legal use. The WHO recommends women-held case notes to improve the quality and continuity of care and pregnancy experience.[6] Women-held case notes may make medical records readily available in settings with no immediate access to documents when women present to other health centers with complications.[19] Health system planners should reflect on the safety and content of women-held case notes to ensure confidentiality and prevent stigma and discrimination.[6] Managing cases of missing women-held case notes could also be challenging. Alternatively, medical records could be built into mobile apps in settings with good mobile phone coverage.

Usually, ANC is offered individually to pregnant women by an HCP, and evidence shows that many of its components are beneficial.[20] However, some parts or all ANC components may be provided to a group of pregnant women. Group ANC can help increase provider availability and women experience, including the time for patient education, and decrease waiting times and health care costs.[21] This may be attractive in resource-limited settings.[22] Compared with individual ANC, group ANC does not seem inferior in improving perinatal outcomes.[20,23] However, it may increase pregnancy knowledge and patient satisfaction and improve mental health, and current evidence suggests it is not associated with adverse consequences.[20,23–25] In women with similar risks such as mellitus, adolescents, and low income, group ANC may be beneficial.[26,2728] Nevertheless, the impact of ANC may vary across settings.[20] Evidence from Nigeria and Kenya showed that women who had group ANC received quality ANC and had a higher frequency of ANC visits compared with individual ANC.[29] A combined approach of individual and group ANC may provide more postnatal information and better prepare women for parenting.[30] Given, the diverse literature on individual vs group ANC, a decision on the primary approach to undertake should be context-specific based on experience, resources, and women's preferences.

Traditionally, in the standard ANC model, a low-risk pregnant woman in which no complications are anticipated has scheduled ANC visits every 4 weeks until 28 weeks of gestation, every 2 weeks until 36 weeks of pregnancy, and then weekly until childbirth.[10,31] With this schedule, a woman who "books" or initiates ANC early, ideally before 10 weeks,[32] and delivers after 40 weeks, would have at least 10 ANC contacts. In contrast, the focused ANC (FANC) model introduced by the WHO in 2002 advocated four scheduled ANC visits for women without complications (basic model).[33] Evidence underpinning FANC was from a WHO multicenter trial and a WHO systematic review of randomized controlled trials of routine ANC showing similar or no in difference in , urinary tract infection, post-partum anemia, low birthweight and maternal mortality with reduced visits.[33] However,more recent evidence indicates that FANC might be associated with more perinatal deaths than a model with at least eight visits that also offers greater maternal satisfaction.[10,34]. A Cochrane review showed no

Table 1
Comparison of the World Health Organization 2002 and 2016 models of antenatal care

	2002 WHO ANC Model	2016 WHO ANC Model
Approach	• Focused or goal-oriented guidance at specific ANC visits	• Individualized, person-centered respectful care at every ANC contact
Number of visits	• Four (basic model)	• At least eight
Schedule of ANC contact	• First visit (8–12 wk) • Second visit (24–26 wk) • Third visit (32 wk) • Fourth visit (36–38 wk) • Return at 41 wk if yet to give birth	• Contact 1 (up to 12 wk) • Contact 2 (20 wk) • Contact 3 (26 wk) • Contact 4 (30 wk) • Contact 5 (34 wk) • Contact 6 (36 wk) • Contact 7 (38 wk) • Contact 8 (40 wk) • Return at 41 wk if yet to give birth
Key considerations	• Potentially more cost-effective because of fewer contacts • Fitting all ANC components into four visits may be difficult to achieve in low-resource settings with overburdened services • Possibly associated with more perinatal deaths	• Offer more contacts to build authentic and supportive relationships with maternity care providers • Valued more by women and associated with greater maternal satisfaction • More contact with knowledgeable, supportive, and respectful health care practitioners likely to lead to a positive pregnancy experience • Potentially improves safety through increased frequency of maternal and fetal assessment

significant differences in maternal and perinatal health outcomes such as maternal death, hypertensive disorders of pregnancy, preterm birth, and small for gestational age between models with at least eight ANC contacts and those with more contacts. **Table 1** compares WHO 2002 and 2016 models of ANC.

Early booking helps establish gestational age using a dating scan, where available. It allows baseline maternal assessment such as blood pressure measurement, weight, and laboratory tests in women with chronic diseases. The booking visit is also where initial risk stratification is carried out. Women are also provided early social service

Thematic areas of Antenatal care

- **Risk assessment or identification of pre-existing diseases**
- **Health education, health promotion, and disease prevention**
- **Early identification and management of pregnancy-related or coexisting disease**
- **Birth preparedness and complication readiness**

Fig. 1. Thematic areas of antenatal care.

Table 2
Suggested list of antenatal care tests[a]

Routine Investigations[b]	Possibly Selective or Context-Specific Investigations[b]
• ABO and Rhesus (Rh) D type (and antibody screen if Rh negative) • Diabetes screening • Full blood count • Tests for key infections: chlamydia, gonorrhea, group B Streptococcus, hepatitis B surface antigen, HIV serology, Rubella serology, serologic screen for syphilis (VDRL or RPR) • Urine culture[d] Urinalysis including proteinuria[c] • Ultrasound: pregnancy dating and fetal anomaly scans	• Breast cancer screening • Cervical cancer screening • Lead level • G6PD screening • Genetic screening • Preeclampsia screening • Screening for sickle cell and thalassemia • Test for infections (based on signs/symptoms, and other individualized considerations): Chagas disease, COVID-19, cytomegalovirus, hepatitis A, hepatitis C, herpes simplex virus, malaria, measles, parvovirus, toxoplasmosis, tuberculosis, Varicella serology, Zika virus • Tests for vaginitis and vaginal discharge: bacterial vaginosis, candidiasis, *Trichomonas vaginalis* • Thyroid function tests • Ultrasound: fetal growth assessment

Abbreviations: G6PD, glucose-6-phosphate dehydrogenase; HIV, human immunodeficiency virus; RPR, rapid plasma reagin; VDRL, venereal disease research laboratory.
   [a] Individual considerations may vary with national antenatal care guidelines.
   [b] May be indicated at different time points in pregnancy.
   [c] Selective proteinuria screening is recommended in some settings because of data showing that it is potentially more cost-effective[38]
   [d] UK recently recommended stopping screening for asymptomatic bacteriuria because screening tests that work and the optimal time to test are unknown (ref. - UK National Screening Committee. Antenatal Screening Programme - Asymptomatic Bacteriuria [Internet]. [London]: UK NSC; 2020 [cited 2022 Aug 29] https://view-health-screening-recommendations.service.gov.uk/asymptomatic-bacteriuria/[38]
   Data from Refs.[6,31,37]

support, prenatal screening, and diagnostic tests when indicated. Although the WHO estimates that 60% of pregnant women register for ANC before 12 weeks globally, geographic and income disparities exist.[8] About 20% of pregnant women in low-income countries registered early for ANC compared with more than 80% in high-income countries (HICs).[8] Adolescents and women with less than high-school education are more likely to start ANC later.[35]

Activities at Antenatal Care Visits

ANC is a planned program to make pregnancy a safe and satisfying experience. Typically, ANC activities are performed under the following themes (**Fig. 1**). ANC aims to implement an appropriate standard of care with guidelines that ensure that crucial examinations, laboratory tests, and interventions are not missed.[36] Nonetheless, the effectiveness of some of the individual components of ANC components have not been assessed through high-quality research.

Risk assessment or identification of pre-existing disease: the booking visit

ANC provides a platform along the reproductive continuum of care for risk assessment and disease diagnosis, treatment, and prevention. Risk assessment helps to identify the potential for complications and the need for specialized care or referral to higher-level health facilities. Thus, the first ANC visit, also known as the booking visit, is critical for assessing the underlying risks to a woman and her baby. The visit documents a woman's relevant obstetric, gynecologic, medical, surgical, drug, allergy, family, and social history. Additionally, a thorough physical examination and appropriate laboratory tests should be conducted to identify the existing conditions that increase maternal or fetal risk of complications during pregnancy. Suggested routine and selective ANC tests are listed in **Table 2**. The laboratory investigations may vary with national guidelines.

Although many checklists and risk assessment tools for a wide range of conditions such as the classifying form of the WHO FANC model exist in many settings,[33] there are no consensus criteria for classifying risks in pregnancy. Risk assessment is dynamic during pregnancy. The ability to systematically identify risks is nuanced by health provider skills, patient characteristics, health system resources for patient examination and laboratory tests, and mechanisms to finance clinical assessment. Checklists and risk assessment tools are practical means of using limited resources, especially in resource-constrained settings, and ensuring that the essential elements of a woman's evaluation are not missed. Nonetheless, antenatal risk assessment tools even with good intentions are not perfect tools.[118] They may either contain irrelevant items or omit critical questions in many settings.[118] Also, they are usually not validated for use in different setting or may exhibit low sensitivity and high specificity in predicting adverse outcomes. Therefore, proof of this approach to reducing pregnancy complications is lacking and using antenatal risk assessment tools requires caution. Classifying a woman high risk might increase anxiety. Conversely, assigning a static low-risk status to women may reduce surveillance for complications and increase the potential of missing conditions associated with adverse outcomes.

A critical activity often performed at the booking visit is determining gestational age. Accurate determination of gestational age is vital for ANC. It is crucial to assess optimal fetal growth, schedule tests and interventions in pregnancy, interpret results, estimate the delivery date, and diagnose and prevent post-term pregnancy complications. A dating scan is helpful to establish when a fetus is viable for independent extrauterine life. The most accurate method to confirm gestational age is an early ultrasound measurement of the embryo or fetus up to and including 13 + 6/7 weeks of gestation.[39] In cases of pregnancies resulting from assisted reproductive technology (ART), an ART-derived gestational age, that is, the date of embryo transfer for in vitro fertilization pregnancies, should be used to assign the estimated delivery date (EDD).[39] Nevertheless, many pregnancies worldwide are dated based on a recall of the first day of a woman's last normal menstrual period (LMP). LMP dates should be confirmed or re-dated using ultrasound. Pregnancy dating is considered suboptimal when ultrasound validation or dating is not performed before 22 + 0/7 weeks.[39] Once determined, the EDD should be communicated and discussed with the woman and documented in the medical records. Additionally, a first-trimester scan can help identify congenital anomalies[40] and it is crucial to determine the number of fetuses, amnionicity, and chorionicity in cases of suspected multiple pregnancies.[41]

Health education, health promotion, and disease prevention

Many pregnant women, especially those expecting their first babies, are concerned about their health and preventing harm to their babies during pregnancy. Health education should be integral to care to counter myths and misinformation. Group ANC typically offers health education activities with facilitated group discussions and skill-building sessions to improve pregnancy knowledge, birth preparedness, complication readiness, and early parenting. Apart from traditional one-on-one and group discussion sessions, other innovative platforms for health education include online courses, apps, credible websites, brochures, and handouts. Topics routinely discussed during ANC classes include food safety and nutrition, family planning including postpartum contraception options, interpregnancy interval, smoking cessation, alcohol abstinence, lowering daily caffeine intake, exercise, sexuality, immunization, substance abuse, medication safety, oral health, prenatal screening, diagnostic tests, danger signs, community support resources, breastfeeding and early parenting, normal labor, and birth including companionship, partner involvement, perinatal grief, birth preparedness, complication readiness, induction of labor, cesarean delivery, pain relief in labor, preterm birth, and neonatal intensive care unit admission. These topics need to be tailored to the woman and setting.

Globally, about one in three pregnant women are anemic,[119] of which majority are nutritional. Therefore, adequate nutrition and evidence-based vitamin and mineral supplementation are critical to optimal pregnancy outcomes. Nutritional intervention includes counseling on a healthy diet containing adequate energy, protein, vitamins, and minerals, including daily supplementation with 400 ug of folic acid and 30 to 60 mg of elemental iron to meet maternal and fetal requirements.[6] Calcium and vitamin A supplementation are recommended only in deficient populations to mitigate the risk of preeclampsia and night blindness, respectively.[6] Routine zinc, multiple micronutrients, and vitamin B6, E, C, or D supplementation are not recommended during pregnancy.[6]

About [120,121,122,123,124] two-thirds or more women take prescription medications during pregnancy,[42] some of which have the potential to induce serious adverse fetal effects, including birth defects. Thus, women should be counseled on the safe use of medications and be involved in the decision to start, stop, or change medications based on their risks and benefits and the presence of safer alternatives.[43] Similar safety considerations apply to over-the-counter medications without prescriptions.

Vaccination protects pregnant women from vaccine-preventable diseases and can transfer antibodies across the placenta to improve fetal and newborn immunity.[44] For instance, vaccination programs reduced the global burden of death from neonatal tetanus deaths by 90% between 1990 and 2015.[45] Generally, vaccines are safe and associated with minimal risks in pregnant women and their fetuses than their corresponding vaccine-preventable diseases. Nonetheless, each case requires consideration of its merits and demerits. Routinely recommended inactivated vaccines in pregnancy include tetanus, diphtheria, and pertussis (Tdap) vaccine[46] and influenza (flu) vaccine.[47,48] Regardless of a woman's history of receiving Tdap, the vaccine should be administered between 27 and 36 weeks of gestation, although it can be offered at any time during pregnancy.[46] If a pregnant woman is unvaccinated or her immunization status is unknown, the 2016 WHO ANC model recommends two doses of a tetanus toxoid–containing vaccine (TT-CV) 1 month apart. The first dose can be given at the first ANC contact, with the second dose administered at least 2 weeks before birth.[6] The ongoing coronavirus (COVID-19) pandemic and evidence that pregnancy increases risk for severe illness if infection occurs makes prevention especially important in this population.[49] With the development of effective COVID-19 vaccines, and evidence of their safety during pregnancy, the WHO recommends COVID-19 vaccination for pregnant women.[49]

Generally, recommended vaccines are inactivated microorganisms or microorganism subunits that contain recombinant, polysaccharide, or conjugate pieces. Thus, they are potentially valuable for almost everyone, including in pregnancy, and growing evidence demonstrates their safety.[46,50] For example, hepatitis B vaccine, a recombinant vaccine can be offered to women completing a vaccination schedule begun before conception, unvaccinated women, and uninfected women at high risk of infection (such as: recent or current injection drug use, exposure to an HBsAg-positive sex partner, more than one sex partner during the previous 6 months, and evaluation or treatment of a sexually transmitted infection).[46,51] A newer hepatitis B vaccine with an adjuvant to boost the immune system (Heplisav-B) is currently not approved for use during pregnancy because safety data is lacking.[52]

Unlike inactivated vaccines that are considered safe during pregnancy, live attenuated vaccines are usually not advised unless there is a risk of contracting an infection that poses risks to a pregnant woman or her fetus or both, and the benefit of vaccination outweighs the risks.[53] Examples include oral polio (inactivated polio vaccine preferred) and yellow fever vaccines. Women should avoid getting pregnant within 4 weeks of receiving a live vaccine and 13 weeks in the case of varicella vaccination.[54] Although if they happen to get pregnant, a termination of pregnancy is not advised because the theoretic risk of adverse outcome is unconfirmed.[54] Also, a large meta-analysis of more than 1 million children reported that vaccines generally are not associated with autism.[55]

Early identification and management of pregnancy-related or coexisting diseases

Many pregnant women experience symptoms or discomfort, such as nausea, vomiting, or pressure symptoms that accompany the physiologic changes during pregnancy. While some symptoms like nausea and vomiting are limited to early pregnancy, others such as pressure symptoms, for example, heartburn, low back and pelvic pain, constipation, varicose vein, and edema, may increase or persist throughout pregnancy.

One of the pillars of ANC is surveillance for new illnesses or worsening prepregnancy diseases. The range of illnesses for which surveillance is mounted differs with geographic settings. While the common illnesses for which surveillance is mounted during pregnancy will include hypertension and diabetes mellitus, one of the less commonly tracked is mental illness. A recent umbrella review of 10 systematic reviews reported that the global prevalence of antenatal depression ranged between 15% and 65%.[56] Despite being very common during pregnancy, many women find it challenging to seek care for mental illnesses due to stigma, cultural conceptions about mental illness, lack of or poor enlightenment about support services, and fear that medication may harm their babies.[57] Without treatment, mental illnesses, especially depression and anxiety, may persist for several years.[58,59] Therefore, many guidelines promote screening for perinatal mental health disorders,[60,61] which can be self- or provider-initiated using paper- or computer-based tools.[62] According to the systematic review by Sambrook-Smith et al., of 76 tools to identify perinatal mental health disorders, the most validated tools were the Edinburgh Postnatal Depression Scale (EPDS), the Beck Depression Inventory (BDI), and the Patient Health Questionnaire (PHQ).[62] Although the review showed that the EPDS, PHQ, and BDI can be used across diverse settings, several considerations such as ethnicity, language, and geographic, cultural, and socioeconomic settings might affect the validity of tools.[62]

With advances in ultrasound and genetic technologies, several guidelines exist for prenatal screening of fetal aneuploidy, neural tube defects, fetal anomalies, and maternal genetic carriers.[63,64] Typically, a routine second-trimester 18- to 22-week ultrasound is recommended for fetal structural abnormality screening and diagnosis, placental localization, amniotic fluid volume assessment, and gestational age (if an earlier dating scan is unavailable).[36,65] In women with a higher risk of congenital anomalies, the structural abnormalities scan can be performed earlier at 13 to 16 weeks gestation.[66] Routine ultrasonography performed before 24 weeks improves the dating

Table 3
WHO antenatal context-specific recommendations

Care Area	Recommendation	Context/Setting
Dietary interventions	• Nutrition education on increasing daily energy and protein intake to reduce the risk of low-birth-weight neonates • Balanced energy and dietary protein supplementation reduce the risk of stillbirths and small-for-gestational-age neonates.	• In undernourished populations
Iron and folic acid supplements	• Intermittent oral iron and folic acid supplementation with 120 mg of elemental iron and 2.8 mg of folic acid once weekly to improve maternal and neonatal outcomes	• If daily iron is not acceptable owing to side effects, and in populations with an anemia prevalence among pregnant women of < 20%.
Calcium supplements	• Daily calcium supplementation (1.5–2.0 g of oral elemental calcium) to reduce the risk of preeclampsia	• In populations with low dietary calcium intake
Vitamin A supplements	• Vitamin A supplementation to prevent night blindness	• Areas whereby vitamin A deficiency is a severe public health problem, that is, if > 5% of women have a history of night blindness in their most recent pregnancy in the previous 3–5 y that ended in a live birth, or if > 20% of pregnant women have a serum retinol level < 0.70 mol/L
Restricting caffeine intake	• For pregnant women with high daily caffeine intake, lowering daily caffeine intake during pregnancy is recommended to reduce the risk of pregnancy loss and low-birth-weight neonates	• Pregnant women with a daily caffeine intake of more than 300 mg per day
Asymptomatic bacteriuria (ASB)	• Midstream urine culture is the recommended method for diagnosing ASB in pregnancy. In settings whereby urine culture is not available, on-site midstream urine Gram staining is recommended over using dipstick tests	• Alternative methods can be considered when urine culture is not available

(continued on next page)

Table 3
(continued)

Care Area	Recommendation	Context/Setting
Intimate partner violence (IPV)	• Clinical inquiry about the possibility of IPV should be strongly considered at antenatal care visits when assessing conditions that may be caused or complicated by IPV to improve clinical diagnosis and subsequent care	• In settings whereby there is the capacity to provide a supportive response, including referral where appropriate
Tuberculosis (TB)	• Systematic screening for active TB should be considered for pregnant women as part of antenatal care	• In settings whereby TB prevalence in the population is $\geq 100/100,000$ population
Preventive anthelmintic treatment	• Preventive anthelmintic treatment is recommended after the first trimester as part of worm infection reduction programs	• Endemic areas with >20% prevalence of infection with any soil-transmitted helminths
Malaria prevention: intermittent preventive treatment in pregnancy (IPTp)	• Intermittent preventive treatment with sulfadoxine–pyrimethamine (IPTp-SP) is recommended. Dosing should start in the 2nd trimester with doses given at least 1 month apart, with goal of at least 3 doses received	• In malaria-endemic areas in Africa
Pre-exposure prophylaxis (PrEP) for HIV prevention	• Oral PrEP containing tenofovir disoproxil fumarate (TDF) should be offered as an additional prevention choice for pregnant women at substantial risk of HIV infection as part of combination prevention approaches	• A substantial risk of HIV infection is an incidence of HIV in the absence of PrEP that is > 3%

Adapted from World Health Organization (WHO). WHO recommendations on antenatal care for a positive pregnancy experience. Published 2016. Available at https://www.who.int/publications/i/item/9789241549912.

and detection of multiple gestations and significant congenital anomalies[41] but showed no significant change in perinatal mortality.[41] After 24 weeks, A Cochrane review by Bricker et. al showed routine ultrasound does not decrease perinatal mortality.[67] Although the review findings have been debated due to its methodological challenges, including being underpowered,[125] its conclusion of the lack of benefit of routine late pregnancy ultrasound remains a gap requiring high-quality research.

In many settings, assessment of fetal growth in the second half of pregnancy involves symphysis-fundal height measurement, abdominal palpation, or both.[36,68] Routine cardiotocography or Doppler ultrasonography is not recommended during pregnancy.[6] Across settings, the WHO recommends provider-initiated testing and counseling forhuman immunodeficiency virus (HIV) (with an opt-out approach),[69,70] maternal assessment for gestational diabetes mellitus, and counseling about exposure to second-hand smoke, tobacco, alcohol, and other substance-use past and present.[6] Many expert groups also advocate for screening for gender-based violence in pregnancy.[71–73]

Other context-specific considerations for preventive management of pregnant women adapted for the WHO 2016 ANC recommendations for a positive pregnancy experience[6] are shown in **Table 3**. Recommendations for screening pregnant women may vary across countries. For instance, the United States Centers for Disease Control and Prevention 2021 Sexually Transmitted Infections Treatment Guidelines specify indications to screen for asymptomatic infections such as chlamydia, gonorrhea, herpes simplex virus, hepatitis C.[74]

Good clinical practice in pregnancy includes gestational weight gain tracking; urinalysis for protein and glucose; blood pressure checks and surveillance for hypertensive disorders in pregnancy, including preeclampsia; and checking for fetal heart sounds when appropriate. Women at high risk for preeclampsia may benefit from daily low-dose aspirin administration. Although prematurity is a prominent cause of newborn morbidity and mortality globally, the best clinical pathways for predicting spontaneous preterm births and mitigating them in at-risk women are uncertain.[31] Details of the care for high-risk pregnancies are beyond the scope of this review and should be in consultation with obstetricians and maternal–fetal specialists.

Birth preparedness and complication readiness

A birth plan helps a woman articulate her preferences for her birth experience. It also helps to identify and arrange resources to support her expectations collaboratively with the care team and family. Due to the diverse sociodemographic characteristics of pregnant women and the wide-ranging health system resources available to help labor and childbirth in different settings, a pragmatic approach is to have flexible plans that aid woman–provider communication and focus on creating a safe and positive birth experience. Some standard birth plan components include where to give birth, transportation to the place of birth, labor companionship, pain relief, anticipated route of delivery (vaginal birth or cesarean section), availability of senior care providers and emergency services, postpartum contraception, and payment mechanisms. Birth plans can help women feel more control over their birth process. However, if they are too detailed, a woman and her family may feel dissatisfied if their expectations are not met.[75] A tour of labor/childbirth facilities may help women feel more relaxed, comfortable, and safe. Some settings support home births for low-risk women in which complications are not anticipated and whereby ambulance and emergency services are of high quality.

The prime goal of ANC is to maximize the potential of a healthy woman and baby and a positive pregnancy experience. Health care providers should provide women with prior information about challenges and expectations and reassure them of "normal" pregnancy symptoms whereby appropriate. However, complications can arise without warning, and birth may be earlier (preterm) or later (postdate) than expected. Women should be counseled on danger signs such as a decreased perception of fetal movement, fever, severe and prolonged headaches, chest pains, visual disturbances, vaginal bleeding, or rupture of membranes, and complication readiness should be ensured. For instance, women may require an emergency visit and admission to the hospital and should have planned transportation and funding mechanisms when needed. The baby may also require specialized neonatal care. Hospitals and health care providers should have written protocols and rehearsed drills to manage complications.

Women who use ANC services frequently belong to a higher financial class and have better social support systems.[76] However, vulnerable pregnant women, including migrants, adolescents, women with disabilities, those in humanitarian settings, ethnic and racial minorities, women with minority sexual orientation, gender identity and expression (including lesbian, bisexual, and other non-heterosexual women), among others often have more needs (physical, emotional, psychological, and social) than other women. Generally, women with meaningful social support systems adjust better to physiologic changes and pregnancy challenges.[77,78] Identifying and acknowledging a woman's support system, including her partner, family, friends, a labor companion or doula, or her spiritual adviser, can potentially mitigate her physical, emotional, and social needs and promote a positive transition to parenthood.[79] These needs extend to her partner and support system, which should be considered and addressed to achieve safe and satisfying adaptations to pregnancy, childbirth, and the baby.

POSTNATAL CARE

PNC describes the care provided to the mother and her newborn baby commencing from the delivery of the baby and the placenta up to 42 days (6 weeks) following child-birth. This includes maternal and newborn care (MNC) to prevent maternal and newborn morbidity and mortality.[80] Common maternal morbidities in the postpartum period include hemorrhage, infections, anemia, and depression, whereas newborn morbidities include neonatal infections, asphyxia, and complications of prematurity. PNC coverage and quality remain largely neglected in the continuum of maternal care, especially in low- and middle-income countries.[81,82] Also, many guidelines, perhaps unnecessarily, limit their scope to a short-term perspective.[83] Although significant success has been achieved globally, there is a substantial unmet need for access to and uptake of PNC in low- and middle-income countries.[80,84,85] Approximately 50% of maternal deaths in the postnatal period occur within the first 24 hours[86]; and 17 infants per 1000 live births die within the first month.[87] There is evidence that suboptimal PNC is associated with maternal and newborn deaths and morbidity and missed opportunities to promote and maintain good health and a positive postnatal experience.[87–89]

The postnatal period is broadly categorized into immediate (first 24 h), early (days 2–7), and late (days 8–42) phases with relatively different maternal and infant needs.[90]

WHO Essential Newborn Care

- Immediate care at birth (delayed cord clamping, thorough drying, assessment of breathing, skin-to-skin contact, early initiation of breastfeeding)
- Thermal care
- Resuscitation when needed
- Support for breast milk feeding
- Nurturing care
- Infection prevention
- Assessment of health problems
- Recognition and response to danger signs
- Timely and safe referral when needed

Fig. 2. Components of essential newborn care. (*Adapted from* World Health Organization. Essential newborn care. Newborn Health. Available at https://www.who.int/teams/maternal-newborn-child-adolescent-health-and-ageing/newborn-health/essential-newborn-care.)

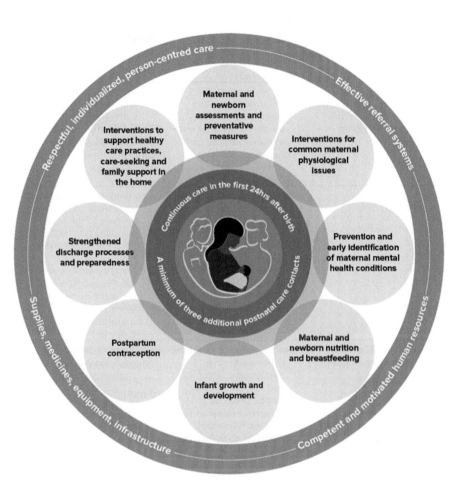

Fig. 3. The WHO postnatal care model from WHO recommendations on maternal and newborn care for a positive postnatal experience. (*From* World Health Organization (WHO). WHO recommendations on maternal and newborn care for a positive postnatal experience. Published 2022. Available at https://www.who.int/publications/i/item/9789240045989.)

Nonetheless, some monitoring and evaluation indicators such as "late maternal deaths" track complications up to one year after termination of pregnancy. In most settings, the provision of care is primarily facility based during the immediate postnatal period. It focuses on critical clinical indicators that assess maternal and newborn health. On the other hand, maternal and infant care during the early and late postnatal periods is primarily community based, focusing on maximizing the health and well-being of the mother and baby.[90] The American College of Obstetricians and Gynecologists advise that PNC should be individualized and all women should have a comprehensive assessment within 12 weeks of birth.[5] Individualized care may involve multiple professionals.

The WHO stated that "high-quality universal newborn health care is the right of every newborn everywhere."[91] This includes the right protection from injury and infection and the right to normal breathing, optimal warmth, and feeding.[91] Essential newborn care (**Fig. 2**) should be available to all newborns immediately after delivery and all through the newborn period, both at health facilities and home settings.[91]

Table 4
WHO maternal and newborn care context-specific postnatal recommendations

Care Area	Recommendation	Context/Setting
Prevention of neonatal infection by application of chlorhexidine to the umbilical cord stump	Daily application of 4% chlorhexidine to the umbilical cord stump in the first week after birth is recommended. Otherwise, clean, dry umbilical cord care is recommended.	Settings whereby harmful traditional substances such as animal dung are commonly used on the umbilical cord.
Neonatal vitamin A supplementation	Providing newborns with a single oral dose of 50,000 IU of vitamin A within the first 3 days after birth may be considered to reduce infant mortality. Otherwise, routine neonatal vitamin A supplementation is not recommended to reduce neonatal and infant mortality.	Settings with recent (<5 y) and reliable data that indicate a high infant mortality rate (>50 per 1000 live births) and a high prevalence of maternal vitamin A deficiency ($\geq$10% of pregnant women with serum retinol concentrations < 0.70 μmol/L)
Postpartum oral iron and folate supplementation	Oral iron supplementation, either alone or in combination with folic acid supplementation, may be provided to postpartum women for 6–12 wk following childbirth to reduce the risk of anemia	Settings whereby gestational anemia is of public health concern
Preventive anthelmintic treatment	Preventive chemotherapy (deworming), using annual or biannual single-dose albendazole (400 mg) or mebendazole (500 mg), is recommended as a public health intervention for all nonpregnant adolescent girls and women of reproductive age, including postpartum and/or lactating women, to reduce the worm burden of soil-transmitted helminths.	Settings whereby the baseline prevalence of any soil-transmitted helminth infection is 20% or more among adolescent girls and women of reproductive age

(continued on next page)

Table 4
(*continued*)

Care Area	Recommendation	Context/Setting
HIV catch-up testing	Catch-up postpartum HIV testing is needed for women of HIV-negative or unknown status who missed early antenatal contact testing or retesting in late pregnancy at a third-trimester visit. Catch-up postpartum HIV testing can be considered for women of HIV-negative or unknown status who missed early antenatal contact testing or retesting in late pregnancy at a third trimester visit as part of the effort to eliminate mother-to-child transmission of HIV.	Settings with a high HIV burden. Settings with low HIV burden: consider for women in serodiscordant relationships, whereby the partner is not virally suppressed on ART, or who had other known ongoing HIV risks in late pregnancy
Screening for tuberculosis disease	Systematic screening for tuberculosis (TB) disease may be conducted among the general population, including women in the postpartum period	Settings with an estimated TB disease prevalence of 0.5% or higher.
	Systematic screening for TB disease may be conducted among women in the postpartum period	Settings whereby TB disease prevalence in the general population is 100/100 000 population or higher
Oral pre-exposure prophylaxis for HIV prevention	Oral pre-exposure prophylaxis (PrEP) containing tenofovir disoproxil fumarate (TDF) should be started or continued as an additional prevention choice	Postpartum and/or lactating women at a substantial risk of HIV infection as part of combination HIV prevention approaches.
Preventive schistosomiasis treatment	Annual preventive chemotherapy with praziquantel in a single dose for $\geq$ 75% up to 100% of pregnant women after the first trimester and nonpregnant adolescent girls and women of reproductive age, including postpartum and/or lactating women	Endemic communities with *Schistosoma spp.* prevalence of 10% or higher

Adapted from World Health Organization (WHO). WHO recommendations on maternal and newborn care for a positive postnatal experience. Published 2022. Available at https://www.who.int/publications/i/item/9789240045989.

Nonetheless, newborn care practices vary widely between countries,[92] and a multi-country study in Ghana, Guinea, and Nigeria showed many newborns did not receive essential care practices.[93] Some newborns also received practices such as separation from mother after birth and delayed initiation of breastfeeding that might constitute mistreatment.[93]

This review discusses maternal and newborn complications during the postnatal period and evidence-based care to improve PNC. PNC provides a conducive environment for maternal–infant bonding, an opportunity for birth registration, and support to the family and community.[80]

The New WHO Postnatal Care Model

On March 30, 2022, the WHO released recommendations to help women, babies, and families have positive postnatal experiences.[80] The new guidelines recommend at least four PNC contacts between women and their newborns to support the WHO's vision for quality care using a human rights–based approach.[80] The guidelines recommend continuous care for healthy women–newborn dyads in the health facility for at least 24 hours after birth or a first postnatal contact within the first 24 hours of home birth.[80] Subsequently, a minimum of three more contacts are recommended, between 48 and 72 hours, 7 and 14 days, and in the sixth week after birth. Implementing the recommendations at postnatal contacts requires considering eight themes within a health system with adequate supplies, medicines, and infrastructure; contented and motivated human resources; effective referral systems; and a focus on respectful, individualized, and person-centered care.[80] These eight themes (**Fig. 3**) are described in the following subsections.

Maternal and newborn assessments and preventative measures

Maternal and newborn assessments during the postnatal period provide health workers an opportunity to assess the well-being of the mother and infant and provide advice on healthy breastfeeding practices, mental health, up-to-date immunization, PNC, and counseling on danger signs and complications as well as family planning. Many maternal complications in the postnatal period are preceded by clinical features that point to the diagnosis. Early and regular postnatal assessment can significantly prevent severe maternal morbidity and mortality during the postnatal period. An essential routine examination of women during the first 24 hours after birth should include assessing vaginal bleeding, uterine tonus, fundal height, temperature, heart rate (pulse), blood pressure, and urinary voiding. After 24 hours, lochia, micturition, urinary incontinence, bowel function, perineal hygiene, wound healing, headache, and back, perineal, breast, and uterine pain should be assessed at each contact. Other context-specific recommendations are included in **Table 4**. Counseling by HCPs should include danger signs that warn them when to limit or terminate physical activity. These signs should be reported to an HCP, especially if childbirth was by cesarean section. Additionally, women should gradually return to regular physical exercise.[80]

Several danger signs indicate neonatal illness.[80] These clinical features include extremes of temperature [fever (temperature $>37.5^0$ C), hypothermia (temperature $<35.5^0$ C)], lack of spontaneous movements, convulsions, severe chest in-drawing or fast breathing (>60 cycles per minute), poor feeding, and jaundice, especially within 24 hours of birth. Ideally, universal screening for neonatal hyperbilirubinemia by a transcutaneous bilirubinometer (TcB) should be done at health facility discharge. Postnatal mothers and caregivers should be educated on these danger signs that indicate impending postnatal complications and the need for urgent assessment by HCPs. The WHO recommends routine newborn eyesight, hearing, and jaundice screening during

PNC. Babies who screen positive should have diagnostic and management services for identified abnormalities.[80] Bathing of a healthy term newborn should not be undertaken for at least 24 hours to mitigate the risk of hypothermia.[80] In contexts whereby harmful traditional substances such as animal dung are commonly used on the umbilical cord, applying 4% chlorhexidine to the umbilical cord stump daily in the first week of birth is advised. Otherwise, the cord stump should be kept clean and dry (see **Table 4**).[80] Putting the baby to sleep in the supine position is recommended to prevent sudden infant death syndrome. Newborn immunization should be promoted as per the latest existing WHO recommendations for routine immunization.

Interventions for common maternal physiologic signs and symptoms

During the postnatal period, maternal anatomic and physiologic changes during pregnancy revert to the prepregnancy state.[94] Reverting to the prepregnancy state may be associated with maternal symptoms and signs that undermine maternal postnatal experience.[80] Many women experience perineal pain,[95] up to half develop breast engorgement,[96] and about one-third have urinary incontinence in the initial months after childbirth.[97] Local cooling, such as with ice packs or cold pads, and oral acetaminophen can be offered to women in the immediate postpartum period for the relief of acute pain from perineal trauma sustained during childbirth. Oral nonsteroidal anti-inflammatory drugs can be used when analgesia is required for the relief of postpartum pain due to uterine cramping. For treatment of breast engorgement in the postpartum period, women should be counseled and supported to practice responsive breast-feeding, good positioning and attachment of the baby to the breast, expression of

Table 5
Maternal and infant benefits of breastfeeding

Infant Benefits	Maternal Benefits
Immediate/short-term	Immediate/short-term
a. Optimal infant nutrition and growth	a. Reduced risk of PPH (improves uterine involution)
b. Reduction in infant infections: otitis media, gastrointestinal infections (diarrhea and vomiting), respiratory tract infections (pneumonia)	b. Reduced risk of postpartum psychological problems (stress and anxiety) and PPD
c. Reductions in necrotizing enterocolitis (preterm infants)	c. Reduced risk of obesity
d. Reductions in sudden infant death syndrome	d. Contraception: lactational amenorrhea (birth spacing)
e. Less frequent hospital admissions	e. Improved infantn–maternal bonding
f. Reduction in infant mortality	
Long-term	Long-term
a. Reduced risk of allergy (atopic dermatitis) and asthma	a. Reduced risk of malignancy (breast, ovarian, and endometrial[a])
b. Higher intelligent quotient and cognitive ability	b. Reduced risk of CVDs (type 2 DM, hypertension, metabolic syndrome)
c. Reduced risk of childhood obesity	c. Reduced risk of osteoporosis*
d. Reduced risk of type 2 DM	d. Reduced risk of endometriosis
e. Reduced risk of metabolic syndrome in adulthood	e. Reduced risk of rheumatoid arthritis
f. Reduced risk of childhood leukemia	

Abbreviations: CVDs, cardiovascular diseases; DM, diabetes mellitus; PPD, postpartum depression; PPH, postpartum.
[a] Mixed evidence.

breastmilk, and the use of warm or cold compresses, based on a woman's preferences. The new guidelines also provide extensive guidance on interventions for constipation and mastitis.[80]

Prevention and identification of maternal mental conditions

Postpartum mental health disorders are notable contributors to the global burden of diseases, affecting approximately one in ten and one in five women during this period in HICs and low- and middle-income countries (LMICs), respectively.[98] Nonetheless, stigma often disincentivizes affected women from seeking clinical care,[99] with only one in five women presenting to health workers with postpartum anxiety and depression.[80] Health workers should inquire about women's emotional well-being at each PNC contact. The WHO recommends screening for postpartum depression and anxiety using validated instruments such as the EPDS or PHQ-9.[80] Screen-positive women should be followed up with referral and appropriate mental health diagnostic and management services. Implementing these services would require significant health system changes such as trained staff, equipment, and infrastructure to integrate perinatal mental health services with PNC, and these changes require further evaluation.[83]

Maternal and newborn nutrition and breastfeeding

Postpartum women require appropriate evidence-based counseling on maternal and newborn nutrition and infant care. In areas with a high burden of anemia during pregnancy, a continuation of the iron supplementation regimen used during pregnancy is advised during the postnatal period.[80] The new WHO recommendation equally advises context-specific interventions (see **Table 4**), including vitamin A administration in newborns.[80]

Exclusive breastfeeding should be initiated within an hour of birth and continued until a minimum of 6 months, except for contraindicated cases such as galactosemia, maple syrup urine disease, and phenylketonuria.[80] In HIV-positive women on antiretroviral therapy, the WHO recommends similar exclusive breastfeeding practices in the first 6 months,[100,101] unlike in the United States where breastfeeding is not recommended.[102] A recent commentary suggested that breastfeeding recommendations focus on infant nutrition without promoting the maternal benefits of breastfeeding.[83] Optimal breastfeeding is associated with recognizable short-term and long-term benefits (**Table 5**) to the infant and mother.[103–107] The recent WHO recommendations on MNC strongly emphasized three care guidelines related to infant feeding, including breastfeeding to encourage positive postnatal experience, as stated in the following:[80]

1. All newborns should receive exclusive breastfeeding from birth until 6 months postnatal. Mothers should receive counseling and support for exclusive breastfeeding during postnatal contacts.[80]
2. There should be a written breastfeeding policy at facilities providing maternity and newborn services, and this should be routinely communicated to staff and parents.[80]
3. Health facility staff involved in providing infant feeding services, including breastfeeding support, should exhibit sufficient knowledge, competence, and skills to facilitate breastfeeding among women.[80]

Infant growth and development

After birth, a newborn usually loses about 5% to 10% of their birth weight within the first 10 days but starts to gain weight at about 2 weeks.[108] Optimal breastfeeding promotes infant growth and development and improves survival.[103,105,107,109] The new WHO recommendation provides guidance on child growth and development for up to 3 years to provide a healthy start.[110] Gentle whole-body massage of the newborn, with or without emollients by rubbing and slow stroking of body parts or a passive range of motion across limb joints, should be considered for healthy newborns delivered at term after initial training of mothers or caregivers.[80] It is an opportunity for parent–infant stimulation to promote early childhood development.[111] Caregivers should respect babies' reactions to massage while providing responsive and respectful care,[80] as excessive distressing massages involving slaps and movements beyond the normal range of movement across limb joints might cause harm. Responsive care is not limited to biological parents and gives anticipatory guidance to a child's safety, education, and development while establishing a caring and understanding child–provider relationship.[80] This involves identifying a child's signals, for example, stress, pain, or readiness for a feed, and responding appropriately to them in communication, play, and feeding.[80]

Postpartum contraception
The postpartum period offers a unique contact opportunity for women. Therefore, client-centered counseling and provision of modern contraception in the postnatal period without discrimination remains an essential component of reproductive health services. In line with previous guidelines, the new WHO postnatal guidelines recommend comprehensive contraceptive information and services during PNC.[80] The main contraceptive options in the postnatal period include progestogen-only pills, progestogen-only injectable contraceptives, levonorgestrel and etonogestrel implants, copper-bearing intrauterine devices, and levonorgestrel-releasing intrauterine devices based on women's medical eligibility criteria.[112] Birth route is not a criterion for selecting a contraceptive method.

Strengthen discharge processes and preparedness
Despite the increasingly shorter duration of facility admission of mother–baby pairs after birth, the range is wide between countries.[80] Early discharge to prevent overmedicalization of birth may contribute to delays in recognizing and managing maternal and newborn complications, particularly in contexts with suboptimal community support.[113] Principally, HCPs must consider the state of the woman and newborn in preparing them for facility discharge, including maternal needs, support, and experience.[114,115] The WHO recommends assessing the physical well-being of the mother–newborn dyad, the woman's emotional well-being, her skills and confidence in caring for herself and the newborn, and the home environment and factors that may influence care and care-seeking behavior.[80] Health care providers should prepare women and provide information before discharge; home visits are encouraged within the first week.[80] To optimize HCP roles, policymakers should consider promoting health-related behaviors and the uptake of postpartum family planning by task sharing to a broad range of HCP cadres.[80,116] Similarly, policies should aim to develop, attract, and retain HCPs in rural and hard-to-reach areas.[80]

Interventions to support healthy care practices, care-seeking, and family support
Evidence shows that men's support is vital for positive experiences.[117] It promotes respect and facilitates a woman's autonomy and choice. The WHO promotes men's involvement during pregnancy, in childbirth, and after birth to support women's facility- and home-based self-care and use of skilled facility-based care for maternal and newborn complications.[80] Complementing facility-based with home-based records can improve provider-held communication, men's involvement, household support,

and care-seeking behavior and is recommended.[80] However, most maternal and newborn interventions are domiciled in health facilities.[117]

SUMMARY

A successful transition from the antenatal to the postnatal period requires early disease detection, management, and prevention; health promotion; birth preparedness; and complication readiness. This review discussed patient-centered ANC and PNC focused on ensuring a culturally sensitive and positive pregnancy and postnatal experience. Maternal and newborn health are dynamic during pregnancy and after birth, and shared decision-making should form an integral component of care. Consequently, women, their newborns, and families require appropriate dignified and evidence-based person-centered care based on a human rights approach. Person-centered care is an enduring process in the continuum of MNC. Context-specific ANC and PNC may be required in some settings. Typically, ANC and PNC are organized during health facility visits in many settings. Services and support are women centered and can be offered as individualized or group-based care. The challenge of ANC and PNC is determining its core components and underpinning them with evidence without overmedicalizing its practice.

CLINICS CARE POINTS

- The ultimate goal of antenatal and postnatal care is to ensure optimal maternal and fetal/newborn health and well-being and a positive experience.
- The WHO recommends models involving at least 8 ANC and 4 PNC contacts for optimal care.
- Health systems should offer respectful, culturally sensitive, evidence-based person-centered antenatal and postnatal care that respects human rights and shared decisions between women and their health care providers.

DISCLOSURE

The authors have nothing to disclose.

We would like to thank Jane Hirst, Daphne DSouza-Akeju and Naima Nasir for reading and providing feedback on the final draft of this review.

REFERENCES

1. Forrester King J. A short history of evidence-based obstetric care. Best Pract Res Clin Obstet Gynaecol 2005;19(1):3–14.
2. Tunçalp, Were WM, Maclennan C, et al. Quality of care for pregnant women and newborns—the WHO vision. BJOG An Int J Obstet Gynaecol 2015;122(8): 1045–9.
3. World Health Organization. *Basic Documents [Internet]*. [Geneva]: WHO; 2020 [49th edition - including amendments adopted up to 31 May 2019; cited 2022 Aug 29]. https://apps.who.int/gb/bd/
4. World Health Organization. *WHO Technical Consultation on Postpartum and Postnatal Care [Internet]*. [Geneva]: WHO; 2010 [cited 2022 Jul 16]. (WHO reference number [WHO/MPS/10.03]) https://www.who.int/publications/i/item/WHO-MPS-10.03

5. ACOG COMMITTEE OPINION No. 736. Optimizing Postpartum Care. Obstet Gynecol 2018;131(5):E140–50.

6. World Health Organization. *WHO Recommendations on Antenatal Care for a Positive Pregnancy Experience [Internet].* [Geneva]: WHO; 2016 [cited 2022 Aug 29] https://www.who.int/publications/i/item/9789241549912

7. World Health Organization. Trends in Maternal Mortality 2000 to 2017: Estimates by WHO, UNICEF, UNFPA, World Bank Group and the United Nations Population Division [Internet]. [Geneva]: WHO; 2019 [cited 2022 Aug 29] https://apps.who.int/iris/handle/10665/327595.

8. Moller AB, Petzold M, Chou D, et al. Early antenatal care visit: a systematic analysis of regional and global levels and trends of coverage from 1990 to 2013. Lancet Glob Heal 2017;5(10):e977–83.

9. Carroli G, Rooney C, Villar J. How effective is antenatal care in preventing maternal mortality and serious morbidity? An overview of the evidence. Paediatr Perinat Epidemiol 2001;15(Suppl 1):1–42.

10. Dowswell T, Carroli G, Duley L, et al. Alternative versus standard packages of antenatal care for low-risk pregnancy. Cochrane Database Syst Rev 2015; 2015(7). https://doi.org/10.1002/14651858.CD000934.PUB3.

11. Homer CS, Bohren MA, Wilson A, Vogel JP. Achieving Inclusive and Respectful Maternity Care. In: Flenady V, ed. The Global Library of Women's Medicine. Vol 3.; 2021. doi:10.3843/GLOWM.411763.

12. Bohren MA, Mehrtash H, Fawole B, et al. How women are treated during facility-based childbirth in four countries: a cross-sectional study with labour observations and community-based surveys. Lancet 2019;394(10210):1750–63.

13. United Nations. *Technical Guidance on the Application of a Human Rights-Based Approach to the Implementation of Policies and Programmes to Reduce Preventable Maternal Morbidity and Mortality [Internet].* [Geneva]: OHCHR; 2012 [cited 2022 August 29] (Report of the Office of the United Nations High Commissioner for Human Rights [A/HRC/21/22]) https://digitallibrary.un.org/record/731068?ln=en

14. World Health Organization. *Standards for Improving Quality of Maternal and Newborn Care in Health Facilities [Internet].* [Geneva]: WHO; 2016 [cited 2022 Aug 29] https://www.who.int/publications/i/item/9789241511216

15. World Health Organization. Continuity and Coordination of Care: A Practice Brief to Support Implementation of the WHO Framework on Integrated People-Centred Health Services [Internet]. [Geneva]. WHO; 2018 [cited 2022 Jul 16] https://apps.who.int/iris/handle/10665/274628.

16. Sandall J, Soltani H, Gates S, et al. Midwife-led continuity models versus other models of care for childbearing women. Cochrane Database Syst Rev 2016; 2016(4):CD004667.

17. Kwame A, Petrucka PM. A literature-based study of patient-centered care and communication in nurse-patient interactions: barriers, facilitators, and the way forward. BMC Nurs 2021;20(1):1–10.

18. King TL, Laros RK, Parer JT. Interprofessional collaborative practice in obstetrics and midwifery. Obstet Gynecol Clin North Am 2012;39(3):411–22.

19. Brown HC, Smith HJ, Mori R, et al. Giving women their own case notes to carry during pregnancy. Cochrane Database Syst Rev 2015;2015(10):CD002856.

20. Ota E, da Silva Lopes K, Middleton P, et al. Antenatal interventions for preventing stillbirth, fetal loss and perinatal death: an overview of Cochrane systematic reviews. Cochrane Database Syst Rev 2020;2020(12):CD009599.

21. ACOG Committee Opinion No. 731: Group Prenatal Care. Obstet Gynecol 2018; 131(3):e104–8.
22. Rowley RA, Phillips LE, O'Dell L, et al. Group Prenatal Care: A Financial Perspective. Matern Child Health J 2016;20(1):1–10.
23. Carter EB, Temming LA, Akin J, et al. Group Prenatal Care Compared With Traditional Prenatal Care: A Systematic Review and Meta-analysis. Obstet Gynecol 2016;128(3):551–61.
24. Catling CJ, Medley N, Foureur M, et al. Group versus conventional antenatal care for women. Cochrane Database Syst Rev 2015;(2):CD007622.
25. Buultjens M, Farouque A, Karimi L, et al. The contribution of group prenatal care to maternal psychological health outcomes: A systematic review. Women Birth 2021;34(6).
26. Ruiz-Mirazo E, Lopez-Yarto M, McDonald SD. Group prenatal care versus individual prenatal care: a systematic review and meta-analyses. J Obstet Gynaecol Can 2012;34(3):223–9.
27. Byerley BM, Haas DM. A systematic overview of the literature regarding group prenatal care for high-risk pregnant women. BMC Pregnancy Childbirth 2017; 17(1):329–39.
28. Malouf R, Redshaw M. Specialist antenatal clinics for women at high risk of preterm birth: a systematic review of qualitative and quantitative research. BMC Pregnancy Childbirth 2017;17(1). https://doi.org/10.1186/S12884-017-1232-9.
29. Grenier L, Suhowatsky S, Kabue MM, et al. Impact of group antenatal care (G-ANC) versus individual antenatal care (ANC) on quality of care, ANC attendance and facility-based delivery: A pragmatic cluster-randomized controlled trial in Kenya and Nigeria. PLoS One 2019;14(10). https://doi.org/10.1371/JOURNAL.PONE.0222177.
30. Swift EM, Zoega H, Stoll K, et al. Enhanced Antenatal Care: Combining one-to-one and group Antenatal Care models to increase childbirth education and address childbirth fear. Women and Birth 2021;34(4):381–8.
31. Silver R (Bob) M, Shea A. Principles of Screening and Disease Prevention in Antenatal Care. In: Flenady V, ed. The Global Library of Women's Medicine. Vol 3.; 2021. doi:10.3843/GLOWM.414613.
32. Quality statement 1: Services – access to antenatal care | Antenatal care | Quality standards | NICE. Available at: https://www.nice.org.uk/guidance/qs22/chapter/Quality-statement-1-Services-access-to-antenatal-care. Accessed April 11, 2022.
33. World Health Organization. WHO Antenatal Care Randomized Trial: Manual for the Implementation of the New Model [Internet]. [Geneva]: WHO; 2002 [cited 2022 Aug 29] (WHO Programme to Map Best Reproductive Health Practices [WHO/RHR/01.30]) https://apps.who.int/iris/bitstream/handle/10665/42513/W?sequence=1.
34. Vogel JP, Habib NA, Souza JP, et al. Antenatal care packages with reduced visits and perinatal mortality: a secondary analysis of the WHO Antenatal Care Trial. Reprod Health 2013;10(1). https://doi.org/10.1186/1742-4755-10-19.
35. Manyeh AK, Amu A, Williams J, et al. Factors associated with the timing of antenatal clinic attendance among first-time mothers in rural southern Ghana. BMC Pregnancy Childbirth 2020;20(1). https://doi.org/10.1186/S12884-020-2738-0.
36. National Institute for Health and Care Excellence. Antenatal Care [Internet]. [London]: NICE; 2021 [cited 2022 Jul 16]. (NICE guideline [NG201]). https://www.nice.org.uk/guidance/ng201.

37. Abalos E, Chamillard M, Diaz V, et al. Antenatal care for healthy pregnant women: a mapping of interventions from existing guidelines to inform the development of new WHO guidance on antenatal care. BJOG 2016;123(4):519–28.

38. Henderson JT, Thompson JH, Burda BU, et al. Preeclampsia Screening: Evidence Report and Systematic Review for the US Preventive Services Task Force. JAMA 2017;317(16):1668–83.

39. Committee Opinion No 700. Methods for Estimating the Due Date. Obstet Gynecol 2017;129(5):E150–4.

40. Karim JN, Roberts NW, Salomon LJ, et al. Systematic review of first-trimester ultrasound screening for detection of fetal structural anomalies and factors that affect screening performance. Ultrasound Obstet Gynecol 2017;50(4):429–41.

41. Whitworth M, Bricker L, Mullan C. Ultrasound for fetal assessment in early pregnancy. Cochrane Database Syst Rev 2015;2015(7). https://doi.org/10.1002/14651858.CD007058.PUB3.

42. Smolina K, Hanley GE, Mintzes B, et al. Trends and Determinants of Prescription Drug Use during Pregnancy and Postpartum in British Columbia, 2002–2011: A Population-Based Cohort Study. PLoS One 2015;10(5):e0128312.

43. Lynch MM, Amoozegar JB, McClure EM, et al. Improving Safe Use of Medications During Pregnancy: The Roles of Patients, Physicians, and Pharmacists. Qual Health Res 2017;27(13):2071.

44. Chu HY, Englund JA. Maternal immunization. Clin Infect Dis 2014;59(4):560–8.

45. Kyu HH, Mumford JE, Stanaway JD, et al. Mortality from tetanus between 1990 and 2015: findings from the global burden of disease study 2015. BMC Public Health 2017;17(1):1–17.

46. Centers for Disease Control and Prevention. Guidelines for Vaccinating Pregnant Women. Available at: https://www.cdc.gov/vaccines/pregnancy/hcp-toolkit/guidelines.html?CDC_AA_refVal=https%3A%2F%2Fwww.cdc.gov%2Fvaccines%2Fpregnancy%2Fhcp%2Fguidelines.html. Accessed May 21, 2022.

47. Influenza Vaccination During Pregnancy | ACOG. Available at: https://www.acog.org/clinical/clinical-guidance/committee-opinion/articles/2018/04/influenza-vaccination-during-pregnancy. Accessed April 11, 2022.

48. Grohskopf LA, Alyanak E, Ferdinands JM, et al. Prevention and Control of Seasonal Influenza with Vaccines: Recommendations of the Advisory Committee on Immunization Practices, United States, 2021-22 Influenza Season. MMWR Recomm Rep Morb Mortal Wkly Rep Recomm Rep 2021;70(5):1–32.

49. World Health Organization. Questions and Answers: COVID-19 vaccines and pregnancy. Available at: https://www.who.int/publications/i/item/WHO-2019-nCoV-FAQ-Pregnancy-Vaccines-2022.1. Accessed May 21, 2022.

50. ACOG Committee Opinion No. 741: Maternal Immunization. Obstet Gynecol 2018;131(6):E214–7.

51. ACOG Practice Bulletin No. 86: Viral hepatitis in pregnancy. Obstet Gynecol 2007;110(4):941–55.

52. Kim DK, Hunter P, Woods LD, et al. Recommended Adult Immunization Schedule, United States, 2019. Ann Intern Med 2019;170(3):182–92.

53. Immunization in pregnancy and breastfeeding: Canadian Immunization Guide - Canada.ca. Available at: https://www.canada.ca/en/public-health/services/publications/healthy-living/canadian-immunization-guide-part-3-vaccination-specific-populations/page-4-immunization-pregnancy-breastfeeding.html. Accessed April 11, 2022.

54. ACIP General Best Practice Guidelines for Immunization | CDC. Available at: https://www.cdc.gov/vaccines/hcp/acip-recs/general-recs/index.html.   Accessed May 21, 2022.

55. Taylor LE, Swerdfeger AL, Eslick GD. Vaccines are not associated with autism: an evidence-based meta-analysis of case-control and cohort studies. Vaccine 2014;32(29):3623–9.

56. Dadi AF, Miller ER, Bisetegn TA, et al. Global burden of antenatal depression and its association with adverse birth outcomes: an umbrella review. BMC Public Heal 2020;20(1):1–16.

57. Hadfield H, Wittkowski A. Women's Experiences of Seeking and Receiving Psychological and Psychosocial Interventions for Postpartum Depression: A Systematic Review and Thematic Synthesis of the Qualitative Literature. J Midwifery Womens Health 2017;62(6):723–36.

58. Biaggi A, Conroy S, Pawlby S, et al. Identifying the women at risk of antenatal anxiety and depression: A systematic review. J Affect Disord 2016;191:62–77.

59. Kingston D, Kehler H, Austin MP, et al. Trajectories of maternal depressive symptoms during pregnancy and the first 12 months postpartum and child externalizing and internalizing behavior at three years. PLoS One 2018;13(4). https://doi.org/10.1371/JOURNAL.PONE.0195365.

60. ACOG Committee Opinion No. 757: Screening for Perinatal Depression. Obstet Gynecol 2018;132(5):E208–12.

61. Austin MP. Marcé International Society position statement on psychosocial assessment and depression screening in perinatal women. Best Pract Res Clin Obstet Gynaecol 2014;28(1):179–87.

62. Sambrook Smith M, Cairns L, Pullen LSW, et al. Validated tools to identify common mental disorders in the perinatal period: A systematic review of systematic reviews. J Affect Disord 2022;298(Pt A):634–43.

63. Screening for Fetal Chromosomal Abnormalities: ACOG Practice Bulletin, Number 226. Obstet Gynecol 2020;136(4):e48–69.

64. Committee Opinion No. 690: Carrier Screening in the Age of Genomic Medicine. Obstet Gynecol 2017;129(3):e35–40.

65. Cargill Y, Morin L. No. 223-Content of a Complete Routine Second Trimester Obstetrical Ultrasound Examination and Report. J Obstet Gynaecol Can 2017; 39(8):e144–9.

66. Nevo O, Brown R, Glanc P, et al. No. 352-Technical Update: The Role of Early Comprehensive Fetal Anatomy Ultrasound Examination. J Obstet Gynaecol Can 2017;39(12):1203–11.

67. Bricker L, Medley N, Pratt JJ. Routine ultrasound in late pregnancy (after 24 weeks' gestation). Cochrane Database Syst Rev 2015;2015(6):CD001451.

68. Update on Prenatal Care - American Family Physician. Available at: https://www.aafp.org/afp/2014/0201/p199.html. Accessed April 11, 2022.

69. ACOG Committee Opinion Number 752 Prenatal and Perinatal Human Immunodeficiency Virus Testing. Obstet Gynecol 2018;132(3):E138–42.

70. Selph SS, Bougatsos C, Dana T, et al. Screening for HIV Infection in Pregnant Women: Updated Evidence Report and Systematic Review for the US Preventive Services Task Force. JAMA 2019;321(23):2349–60.

71. ACOG Committee Opinion No. 518: Intimate partner violence. Obstet Gynecol 2012;119(2 Pt 1):412–7.

72. ACOG Committee opinion no. 554: reproductive and sexual coercion. Obstet Gynecol 2013;121(2 Pt 1):411–5.

73. Committee opinion no. 498: Adult manifestations of childhood sexual abuse. Obstet Gynecol 2011;118(2 Pt 1):392–5.
74. Workowski KA, Bachmann LH, Chan PA, et al. Sexually Transmitted Infections Treatment Guidelines, 2021. MMWR Recomm Rep Morb Mortal Wkly Rep Recomm Rep 2021;70(4):1–187.
75. Mei JY, Afshar Y, Gregory KD, et al. Birth Plans: What Matters for Birth Experience Satisfaction. Birth 2016;43(2):144–50.
76. Ali N, Sultana M, Sheikh N, et al. Predictors of Optimal Antenatal Care Service Utilization Among Adolescents and Adult Women in Bangladesh. Heal Serv Res Manag Epidemiol 2018;5. 233339281878172.
77. Bedaso A, Adams J, Peng W, et al. The relationship between social support and mental health problems during pregnancy: a systematic review and meta-analysis. Reprod Heal 2021;18(1):1–23.
78. Battulga B, Benjamin MR, Chen H, et al. The Impact of Social Support and Pregnancy on Subjective Well-Being: A Systematic Review. Front Psychol 2021;12. https://doi.org/10.3389/FPSYG.2021.
79. McLeish J, Redshaw M. Mothers' accounts of the impact on emotional wellbeing of organised peer support in pregnancy and early parenthood: A qualitative study. BMC Pregnancy Childbirth 2017;17(1):1–14.
80. World Health Organization. WHO Recommendations on Maternal and Newborn Care for a Positive Postnatal Experience [Internet]. [Geneva]: WHO; 2022 [Cited 2022 August 29] https://www.who.int/publications/i/item/9789240045989.
81. Langlois É V, Miszkurka M, Zunzunegui MV, et al. Inequities in postnatal care in low- and middle-income countries: a systematic review and meta-analysis. Bull World Health Organ 2015;93(4):259.
82. Requejo J, Diaz T, Park L, et al. Assessing coverage of interventions for reproductive, maternal, newborn, child, and adolescent health and nutrition. BMJ 2020;368. https://doi.org/10.1136/BMJ.L6915.
83. Bick D, Ram U, Saravanan P, et al. New global WHO postnatal guidance is welcome but misses the long-term perspective. Lancet 2022;0(0). https://doi.org/10.1016/S0140-6736(22)00616-X.
84. Gresh A, Cohen M, Anderson J, et al. Postpartum care content and delivery throughout the African continent: An integrative review. Midwifery 2021;97. https://doi.org/10.1016/J.MIDW.2021.102976.
85. Nasir N, Aderoba AK, Ariana P. Scoping review of maternal and newborn health interventions and programmes in Nigeria. BMJ Open 2022;12(2):e054784.
86. World Health Organization. WHO technical consultation on postpartum and postnatal care. Published online 2010;57.
87. Hug L, Alexander M, You D, et al. National, regional, and global levels and trends in neonatal mortality between 1990 and 2017, with scenario-based projections to 2030: a systematic analysis. Lancet Glob Heal 2019;7(6):e710–20.
88. Gon G, Leite A, Calvert C, et al. The frequency of maternal morbidity: A systematic review of systematic reviews. Int J Gynecol Obstet 2018;141:20–38.
89. Kassebaum NJ, Bertozzi-Villa A, Coggeshall MS, et al. Global, regional, and national levels and causes of maternal mortality during 1990-2013: a systematic analysis for the Global Burden of Disease Study 2013. Lancet 2014;384(9947):980–1004.
90. Finlayson K, Crossland N, Bonet M, et al. What matters to women in the postnatal period: A meta-synthesis of qualitative studies. PLoS One 2020;15(4). https://doi.org/10.1371/JOURNAL.PONE.0231415.

91. World Health Organization. Essential newborn care. Newborn Health. Available at: https://www.who.int/teams/maternal-newborn-child-adolescent-health-and-ageing/newborn-health/essential-newborn-care. Accessed July 13, 2022.

92. Bee M, Shiroor A, Hill Z. Neonatal care practices in sub-Saharan Africa: A systematic review of quantitative and qualitative data. J Health Popul Nutr 2018; 37(1):1–12.

93. Sacks E, Mehrtash H, Bohren M, et al. The first 2 h after birth: prevalence and factors associated with neonatal care practices from a multicountry, facility-based, observational study. Lancet Glob Heal 2021;9(1):e72–80.

94. Gonzalo-Carballes M, Ríos-Vives MÁ, Fierro EC, et al. A pictorial review of postpartum complications. Radiographics 2020;40(7):2117–41.

95. Manresa M, Pereda A, Bataller E, et al. Incidence of perineal pain and dyspareunia following spontaneous vaginal birth: a systematic review and meta-analysis. Int Urogynecol J 2019;30(6):853–68.

96. Zakarija-Grkovic I, Stewart F. Treatments for breast engorgement during lactation. Cochrane Database Syst Rev 2020;2020(9). SVG.

97. Altman D, Cartwright R, Lapitan MC, et al. Epidemiology of urinary incontinence (UI) and other lower urinary tract symptoms (LUTS), pelvic organ prolapse (POP) and anal incontinence (AI). In: Abrams P, Cardozo L, Wagg A, et al, editors. Incontinence : 6th international consultation on incontinence. International Continence Society; 2017. p. 141.

98. Fisher J, de Mello MC, Patel V, et al. Prevalence and determinants of common perinatal mental disorders in women in low- and lower-middle-income countries: a systematic review. Bull World Health Organ 2012;90(2):139–49.

99. Smith MS, Lawrence V, Sadler E, et al. Barriers to accessing mental health services for women with perinatal mental illness: systematic review and meta-synthesis of qualitative studies in the UK. BMJ Open 2019;9(1):e024803.

100. World Health Organization. Guideline: Updates on HIV and Infant Feeding: The Duration of Breastfeeding, and Support from Health Services to Improve Feeding Practices among Mothers Living with HIV [Internet]. [Geneva]: WHO; 2016 [cited 2022 Aug 29].

101. World Health Organization, United Nations Children's Fund. Frequently Asked Questions: Protecting, Promoting, and Supporting Breastfeeding in Facilities Providing Maternity and Newborn Services: The Revised Baby-Friendly Hospital Initiative 2018 [Internet]. [Geneva]: WHO; 2020 [cited 2022 Aug 29] https://www. who.int/publications/i/item/9789241513807

102. Human Immunodeficiency Virus (HIV) | Breastfeeding | CDC. Available at: https://www.cdc.gov/breastfeeding/breastfeeding-special-circumstances/ maternal-or-infant-illnesses/hiv.html. Accessed May 22, 2022.

103. North K, Gao M, Allen G, et al. Breastfeeding in a Global Context: Epidemiology, Impact, and Future Directions. Clin Ther 2022;44(2):228–44.

104. Del Ciampo L, Del Ciampo I. Breastfeeding and the Benefits of Lactation for Women's Health. Rev Bras Ginecol e Obs/RBGO Gynecol Obstet 2018; 40(06):354–9.

105. Lackey KA, Fehrenkamp BD, Pace RM, et al. Breastfeeding Beyond 12 Months: Is There Evidence for Health Impacts? Annu Rev Nutr 2021;41(1):283–308.

106. Allen J, Hector D. Benefits of breastfeeding. N S W Public Health Bull 2005; 16(4):42.

107. Binns C, James J. Infant feeding guidelines: Updating the evidence 2022. Breastfeed Rev 2022;30(1):19–26.

108. Noel-Weiss J, Courant G, Woodend AK. Physiological weight loss in the breastfed neonate: a systematic review. Open Med 2008;2(4):e99.

109. Pereyra-Elías R, Quigley MA, Carson C. To what extent does confounding explain the association between breastfeeding duration and cognitive development up to age 14? Findings from the UK Millennium Cohort Study. Kalk EK, ed. PLoS One. 2022;17(5):e0267326. doi:10.1371/journal.pone.0267326.

110. World Health Organization. Improving Early Childhood Development: WHO Guideline [Internet]. [Geneva]: WHO; 2020 [cited 2022 Aug 29] https://apps.who.int/iris/bitstream/handle/10665/331306/9789240002098-eng.pdf

111. Bennett C, Underdown A, Barlow J. Massage for promoting mental and physical health in typically developing infants under the age of six months. Cochrane Database Syst Rev 2013;2013(4):CD005038.

112. World Health Organization. Medical Eligibility Criteria for Contraceptive Use [Internet]. [Geneva]: WHO; 2015 [5th edition; cited 2022 Aug 29] https://www.who.int/publications/i/item/9789241549158

113. Jones E, Stewart F, Taylor B, et al. Early postnatal discharge from hospital for healthy mothers and term infants. Cochrane Database Syst Rev 2021;(6):2021.

114. Malagon-Maldonado G, Connelly CD, Bush RA. Predictors of Readiness for Hospital Discharge After Birth: Building Evidence for Practice. Worldviews Evidence-based Nurs 2017;14(2):118–27.

115. Dol J, Kohi T, Campbell-Yeo M, et al. Exploring maternal postnatal newborn care postnatal discharge education in Dar es Salaam, Tanzania: Barriers, facilitators and opportunities. Midwifery 2019;77:137–43.

116. World Health Organization. WHO recommendations: Optimizing health worker roles for maternal and newborn health through task shifting - WHO OptimizeMNH. Available at: https://optimizemnh.org/optimizing-health-worker-roles-maternal-newborn-health/. Accessed June 15, 2021.

117. Tokhi M, Comrie-Thomson L, Davis J, et al. Involving men to improve maternal and newborn health: A systematic review of the effectiveness of interventions. PLoS One 2018;13(1). https://doi.org/10.1371/JOURNAL.PONE.0191620.

118. Ekele BA, Villar J, Bergsjo P, Carroli G, Gulmezoglu M. The WHO antenatal care model: the defects. Acta Obstet Gynecol Scand. 2003;82(11):1063-1064. doi:10.1034/J.1600-0412.2003.00330.X.

119. Karami M, Chaleshgar M, Salari N, Akbari H, Mohammadi M. Global Prevalence of Anemia in Pregnant Women: A Comprehensive Systematic Review and Meta-Analysis. Matern Child Health J. 2022;26(7):1473-1487. doi:10.1007/S10995-022-03450-1/TABLES/2.

120. Smolina K, Hanley GE, Mintzes B, Oberlander TF, Morgan S. Trends and Determinants of Prescription Drug Use during Pregnancy and Postpartum in British Columbia, 2002-2011: A Population-Based Cohort Study. PLoS One. 2015;10(5):e0128312. doi:10.1371/JOURNAL.PONE.0128312.

121. Engeland A, Bjørge T, Klungsøyr K, Hjellvik V, Skurtveit S, Furu K. Trends in prescription drug use during pregnancy and postpartum in Norway, 2005 to 2015. Pharmacoepidemiol Drug Saf. 2018;27(9):995-1004. doi:10.1002/PDS.4577

122. Fortinguerra F, Belleudi V, Poggi FR, et al. Medication prescriptions before, during and after pregnancy in Italy: a population-based study. Ann Ist Super Sanita. 2021;57(3):249-258. doi:10.4415/ANN_21_03_09

123. Irvine L, Flynn RWV, Libby G, Crombie IK, Evans JMM. Drugs dispensed in primary care during pregnancy: a record-linkage analysis in Tayside, Scotland. Drug Saf. 2010;33(7):593-604. doi:10.2165/11532330-000000000-00000.

124. Ayele Y, Mekuria AN, Tola A, Mishore KM, Geleto FB. Prescription drugs use during pregnancy in Ethiopia: A systematic review and meta-analysis. SAGE open Med. 2020;8:205031212093547. doi:10.1177/2050312120935471

125. Smith G. A critical review of the Cochrane meta-analysis of routine late-pregnancy ultrasound. BJOG An Int J Obstet Gynaecol. 2021;128(2):207-213. doi:10.1111/1471-0528.16386.

Human Immunodeficiency Virus Treatment and Prevention for Pregnant and Postpartum Women in Global Settings

Friday Saidi, MBBS, MMed[a,b,*], Benjamin H. Chi, MD, MSc[b]

KEYWORDS

- HIV treatment • Antiretroviral regimens • HIV prevention • Pre-exposure prophylaxis
- Birth outcomes • Pregnancy • Breastfeeding

KEY POINTS

- Efforts to prevent mother-to-child transmission (PMTCT) of human immunodeficiency virus (HIV) have led to dramatic reductions in new pediatric HIV cases. New approaches and strategies are needed to eliminate pediatric acquired immune deficiency syndrome.
- Antiretroviral therapy for pregnant and breastfeeding women living with HIV and antiretroviral prophylaxis for their infants remains the cornerstone of PMTCT programs and to optimize maternal health. Regimens have evolved over time and are now safer, simpler, and better integrated with long-term HIV treatment.
- HIV prevention also has an important role for pregnant and breastfeeding women. HIV pre-exposure prophylaxis is an effective intervention that can reduce new maternal HIV infections, which has important long-term consequences for mother and child.
- While important advances have been made in HIV treatment and prevention, the delivery of these services has lagged. Greater attention is needed to the implementation of these evidence-based interventions, with approaches that consider contextual factors and individual patient priorities.

BACKGROUND

Efforts to prevent mother-to-child transmission (PMTCT) of human immunodeficiency virus (HIV) have led to dramatic reductions in pediatric HIV worldwide—from an estimated 320,000 new cases in 2010 to 150,000 in 2020.[1] These gains have been driven by a confluence of factors, including transformative biomedical advances, expanded

[a] UNC Project Malawi, Private Bag A-104, Lilongwe, Malawi; [b] Department of Obstetrics and Gynecology, University of North Carolina at Chapel Hill, Chapel Hill, NC, USA
* Corresponding author.
E-mail address: fsaidi@unclilongwe.org

Obstet Gynecol Clin N Am 49 (2022) 693–712
https://doi.org/10.1016/j.ogc.2022.07.002
0889-8545/22/© 2022 Elsevier Inc. All rights reserved.

health care access, strong political will, and increased donor funding. Once a seemingly intractable problem—especially in settings of high HIV prevalence and limited resources—national programs are now discussing the elimination of mother-to-child HIV transmission.[2]

Towing to the nature of vertical transmission, efforts to reduce pediatric HIV are inextricably linked to the care of pregnant and breastfeeding women. Absent any intervention, as many as 40% of infants born to women living with HIV (WLHIV) will acquire HIV.[3] Antiretroviral drugs, taken by pregnant or breastfeeding WLHIV, and as prophylaxis for their infants, can significantly reduce HIV transmission. With early initiation and consistent adherence, for example, combination antiretroviral therapy (ART) for the pregnant woman and 4 to 6 weeks of infant prophylaxis with nevirapine or zidovudine results in infant HIV transmission rates of less than 2%.[4] Lifelong treatment for women with these regimens—as recommended by the World Health Organization (WHO)[5]—also decreases HIV-associated morbidity and horizontal HIV transmission,[6,7] in ways that promote the health of mother and child.

Primary HIV prevention plays an important role during pregnancy and breastfeeding as well. In 2018, the Joint United Nations Programme on HIV/AIDS (UNAIDS) estimated that about 140,000 women acquire HIV during pregnancy each year.[8] These figures are consistent with the high HIV incidence observed during these periods across many studies,[9,10] likely resulting from different biological and behavioral factors.[11] Because most new cases of HIV remain undiagnosed through antenatal care, few of these women receive PMTCT services, with negative downstream consequences for maternal health, vertical transmission, and horizontal transmission. As the armamentarium of HIV prevention interventions continues to grow—including HIV pre-exposure prophylaxis (PrEP)[12]—tailored approaches are needed to support their use in clinical practice and public health programs.[13,14] With expanding coverage of HIV treatment programs worldwide, the contribution of new but undiagnosed maternal HIV infections to the global pediatric HIV burden will only increase.

We developed a framework for HIV prevention during pregnancy and breastfeeding.[15] Rather than focusing on the WLHIV and their newborns alone,[16–18] our broadened scope considers the family unit (ie, parents and child) to better individualize HIV services for all. The framework itself is shown in **Fig. 1**. In most countries worldwide, a large proportion of pregnant women are offered HIV testing at the first antenatal visit (or are already aware of their positive status).[19] By encouraging HIV testing and disclosure of partner HIV status, it is possible to further tailor HIV services for both members of the couple. For those living with HIV, for example, this includes initiation of and adherence to lifelong HIV treatment (ie, ART). For those who are HIV-negative, knowledge of the partner's status can help to stratify the risk for HIV acquisition and identify groups in need of targeted HIV prevention services (eg, PrEP). In our prior work, we identified three potential leverage points to reduce the overall HIV burden through antenatal/postnatal settings (labeled 1–3 in **Fig. 1**). Mathematical modeling indicates that, with moderate gains in all three areas, nearly one-third of maternal and pediatric HIV infections can be averted.[20]

In this review, we use this approach to discuss key issues related to HIV in pregnant and breastfeeding women in global settings. We focus narrowly on these distinct periods, because of their unique considerations, opportunities, and risks. [In this paper we do not discuss antiretroviral prophylaxis for HIV-exposed infants, which is an important part of the strategy for prevention of perinatal transmission, and refer the reader to the 2021 WHO Consolidated Guidelines on HIV Prevention, Testing, Treatment, Service Delivery and Monitoring (https://www.who.int/publications/i/item/9789240031593) for details and recommendations]. At the same time, we broaden

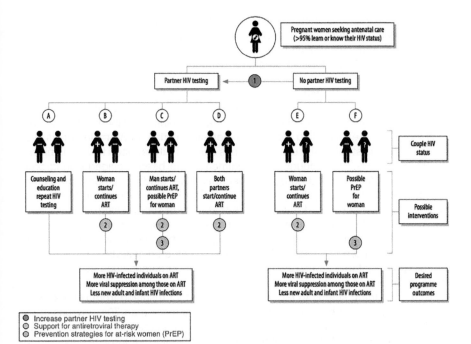

Fig. 1. Proposed couples-based framework for HIV prevention for pregnant or breastfeeding women and their partners. This figure focuses on prevention interventions for the woman as the index patient, though HIV-negative men in HIV serodifferent relationships may also initiate PrEP. In addition, in serodifferent relationships where the HIV-positive individual is on ART and is known to be virologically suppressed, PrEP can be stopped for the HIV-negative member of the couple. However, the decision should be carefully considered and monitored, especially if ART adherence for the HIV-positive individual changes over time. ART, antiretroviral therapy; PrEP: pre-exposure prophylaxis. (*From* Chi BH, Rosenberg NE, Mweemba O, et al. Involving both parents in HIV prevention during pregnancy and breastfeeding. Bull World Health Organ. 2018;96(1):69-71. https://doi.org/10.2471/BLT.17. 200139 with permission.)

our scope to encompass both HIV treatment *and* prevention. Such coordinated approaches—"status neutral"[21] strategies that provide HIV services to all pregnant women in need—will be critical as we seek to comprehensively address the HIV epidemic at scale.

DISCUSSION
Human Immunodeficiency Virus Treatment in Pregnancy

Evidence for maternal and infant benefit
HIV has been shown to increase the risk of morbidity and mortality among pregnant and postpartum women. HIV-related immunosuppression can adversely affect the frequency and course of many viral and bacterial infections in pregnancy, including genital herpes simplex, human papillomavirus, bacterial vaginosis, syphilis, and bacterial pneumonia.[22] Parasitic infestations and HIV-related opportunistic infections (eg, tuberculosis, pneumocystis pneumonia) also appear more frequently during this period.[22,23] Because of access to specialized health care services, HIV rarely causes maternal mortality in high-income countries. However, in low-income countries—

including those in sub-Saharan Africa—it has been a major contributor to maternal illness and death. Maternal HIV infection has also been associated with an increased risk of adverse pregnancy outcomes.[24,25]

The benefits of ART—three-drug antiretroviral regimens for long-term HIV treatment—are well documented in pregnant and breastfeeding women. ART suppresses circulating HIV viral load, with measurable improvements in the individual's immune status and clinical status.[7,26,27] With good adherence, individuals on ART are dramatically less likely to transmit HIV to sexual partners.[28–30] HIV treatment during pregnancy and breastfeeding has direct benefits to the newborn infant as well. Across numerous studies, the use of ART has significantly reduced HIV transmission rates to below 2%.[5,31] Although such regimens have been provided during pregnancy in North America and Europe for decades, later studies demonstrated effectiveness and safety during breastfeeding too.[32] ART can reduce mother-to-child transmission by a number of mechanisms that include suppressing maternal antepartum HIV viral load and pre-exposure and post-exposure prophylaxis of the infant.[33] Initiation of maternal ART before pregnancy has been shown to lower the rates of hospitalization among HIV-exposed uninfected infants compared with HIV-unexposed infants.[34] Interestingly, while infant outcomes such as survival and severe co-morbidity are dramatically reduced with exposure to maternal and neonatal ART, there seems to be some residual effect resulting from HIV exposure in utero. HIV-exposed but uninfected children have more than 70% increased risk of mortality compared with their HIV-unexposed counterparts,[35] emphasizing the importance of primary HIV prevention in women of child-bearing age—even in the context of universal HIV treatment.

Toward universal human immunodeficiency virus treatment for pregnant and breastfeeding women

There has been a rapid evolution in the recommended antiretroviral regimens during pregnancy. While combination three-drug regimens have been available in North America and Europe for decades, for much of that time similar interventions were not readily accessible in most low-income settings. As HIV services have expanded globally, there has been a shift to more efficacious and complex regimens to reduce mother-to-child HIV transmission. In July 2011, Malawi became the first country to adopt a policy of lifelong HIV treatment—in the form of ART—for all pregnant and breastfeeding women regardless of HIV disease stage or CD4 count.[36] Known as the "Option B+" strategy (in reference to the WHO guidelines at the time[37]), this innovative strategy sought to streamline the operational demands of HIV triage which, -at the time included CD4 testing and clinical staging. The approach was designed for earlier initiation of ART during pregnancy—a key factor in vertical HIV transmission rates—and minimized interruptions in settings where breastfeeding was prevalent and fertility was high.[38] The Option B+ strategy resulted in a dramatic increase in the number of pregnant or breastfeeding women on ART in Malawi,[39] and in 2012 the WHO endorsed the strategy as the preferred PMTCT approach in settings with high HIV prevalence, short durations between pregnancies, and extended breastfeeding.[37] By 2015, the implementation of Option B+ had resulted in a more than 90% increase in the number of women receiving ART as part of PMTCT services. Beginning in 2016, these efforts have converged with new recommendations for universal "test and treat" strategies for all individuals living with HIV.[40] As a result, increasing numbers of women are conceiving while on ART and additional women are newly diagnosed and initiated on ART when they attend antenatal care.[19,41] This has led to a rapid rise in fetal exposure to antiretroviral drugs.[42]

Antiretroviral regimens for human immunodeficiency virus treatment

The first- and second-line ART regimens for pregnant and breastfeeding WLHIV, as recommended by the WHO,[43] have evolved over time (**Table 1**). To promote continuity and minimize regimen changes, there has been an effort to align these with general adult guidelines for HIV treatment. However, the choice of drugs for any individual depends on contextual factors, including toxicities and tolerance, possible HIV resistance (for those with prior ART experience), and co-morbidities, such as hepatitis B virus and hepatitis C infection.[44] The wide availability of fixed-dose ART combinations (ie, multiple drugs co-formulated in a single tablet) has provided efficacious yet simpler and less toxic options over time. First-line regimens are now taken once daily, which has greatly enhanced the coverage of and adherence to ART.

Pregnancy presents unique challenges in terms of safety assessment related to drug exposure. Congenital anomalies, resulting from in utero exposure to antiretroviral drugs, could potentially lead to significant morbidity and mortality; however, such events are rare. However, because pregnant and breastfeeding women are often excluded from efficacy trials,[45] there are limited safety data to guide the use of specific antiretroviral drugs at scale. In some cases, this can unnecessarily restrict the use of otherwise safe and effective drugs for HIV treatment during pregnancy. For example, the non-nucleoside reverse transcriptase inhibitor efavirenz was considered a Category D drug for years because of reported cases of neural tube defects as suggested by animal teratology studies.[46] Following a series of systematic reviews and empiric studies demonstrating safety in humans,[47–49] the WHO endorsed its use during pregnancy in 2013, listing it among recommended first-line ART regimens.

Limited safety data in pregnancy can also complicate clinical guidelines and public health recommendations. This was observed most recently with dolutegravir, an integrase strand transfer inhibitor that is taken once daily results in rapid suppression of HIV and is associated with lower rates of HIV drug resistance. In 2019, the WHO endorsed dolutegravir as the preferred HIV treatment option in all populations.[50] However, soon after, this recommendation was temporarily suspended for pregnant and breastfeeding women after surveillance data suggested higher rates of neural tube defects among women taking dolutegravir-based regimens periconceptually versus those who had taken other regimens (3.0 per 1000 deliveries vs 1.0 per 1000 deliveries).[51] Ongoing follow-up eventually cleared the drug: WLHIV starting dolutegravir before pregnancy (5 of 1683, 0.3%) or during pregnancy (0 of 2812) did not have substantially higher rates of fetal neural tube defects compared with those on other regimens (15 of 14,792, 0.1%). While these results are reassuring—and certainly supported the WHO's original recommendations about dolutegravir[44]—the narrative highlights the potential challenges of ART recommendations, when only partial and/or incomplete safety data are available during pregnancy. There is growing consensus about the need for early inclusion of pregnant and breastfeeding women in safety and efficacy trials of new antiretroviral agents and the need for new research, regulatory, and policy frameworks in this area.[52] At the present time, based on the currently available evidence, WLHIV can be counseled that the recommended antiretroviral drugs are taken during pregnancy generally do not increase the risk of birth defects.[44]

Other interventions

Labor and delivery represent periods of high potential risk for vertical HIV transmission. In the United States, HIV viral load is used as a triage tool, and for women with concentrations >1000 copies/mL in the late third trimester, elective cesarean delivery at 38 weeks gestation is recommended.[53] Management of patients originally scheduled for cesarean delivery because of elevated HIV viral load who present in

Table 1
World Health Organization-recommended regimens for antiretroviral therapy in pregnancy and breastfeeding since 2013

	2013 Guidelines	2016 Guidelines	2018 and 2021 Guidelines
First-line regimens	Tenofovir + Lamivudine (or Emtricitabine) + Efavirenz Zidovudine + Lamivudine + Efavirenz (or Nevirapine) Tenofovir + Lamivudine (or Emtricitabine) + Nevirapine	Tenofovir + Lamivudine (or Emtricitabine) + Efavirenz Tenofovir + Lamivudine (or Emtricitabine) + Dolutegravir Tenofovir + Lamivudine (or Emtricitabine) + Nevirapine	Tenofovir + Lamivudine (or Emtricitabine) + Dolutegravir Tenofovir + Lamivudine (or Emtricitabine) + Efavirenz Zidovudine + Lamivudine + Dolutegravir
Second-line regimens	Tenofovir + Lamivudine (or Emtricitabine) + Lopinavir/r (or Atazanavir/r) Zidovudine + Lamivudine (or Emtricitabine) + Lopinavir/r (or Atazanavir/r)	Tenofovir + Lamivudine (or Emtricitabine) + Lopinavir/r (or Atazanavir/r) Zidovudine + Lamivudine (or Emtricitabine) + Lopinavir/r (or Atazanavir/r) Darunavir/r + Dolutegravir (or Raltegravir) + 1–2 NRTIs	Zidovudine + Lamivudine (or Emtricitabine) + Lopinavir/r (or Atazanavir/r) Tenofovir + Lamivudine (or Emtricitabine) + Dolutegravir
Third-line regimens			Darunavir/r + Dolutegravir (or Raltegravir) + 1–2 NRTIs

Preferred first-line regimens noted in *italics*./r = in combination with ritonavir.

labor or with ruptured membranes is individualized at the time of presentation since the evidence is insufficient to determine if cesarean delivery reduces the risk of transmission in those situations. When HIV viral load is ≤ 1000 copies/mL, the available evidence suggests that cesarean delivery may not confer additional benefit[54] and therefore does not justify the additional surgical risks to the mother. In many low- and middle-income settings, local infrastructure is often unable to support this standard of care. Routine HIV viral load in the third trimester is often not available; health systems may not have the capacity to provide safe, elective cesarean delivery, especially where HIV prevalence is high. In such places, there is greater reliance on HIV viral suppression as the primary means of minimizing vertical HIV transmission. This includes earlier initiation of ART and the incorporation of antiretroviral drugs—like integrase strand transfer inhibitor—that can rapidly reduce HIV viral load.[55]

Primary Human Immunodeficiency Virus Prevention in Pregnancy

Human immunodeficiency virus incidence during pregnancy and breastfeeding

A growing body of evidence suggests that HIV acquisition is increased during pregnancy and breastfeeding, especially in generalized HIV epidemics. A series of systematic reviews demonstrated high HIV incidence during these periods,[9,10] at levels that approximate—or even exceed—WHO thresholds for HIV risk populations (ie, ≥3.0 per 100 person-years).[56] Thomson and colleagues showed that the per-coital-act rates of HIV acquisition varied over a woman's antenatal/postnatal course, with elevated risk noted late in pregnancy (adjusted relative risk: 2.82, P = .01) and in the postpartum period (adjusted relative risk: 3.97; P = .01) when compared with the nonpregnant state.[57] A new maternal HIV infection has obvious consequences for long-term health. In addition, because of low repeat HIV testing in many resource-limited settings,[58] women who acquire HIV over the course of pregnancy often go undiagnosed; as a result, they receive few to no interventions to reduce vertical HIV transmission. In the latest modeling estimates from UNAIDS, as high as 23% of new infant HIV cases were in the context of new maternal HIV infections worldwide.[59,60] To eliminate mother-to-child HIV transmission at a population level, efforts to prevent new maternal HIV infections are critical.

Human immunodeficiency virus pre-exposure prophylaxis

PrEP represents an important intervention in the growing armamentarium for HIV prevention. With adequate adherence, daily oral emtricitabine/tenofovir disoproxil fumarate (FTC/TDF) has been shown to reduce new HIV infections by as much as 44% in randomized trials.[61,62] FTC/TDF has been shown to be safe in pregnancy, across numerous trials in the HIV and hepatitis B treatment literature.[61] Although several studies show that drug concentrations may be lowered in the antenatal period— including the recent IMPAACT 2009 trial, which directly observed PrEP ingestion to ensure near-perfect to perfect adherence[63]—there is currently no evidence that suggests PrEP efficacy is lowered during pregnancy. In 2016, the WHO recommended PrEP for pregnant and breastfeeding women at elevated risk for new HIV infection and many national HIV programs have incorporated it into their clinical guidelines.[64] In addition, PrEP may also have an important role peri-conceptionally, for HIV-negative partners in HIV serodifferent relationships.[65] Several large-scale programs have been implemented, including in Kenya[66] and South Africa.[67]

At present, daily oral FTC/TDF is the only antiretroviral regimen approved for PrEP in women; however, several promising agents are under evaluation. For example, the dapivirine vaginal ring demonstrated a 30% reduction in HIV acquisition in clinical trials,[68,69] with even greater effectiveness in open-label studies.[70,71] The MTN-042 trial (ie, DELIVER) is currently underway to assess its safety during pregnancy and breast-feeding.[72] Long-acting injectable cabotegravir has been shown to be superior to daily oral FTC/TDF in men and women,[73,74] but studies in pregnant and breastfeeding women are still ongoing. Finally, tenofovir alafenamide (TAF), a prodrug analog of TDF, is the Food and Drug Administration-approved as an ART component in HIV treatment in men and women, and as part of PrEP for men.[75,76] Studies of TAF-based PrEP in women—and pregnant women in particular—are currently planned.[77] As the pipeline of PrEP agents continues to grow, the early inclusion of pregnant and breastfeeding women in clinical trials is needed to ensure their safety and shorten the period of availability.[78]

Other human immunodeficiency virus prevention strategies

Despite its demonstrated efficacy, the uptake of and persistence of oral PrEP—even among women at high risk for acquiring HIV—remains suboptimal.[66] However, there may be an important role for PrEP in combination with other HIV prevention strategies. Data about behavioral interventions for HIV prevention during pregnancy and breast-feeding have been limited and results to date have been mixed.[79–81] The addition of PrEP (or other biomedical intervention) may enhance the effectiveness of these combi-nation HIV prevention strategies, though there is currently limited data available. Our team is currently studying one such strategy—a combination of intensive patient coun-seling and self-identified peer supporters—to improve PrEP adherence in pregnant and breastfeeding women.[82,83] Condoms remain an effective strategy for the prevention of HIV and can also reduce the risk of other sexually transmitted infections, but can be a challenge for women to control and are often not thought about during pregnancy.

Birth outcomes and antiretroviral regimens

Untreated maternal HIV infection has been associated with an increased risk of adverse birth outcomes that include preterm birth, stillbirth, low birth weight, or small-for-gestational-age infants.[84] While the benefits of ART for PMTCT are undis-puted and well documented, the effect of antiretroviral drugs on pregnancy outcomes is not fully understood. However, there is growing consensus that, while ART improves adverse birth outcomes among pregnant WLHIV, it does not restore it to the baseline levels seen in HIV-uninfected women.[85–87]

Studies in both high-income and low-income countries have reported mixed—and at times conflicting—evidence about maternal ART exposure and adverse pregnancy outcomes. Across studies, ART has been associated with lower risk,[47,88,89] higher risk[42,86,90,91] or no effect on adverse birth outcomes.[92–95] Timing of ART exposure (pre- or post-conception) during pregnancy, methodological pitfalls in conducting pre-term birth research,[96] and specific antiretroviral drug regimens may help to explain these differing results, particularly for preterm birth.[4,97–99] The different regimens have been shown to have varying rates of preterm birth. For example, results from the multicenter PROMISE trial showed higher rates of preterm delivery and low birth weight among women initiating ART during pregnancy, compared with those starting zidovudine monotherapy plus intrapartum nevirapine (6.0% vs 2.6%, $P = .04$).[4] The IMPAACT 2010 trial found lower composite adverse birth outcomes among women receiving dolutegravir + FTC/TAF, compared with those who received dolutegravir + FTC/TDF or efavirenz + FTC/TDF (24.1% vs 32.7%, $P = .047$).[99]

New interventions are needed to reduce adverse birth outcomes among WLHIV on ART; however, such evidence is only beginning to emerge. For example, weekly inject-able 17-alpha-hydroxyprogesterone caproate has been shown to be effective in trials of women who had a previous spontaneous preterm birth of a singleton infant.[100] In a randomized trial of 800 pregnant WLHIV in Zambia, weekly administration of the drug did not result in lower preterm birth rates or stillbirth compared with placebo (9.0% vs 9.0% $P = .98$).[101] Given the obvious benefits of ART for pregnant and breastfeeding WLHIV, approaches that mitigate these risks are urgently needed.

Safety data for PrEP—in the form of oral daily FTC/TDF—has likewise been reassuring, both in early clinical trials[102] and in larger public health initiatives. In the evaluation of the PrEP Implementation in Young Women and Adolescents (PrIYA) program, for example, no major differences in preterm birth or low birth weight were observed, when women with and without FTC/TDF exposure were compared.[103] These findings are consistent with other studies as well.[104] Safety monitoring and surveillance are essential, especially with the availability of newer PrEP agents. Unlike ART, most women taking PrEP are otherwise healthy and this must be considered when weighing safety risks. A number of ongoing studies is exploring these questions in greater depth, with more data available in the coming years.[104]

Bringing services to scale

In this article, we focus primarily on biomedical interventions for HIV prevention in pregnant and breastfeeding WLHIV and their infants. These evidence-based practices are supported by the medical literature and recommended by national and international guidelines. However, implementation has lagged, particularly in settings where the burden of HIV is high and resources are limited.

To bring HIV prevention to scale, new and novel strategies are needed to support health delivery. For example, "opt-out" approaches that incorporate HIV testing into routine antenatal care have increased uptake of HIV testing in pregnancy and are now the standard of care in many settings.[105] The integration of PMTCT services within maternal and child health platforms has improved the coverage and timeliness of ART initiation[106,107] and led to better continuity of care over the course of pregnancy and postpartum. Such integrated approaches have been adapted for PrEP delivery in antenatal/postnatal settings as well.[66] Differentiated care models also appear promising. Such approaches recognize the differences in patient priorities and provide alternatives for service delivery, including the venue (eg, facility-based vs community-based) and management structure (eg, health care-led vs client-led). Several approaches—including postnatal adherence clubs—are being evaluated as differentiated care strategies to increase patient engagement.[108–110]

While programs have emphasized the uptake of specific interventions, support is needed to promote their continued use. For HIV treatment, HIV viral suppression is a reliable indicator of adherence. HIV viremia is independently associated with vertical HIV transmission[111,112] and can be used to guide intrapartum and early postnatal management.[111] In contrast, the measurement of persistence and adherence to PrEP can present unique challenges. Unlike ART, which treats a chronic condition, prevention-focused interventions like PrEP are only needed at times of increased risk of HIV acquisition. This is the paradigm of "prevention-effective adherence," which considers dynamic HIV risk behaviors and the use of alternate HIV prevention modalities.[113] Unfortunately, such approaches may be difficult to apply in a public health setting. Self-reported HIV risk is often unreliable, making it difficult for individuals to identify instances in which PrEP is most suitable.[114] In addition, more consistent use of FTC/TDF and lengthier "lead-in" periods may be needed to reach protective drug concentrations in the vaginal mucosa, compared with other biological compartments.[115–117] In the absence of instruments to better measure and/or anticipate HIV risk, most programs rely on individual self-assessments to guide PrEP use.[114] If the use of PrEP is to be optimized in this population, however, better approaches are needed.

Social and cultural contexts should be considered as HIV services are brought to scale. Across sub-Saharan Africa, for example, gender can play an important role in health care access, especially in the context of pregnancy.[118] For some women, the engagement of male partners provides a permission structure that facilitates the uptake and adherence to HIV interventions (ie, ART or PrEP). When accompanied by male partner HIV testing, it can also guide HIV treatment and prevention services (see **Fig. 1**).[15] However, male partner involvement may be challenging if there is a lack of disclosure due to stigma and fear of abandonment. Similarly, stigma directly impacts the scalability of PrEP as a prevention strategy, including the pace of uptake, rates of adherence and persistence, and disparities in dissemination among highest priority populations.[119] Fostering greater social support—including through male partners and disclosure assistance if needed—can help to reduce the barriers resulting from real and perceived stigma, and improve health outcomes among pregnant and breastfeeding women.

Data-driven approaches to monitoring and evaluation can optimize PMTCT services. The concept of the "PMTCT cascade" (ie, the sequence of steps needed for a mother and infant to receive maximum benefit from HIV services) is well established in the medical literature.[16–18] Routinely collected and evaluated, such frameworks help to identify existing gaps and inform programmatic efforts to address them via quality improvement methods.[120–122] In a cluster-randomized trial in Cote d'Ivoire, Kenya, and Mozambique ($n = 36$ sites), Rustagi and colleagues found that a structured systems engineering intervention led to significant improvements in ART uptake and early infant HIV testing.[123] Iterative, data-driven approaches may have an important role in program improvement at the national level as well.[124]

Finally, we have focused narrowly on HIV in the context of the mother–infant dyad; however, antenatal platforms can be an important entry point for family based care.[125] Engagement of male partners is critical and can lead to earlier access to HIV testing, prevention, and treatment services for both members of the couple.[126] An integrated view of HIV across a woman's lifespan is also needed. For many women, antenatal care represents an early—maybe even the first—encounter with HIV services, due to the universal nature of HIV testing in pregnancy. However, continued engagement is important and should continue well after delivery and the postpartum period. In its framework for PMTCT, the WHO describes four pillars: (1) primary prevention of HIV infection among women of childbearing age; (2) preventing unintended pregnancies among WLHIV; (3) preventing HIV transmission from a woman living with HIV to her infant; and (4) providing appropriate treatment, care, and support to mothers living with HIV and their children and families.[127] Such linkages between HIV and reproductive health services can lead to fewer maternal and infant HIV infections globally.

SUMMARY

In this review, we have discussed key issues related to HIV in pregnant and breastfeeding women in global settings. We have highlighted the global achievements that have been made in PMTCT and the ongoing challenges that still need to be addressed to achieve zero HIV transmission during pregnancy and breastfeeding. The combination of different evidence-based strategies could further enhance uptake of ART among pregnant and breastfeeding WLHIV, as well as PrEP uptake among HIV-uninfected women at high risk of HIV acquisition. The needs and perspectives of pregnant and breastfeeding women and their families are critical to the effective delivery of care and the design and implementation of integrated HIV treatment/prevention programs and services.

CLINICS CARE POINTS

- Lifelong antiretroviral therapy is now recommended for all pregnant and breastfeeding women living with human immunodeficiency virus (HIV). This represents an important entry point into long-term care, but additional support may be needed to sustain adherence, retention, and engagement in care over time.

- Accurate and reliable assessment of HIV risk is essential for HIV prevention services. Initiatives should consider HIV risk in their recommendation and support for such services, including HIV pre-exposure prophylaxis.

- New antiretroviral drugs show promise, especially in the context of HIV prevention. However, the exclusion of pregnant and breastfeeding women from clinical trials has delayed their availability for these important at-risk populations.

ACKNOWLEDGMENTS

This work was supported in part by the National Institute of Allergy and Infectious Diseases (R01 AI131060, R01 AI157859, K24 AI120796, and P30 AI50410) and the Fogarty International Center of the National Institutes of Health (D43-TW009340, D43-TW010060).The content is solely the responsibility of the authors and does not necessarily represent the official views of the funders.

DISCLOSURE

The authors have nothing to disclose.

REFERENCES

1. Kourtis AP, Ellington S, Pazol K, et al. Complications of cesarean deliveries among HIV-infected women in the United States. AIDS 2014;28(17):2609–18. https://doi.org/10.1097/QAD.0000000000000474.
2. UNAIDS. Fast-Track - Ending the AIDS Epidemic by 2030. UNAIDS 2014;. https://www.unaids.org/en/resources/documents/2014/JC2686_ WAD2014report. Accessed April 4, 2020.
3. Teasdale CA, Marais BJ, Abrams EJ. HIV: prevention of mother-to-child transmission. BMJ Clin Evid 2011;2011:0909.
4. Fowler MG, Qin M, Fiscus SA, et al. Benefits and Risks of Antiretroviral Therapy for Perinatal HIV Prevention. N Engl J Med 2016;375(18):1726–37.
5. World Health Organization. World Health Organization HIV/AIDS. WHO 2018;. https://www.who.int/news-room/fact-sheets/detail/hiv-aids. Accessed March 1, 2022.
6. Cohen MS, Chen YQ, McCauley M, et al. Prevention of HIV-1 Infection with Early Antiretroviral Therapy | NEJM. https://www.nejm.org/doi/full/10.1056/ nejmoa1105243. Accessed April 15, 2022.
7. Hoffman RM, Angelidou KN, Brummel SS, et al. Maternal health outcomes among HIV-infected breastfeeding women with high CD4 counts: results of a treatment strategy trial. HIV Clin Trials 2018;19(6):209–24.
8. UNAIDS DATA. 2019. https://www.unaids.org/sites/default/files/media_asset/ 2019-UNAIDS-data_en.pdf. Accessed April 21, 2022.
9. Graybill LA, Kasaro M, Freeborn K, et al. Incident HIV among pregnant and breast-feeding women in sub-Saharan Africa: a systematic review and meta-

analysis. AIDS 2020;34(5):761–76. https://doi.org/10.1097/QAD. 0000000000002487.

10. Drake AL, Wagner A, Richardson B, et al. Incident HIV during pregnancy and postpartum and risk of mother-to-child HIV transmission: a systematic review and meta-analysis. Plos Med 2014;e1001608. https://doi.org/10.1371/journal. pmed.1001608. Mofenson LM, ed.

11. Abbai NS, Wand H, Ramjee G. Biological factors that place women at risk for HIV: evidence from a large-scale clinical trial in Durban. BMC Women's Health 2016;16(1):19. https://doi.org/10.1186/s12905-016-0295-5.

12. Fonner VA, Dalglish SL, Kennedy CE, et al. Effectiveness and safety of oral HIV preexposure prophylaxis for all populations. AIDS 2016;30(12):1973–83. https:// doi.org/10.1097/QAD.0000000000001145.

13. Pintye J, Davey DLJ, Wagner AD, et al. Defining gaps in pre-exposure prophy- laxis delivery for pregnant and post-partum women in high-burden settings us- ing an implementation science framework - PubMed. Available at: https:// pubmed.ncbi.nlm.nih.gov/32763221/. Accessed April 15, 2022.

14. Joseph Davey DL, Bekker LG, Gorbach PM, et al. Delivering preexposure pro- phylaxis to pregnant and breastfeeding women in Sub-Saharan Africa: the im- plementation science frontier. AIDS 2017;31(16):2193–7. https://doi.org/10. 1097/QAD.0000000000001604.

15. Chi BH, Rosenberg NE, Mweemba O, et al. Involving both parents in HIV pre- vention during pregnancy and breastfeeding. Bull World Health Organ 2018; 96(1):69–71. https://doi.org/10.2471/BLT.17.200139.

16. Stringer EM, Chi BH, Chintu N, et al. Monitoring effectiveness of programmes to prevent mother-to-child HIV transmission in lower-income countries. Bull World Health Organ 2008;86(1):57–62. https://doi.org/10.2471/BLT.07.043117.

17. Hamilton E, Bossiky B, Ditekemena J, et al. Using the PMTCT Cascade to Accel- erate Achievement of the Global Plan Goals - PubMed. Available at: https:// pubmed.ncbi.nlm.nih.gov/28398994/. Accessed April 15, 2022.

18. McNairy ML, Lamb MR, Abrams EJ, et al. Use of a Comprehensive HIV Care Cascade for Evaluating HIV Program Performance: Findings From 4 Sub- Saharan African Countries. J Acquir Immune Defic Syndr 2015;70(2):e44–51. https://doi.org/10.1097/QAI.0000000000000745.

19. Awopegba OE, Kalu A, Ahinkorah BO, et al. Prenatal care coverage and corre- lates of HIV testing in sub-Saharan Africa: insight from demographic and health surveys of 16 countries. PLoS One 2020;e0242001. https://doi.org/10.1371/ journal.pone.0242001. Kalk EK, ed.

20. Powers KA, Orroth K, Rosenberg NE, et al. A mathematical modeling analysis of combination HIV prevention in antenatal clinics. Presented at: conference on Retroviruses and Opportunistic Infections2019 2019. Paper presented at: 2019 Conference on Retroviruses and Opportunistic Infections2019.

21. Myers JE, Braunstein SL, Xia Q, et al. Redefining Prevention and Care: A Status- Neutral Approach to HIV. Open Forum Infect Dis 2018;5(6):ofy097. https://doi. org/10.1093/ofid/ofy097.

22. Magiorkinis G, Angelis K, Mamais I, et al. The global spread of HIV-1 subtype B epidemic -. Infect Genet Evol. doi:10.1016/j.meegid.2016.05.041.

23. Chilaka VN, Konje JC. HIV in pregnancy – An update. Eur J Obstet Gynecol Re- prod Biol 2021;256:484–91. https://doi.org/10.1016/j.ejogrb.2020.11.034.

24. Brocklehurst P, French R. The association between maternal HIV infection and perinatal outcome: a systematic review of the literature and meta-analysis. Br

J Obstet Gynaecol 1998;105(8):836–48. https://doi.org/10.1111/j.1471-0528. 1998.tb10227.x.

25. Twabi HS, Manda SO, Small DS. Assessing the effects of maternal HIV infection on pregnancy outcomes using cross-sectional data in Malawi. BMC Public Health 2020;20(1):974. https://doi.org/10.1186/s12889-020-09046-0.

26. Kim MH, Ahmed S, Hosseinipour MC, et al. The Impact of Option B+ on the Antenatal PMTCT Cascade in Lilongwe, Malawi. J Acquir Immune Defic Syndr 2015;68(5):7.

27. Miro JM, Manzardo C, Mussini C, et al. Survival Outcomes and Effect of Early vs. Deferred cART Among HIV-Infected Patients Diagnosed at the Time of an AIDS-Defining Event: A Cohort Analysis - PMC. Available at: https://www.ncbi.nlm.nih. gov/labs/pmc/articles/PMC3197144/. Accessed March 17, 2022.

28. Becquet R, Bland R, Ekouevi DK, et al. Universal antiretroviral therapy among pregnant and postpartum HIV-infected women would improve maternal health and decrease postnatal HIV transmission. AIDS 2010;24(8):1239–41. https:// doi.org/10.1097/QAD.0b013e328338b791.

29. Cohen MS, Chen YQ, McCauley M, et al. Antiretroviral Therapy for the Prevention of HIV-1 Transmission | NEJM. Available at: https://www.nejm.org/doi/full/10. 1056/nejmoa1600693. Accessed March 1, 2022.

30. World Health Organization. Prevention of mother-to-child transmission - Estimates by WHO region. WHO. Available at: https://apps.who.int/gho/data/view. main.23500REG?lang=en. Accessed February 27, 2022.

31. The INSIGHT START Study Group. Initiation of Antiretroviral Therapy in Early Asymptomatic HIV Infection. N Engl J Med 2015;373(9):795–807. https://doi. org/10.1056/NEJMoa1506816.

32. Bispo S, Chikhungu L, Rollins N, et al. Postnatal HIV transmission in breastfed infants of HIV-infected women on ART: a systematic review and meta-analysis. J Int AIDS Soc 2017;20(1):21251. https://doi.org/10.7448/IAS.20.1.21251.

33. Choudhary Madhu Chhanda. Antiretroviral Therapy (ART) in Pregnant Women With HIV Infection: Overview of HIV Antiretroviral Therapy (ART) in Pregnancy, Clinical Data on HIV Antiretroviral Therapy (ART) in Pregnancy, Factors for HIV Antiretroviral Therapy (ART) Selection in Pregnancy. 2021. Available at: https://emedicine.medscape.com/article/2042311-overview. Accessed March 15, 2022.

34. Goetghebuer T, Smolen KK, Adler C, et al. Initiation of Antiretroviral Therapy Before Pregnancy Reduces the Risk of Infection-related Hospitalization in Human Immunodeficiency Virus–exposed Uninfected Infants Born in a High-income Country. Clin Infect Dis 2019;68(7):1193–203. https://doi.org/10.1093/ cid/ciy673.

35. Brennan AT, Bonawitz R, Gill CJ, et al. A meta-analysis assessing all-cause mortality in HIV-exposed uninfected compared with HIV-unexposed uninfected infants and children. AIDS 2016;30(15):2351–60. https://doi.org/10.1097/QAD. 0000000000001211.

36. Schouten EJ, Jahn A, Midiani D, et al. Prevention of mother-to-child transmission of HIV and the health-related Millennium Development Goals: time for a public health approach. Lancet 2011;378(9787):282–4. https://doi.org/10.1016/ S0140-6736(10)62303-3.

37. World Health Organization. WHO. Programmatic update guidelines use of antiretroviral drugs for treating pregnant women and preventing HIV infection in infants. Executive summary 2012. Available at: www.who.int/hiv/PMTCT_ update.pdf.

38. Stover J, Bollinger L, Izazola JA, et al. What is required to end the AIDS epidemic as a public health threat by 2030? The cost and impact of the fast-track approach. Available at: https://doi.org/10.1371/journal.pone.0213970. Accessed April 13, 2022.

39. CDC. Impact of an innovative approach to prevent mother-to-child transmission of HIV — Malawi 2011. Available at: https://www.cdc.gov/mmwr/preview/mmwrhtml/mm6208a3.htm. Accessed March 17, 2022.

40. World Health Organization. Consolidated guidelines on the use of antiretroviral drugs for treating and preventing HIV infection: recommendations for a public health approach. World Health Organization; 2016. Available at: https://apps.who.int/iris/handle/10665/208825. Accessed February 25, 2022.

41. Astawesegn FH, Stulz V, Conroy E, et al. Trends and effects of antiretroviral therapy coverage during pregnancy on mother-to-child transmission of HIV in Sub-Saharan Africa. Evidence from panel data analysis. BMC Infect Dis 2022;22(1):134. https://doi.org/10.1186/s12879-022-07119-6.

42. Uthman OA, Nachega JB, Anderson J, et al. Timing of initiation of antiretroviral therapy and adverse pregnancy outcomes: a systematic review and meta-analysis. Lancet HIV 2017;4(1):e21–30. https://doi.org/10.1016/S2352-3018(16)30195-3.

43. World Health Organization. Consolidated guidelines on HIV prevention, testing, treatment, service delivery and monitoring: recommendations for a public health approach. 2021. Available at: https://reliefweb.int/sites/reliefweb.int/files/resources/9789240031593-eng.pdf.

44. Recommendations NIH. for the Use of Antiretroviral Drugs During Pregnancy and Interventions to Reduce Perinatal HIV Transmission in the United States. Available at: https://clinicalinfo.hiv.gov/en/guidelines/perinatal/whats-new-guidelines. Accessed February 26, 2022.

45. Sheth AN, Rolle CP, Gandhi M. HIV pre-exposure prophylaxis for women. J Virus Eradication 2016;2(3):149–55. https://doi.org/10.1016/S2055-6640(20)30458-1.

46. Chersich MF, Urban MF, Venter FW, et al. Efavirenz use during pregnancy and for women of child-bearing potential. AIDS Res Ther 2006;3:11. https://doi.org/10.1186/1742-6405-3-11.

47. Zash R, Souda S, Chen JY, et al. Reassuring Birth Outcomes With Tenofovir/Emtricitabine/Efavirenz Used for Prevention of Mother-to-Child Transmission of HIV in Botswana. JAIDS J Acquired Immune Deficiency Syndromes 2016;71(4):428–36. https://doi.org/10.1097/QAI.0000000000000847.

48. Ford N, Calmy A, Mofenson L. Safety of efavirenz in the first trimester of pregnancy: an updated systematic review and meta-analysis. AIDS 2011;25(18):2301–4. https://doi.org/10.1097/QAD.0b013e32834cdb71.

49. Ford N, Mofenson L, Shubber Z, et al. Safety of efavirenz in the first trimester of pregnancy: an updated systematic review and meta-analysis. AIDS 2014;28(Suppl 2):S123–31. https://doi.org/10.1097/QAD.0000000000000231.

50. World Health Organization. WHO recommends dolutegravir as preferred HIV treatment option in all populations. Available at: https://www.who.int/news/item/22-07-2019-who-recommends-dolutegravir-as-preferred-hiv-treatment-option-in-all-populations. Accessed March 19, 2022.

51. Zash R, Holmes L, Diseko M, et al. Neural-Tube Defects and Antiretroviral Treatment Regimens in Botswana. N Engl J Med 2019;381(9):827–40. https://doi.org/10.1056/NEJMoa1905230.

52. Lyerly AD, Beigi R, Bekker LG, et al. Ending the evidence gap for pregnancy, HIV and co-infections: ethics guidance from the PHASES project. J Int AIDS Soc 2021;24(12):e25846. https://doi.org/10.1002/jia2.25846.

53. American College of Obstetricians and Gynecologists (ACOG). Labor and Delivery Management of Women With Human Immunodeficiency Virus Infection. 2018. Available at: https://www.acog.org/en/clinical/clinical-guidance/committee-opinion/articles/2018/09/labor-and-delivery-management-of-women-with-human-immunodeficiency-virus-infection. Accessed June 28, 2022.

54. Andiman W, Bryson Y, de Martino M, Fowler M, Harris D, et al. The mode of delivery and the risk of vertical transmission of human immunodeficiency virus type 1–a meta-analysis of 15 prospective cohort studies. Available at: https://read.qxmd.com/read/10099139/the-mode-of-delivery-and-the-risk-of-vertical-transmission-of-human-immunodeficiency-virus-type-1-a-meta-analysis-of-15-prospective-cohort-studies. Accessed June 28, 2022.

55. João EC, Morrison RL, Shapiro DE, et al. Raltegravir versus efavirenz in antiretroviral-naive pregnant women living with HIV (NICHD P1081): an open-label, randomised, controlled, phase 4 trial. Lancet HIV 2020;7(5):e322–31. https://doi.org/10.1016/S2352-3018(20)30038-2.

56. World Health Organization. World Health Organization. WHO technical brief: preventing HIV during pregnancy and breastfeeding in the context of pre-exposure prophylaxis (PrEP). Geneva: World Health Organization; 2017. Available at: https://www.google.com/search?client=firefox-b-d&q=World+Health+Organization.+WHO+technical+brief%3A+preventing+HIV+during+pregnancy+and+breastfeeding+in+the+context+of+pre-exposure+prophylaxis+%28PrEP%29.+Geneva%3A+World+Health+Organization%2C+2017. Accessed April 8, 2020.

57. Thomson KA, Hughes J, Baeten JM, et al. Increased Risk of HIV Acquisition Among Women Throughout Pregnancy and During the Postpartum Period: A Prospective Per-Coital-Act Analysis Among Women With HIV-Infected Partners. J Infect Dis 2018;218(1):16–25. https://doi.org/10.1093/infdis/jiy113.

58. Mushamiri I, Adudans M, Apat D, et al. Optimizing PMTCT efforts by repeat HIV testing during antenatal and perinatal care in resource-limited settings: A longitudinal assessment of HIV seroconversion. PLOS ONE 2020;15(5):e0233396. https://doi.org/10.1371/journal.pone.0233396.

59. UNAIDS DATA 2021. Available at: https://www.unaids.org/sites/default/files/media_asset/JC3032_AIDS_Data_book_2021_En.pdf. Accessed April 16, 2022.

60. Global HIV & AIDS statistics — Fact sheet. Available at: https://www.unaids.org/en/resources/fact-sheet. Accessed April 16, 2022.

61. Mofenson L, Baggaley R, Mameletzis I. Tenofovir disoproxil fumarate safety for women and their infants during pregnancy and breastfeeding. Aids 2017;31(2):213–32. https://doi.org/10.1097/QAD.0000000000001313.

62. Grant RM, Lama JR, Anderson PL, et al. Preexposure Chemoprophylaxis for HIV Prevention in Men Who Have Sex with Men. N Engl J Med 2010;363(27):2587–99. https://doi.org/10.1056/NEJMoa1011205.

63. Stranix-Chibanda L, Anderson PL, Kacanek D, et al, IMPAACT. Tenofovir Diphosphate Concentrations in Dried Blood Spots From Pregnant and Postpartum Adolescent and Young Women Receiving Daily Observed Preexposure Prophylaxis in Sub-Saharan Africa - PubMed. 2009. Available at: https://pubmed.ncbi.nlm.nih.gov/33341883/. Accessed April 15, 2022.

64. Davies N, Heffron R. Global and national guidance for the use of pre-exposure prophylaxis during peri-conception, pregnancy and breastfeeding. Sex Health 2018;15(6):501. https://doi.org/10.1071/SH18067.

65. Hanscom B, Janes HE, Guarino PD, et al. Preventing HIV-1 Infection in Women using Oral Pre-Exposure Prophylaxis: A Meta-analysis of Current Evidence. J Acquir Immune Defic Syndr 2016;73(5):606–8. https://doi.org/10.1097/QAI. 0000000000001160.

66. Kinuthia J, Pintye J, Abuna F, et al. Pre-exposure prophylaxis uptake and early continuation among pregnant and post-partum women within maternal and child health clinics in Kenya: results from an implementation programme. Lancet HIV 2020;7(1):e38–48. https://doi.org/10.1016/S2352-3018(19)30335-2.

67. Joseph Davey DL, Mvududu R, Mashele N, et al. Early pre-exposure prophylaxis (PrEP) initiation and continuation among pregnant and postpartum women in antenatal care in Cape Town, South Africa. J Int AIDS Soc 2022;25(2):e25866. https://doi.org/10.1002/jia2.25866.

68. Baeten JM, Palanee-Phillips T, Brown ER, et al. Use of a Vaginal Ring Containing Dapivirine for HIV-1 Prevention in Women. New Engl J Med 2016;375(22): 2121–32. https://doi.org/10.1056/NEJMoa1506110.

69. Nel A, van Niekerk N, Kapiga S, et al. Safety and Efficacy of a Dapivirine Vaginal Ring for HIV Prevention in Women - PubMed. Available at: https://pubmed.ncbi. nlm.nih.gov/27959766/. Accessed April 15, 2022.

70. Nel A, van Niekerk N, Van Baelen B, et al. HIV incidence and adherence in DREAM: an open-label trial of dapivirine vaginal ring [Abstract #144LB]. Presented at: 2018; Conference on Retroviruses and Opportunistic Infections2018. Available at: https://www.croiconference.org/abstract/hiv-incidence-and-adherence-dream-open-label-trial-dapivirine-vaginal-ring/. Accessed April 15, 2022.

71. Brown ER, Hendrix CW, van der Straten A, et al. Greater dapivirine release from the dapivirine vaginal ring is correlated with lower risk of HIV-1 acquisition: a secondary analysis from a randomized, placebo-controlled trial. J Int AIDS Soc 2020;23(11):e25634. https://doi.org/10.1002/jia2.25634.

72. Where we are with the DELIVER and B-PROTECTED studies. Available at: https://www.mtnstopshiv.org/sites/default/files/mtn4433_infographic_r7_web. pdf. Accessed April 17, 2022.

73. Delany-Moretlwe S, Hughes JP, Bock P, et al. Cabotegravir for the prevention of HIV-1 in women: results from HPTN 084, a phase 3, randomised clinical trial. Lancet. Published online April 1, 2022. doi:10.1016/S0140-6736(22)00538-4.

74. Landovitz RJ, Donnell D, Clement ME, et al. Cabotegravir for HIV Prevention in Cisgender Men and Transgender Women. N Engl J Med 2021;385(7):595–608. https://doi.org/10.1056/NEJMoa2101016.

75. Commissioner O of the. FDA Approves First Injectable Treatment for HIV Pre-Exposure Prevention. FDA. Published December 20, 2021. Available at: https://www.fda.gov/news-events/press-announcements/fda-approves-first-injectable-treatment-hiv-pre-exposure-prevention. Accessed April 15, 2022.

76. Mayer KH, Molina JM, Thompson MA, et al. Emtricitabine and tenofovir alafenamide vs emtricitabine and tenofovir disoproxil fumarate for HIV pre-exposure prophylaxis (DISCOVER): primary results from a randomised, double-blind, multicentre, active-controlled, phase 3, non-inferiority trial. Lancet 2020;396(10246): 239–54. https://doi.org/10.1016/S0140-6736(20)31065-5.

77. HIV prevention options during pregnancy and breastfeeding – what's in the pipeline?. Available at: https://www.prepwatch.org/wp-content/uploads/2021/08/AVAC-R4P-Noguchi-05FEB2021_REV.pdf. Accessed April 17, 2022.

78. Joseph Davey DL, Bekker LG, Bukusi EA, et al. Where are the pregnant and breastfeeding women in new pre-exposure prophylaxis trials? The imperative to overcome the evidence gap. Lancet HIV 2022;9(3):e214–22. https://doi.org/10.1016/S2352-3018(21)00280-0.

79. Jones DL, Peltzer K, Villar-Loubet O, et al. Reducing the risk of HIV infection during pregnancy among South African women: a randomized controlled trial. AIDS Care 2013;25(6):702–9. https://doi.org/10.1080/09540121.2013.772280.

80. Homsy J, King R, Bannink F, et al. Primary HIV prevention in pregnant and lactating Ugandan women: A randomized trial. PLOS ONE 2019;14(2): e0212119. https://doi.org/10.1371/journal.pone.0212119.

81. Fatti G, Shaikh N, Jackson D, et al. Low HIV incidence in pregnant and postpartum women receiving a community-based combination HIV prevention intervention in a high HIV incidence setting in South Africa. Available at: https://journals.plos.org/plosone/article?id=10.1371/journal.pone.0181691. Accessed April 15, 2022.

82. Saidi F, Mutale W, Freeborn K, et al. Combination adherence strategy to support HIV antiretroviral therapy and pre-exposure prophylaxis adherence during pregnancy and breastfeeding: protocol for a pair of pilot randomised trials. BMJ Open 2021;11(6):e046032. https://doi.org/10.1136/bmjopen-2020-046032.

83. Hill LM, Saidi F, Freeborn K, et al. Tonse Pamodzi: Developing a combination strategy to support adherence to antiretroviral therapy and HIV pre-exposure prophylaxis during pregnancy and breastfeeding. 2021. Available at: https://journals.plos.org/plosone/article?id=10.1371/journal.pone.0253280. Accessed April 15, 2022.

84. Turner BJ, McKee LJ, Silverman NS, et al. Prenatal Care and Birth Outcomes of a Cohort of HIV-Infected Women. JAIDS J Acquired Immune Deficiency Syndromes 1996;12(3):259–67.

85. Cowdell I, Beck K, Portwood C, et al. Adverse perinatal outcomes associated with protease inhibitor-based antiretroviral therapy in pregnant women living with HIV: A systematic review and meta-analysis. eClinicalMedicine 2022;0(0). https://doi.org/10.1016/j.eclinm.2022.101368.

86. Tukei VJ, Hoffman HJ, Greenberg L, et al. Adverse Pregnancy Outcomes Among HIV-positive Women in the Era of Universal Antiretroviral Therapy Remain Elevated Compared With HIV-negative Women. Pediatr Infect Dis J 2021;40(9):821–6. https://doi.org/10.1097/INF.0000000000003174.

87. Perinatal outcomes in women living with HIV-1 and receiving antiretroviral therapy—a systematic review and meta-analysis - Shinar - 2022 - Acta Obstetricia et Gynecologica Scandinavica - Wiley Online Library. Available at: https://obgyn.onlinelibrary.wiley.com/doi/full/10.1111/aogs.14282. Accessed April 20, 2022.

88. Moodley T, Moodley D, Sebitloane M, et al. Improved pregnancy outcomes with increasing antiretroviral coverage in South Africa. BMC Pregnancy Childbirth 2016;16(1):35. https://doi.org/10.1186/s12884-016-0821-3.

89. Dadabhai S, Gadama L, Chamanga R, et al. Pregnancy Outcomes in the Era of Universal Antiretroviral Treatment in Sub-Saharan Africa (POISE Study). JAIDS J Acquired Immune Deficiency Syndromes 2019;80(1):7–14. https://doi.org/10.1097/QAI.0000000000001875.

90. Hoffman RM, Brummel SS, Britto P, et al. Adverse Pregnancy Outcomes Among Women Who Conceive on Antiretroviral Therapy. Clin Infect Dis 2019;68(2): 273–9. https://doi.org/10.1093/cid/ciy471.

91. Stringer EM, Kendall MA, Lockman S, et al. Pregnancy outcomes among HIV-infected women who conceived on antiretroviral therapy. PLoS ONE 2018;e0199555. https://doi.org/10.1371/journal.pone.0199555. Law M, ed.

92. Malaba TR, Phillips T, Le Roux S, et al. Antiretroviral therapy use during pregnancy and adverse birth outcomes in South African women. Int J Epidemiol 2017;46(5):1678–89. https://doi.org/10.1093/ije/dyx136.

93. Maswime S, Pule C, Bebell LM, et al. Stillbirth rate by maternal HIV serostatus and antiretroviral use in pregnancy in South Africa: An audit - PMC. Available at: https://www.ncbi.nlm.nih.gov/labs/pmc/articles/PMC8713459/. Accessed February 27, 2022.

94. Rempis EM, Schnack A, Decker S, et al. Option B+ for prevention of vertical HIV transmission has no influence on adverse birth outcomes in a cross-sectional cohort in Western Uganda. BMC Pregnancy Childbirth 2017;17(1):82. https://doi.org/10.1186/s12884-017-1263-2.

95. Chagomerana MB, Miller WC, Pence BW, et al. PMTCT Option B+ Does Not Increase Preterm Birth Risk and May Prevent Extreme Prematurity: A Retrospective Cohort Study in Malawi. J Acquir Immune Defic Syndr 2017;74(4):367–74. https://doi.org/10.1097/qai.0000000000001253.

96. Malaba TR, Newell ML, Myer L, et al. Methodological Considerations for Preterm Birth Research. Front Glob Women's Health 2022;2. Available at: https://www.frontiersin.org/article/10.3389/fgwh.2021.821064. Accessed April 20, 2022.

97. Zash R, Jacobson DL, Diseko M, et al. Comparative Safety of Antiretroviral Treatment Regimens in Pregnancy. JAMA Pediatr 2017;171(10). https://doi.org/10.1001/jamapediatrics.2017.2222.

98. Veroniki AA, Antony J, Straus SE, et al. Comparative safety and effectiveness of perinatal antiretroviral therapies for HIV-infected women and their children: systematic review and network meta-analysis including different study designs. PLoS ONE 2018;e0198447. https://doi.org/10.1371/journal.pone.0198447. Kanters S, ed.

99. Lockman S, Brummel SS, Ziemba L, et al. Efficacy and safety of dolutegravir with emtricitabine and tenofovir alafenamide fumarate or tenofovir disoproxil fumarate, and efavirenz, emtricitabine, and tenofovir disoproxil fumarate HIV antiretroviral therapy regimens started in pregnancy (IMPAACT 2010/VESTED): a multicentre, open-label, randomised, controlled, phase 3 trial. The Lancet 2021;397(10281):1276–92. https://doi.org/10.1016/S0140-6736(21)00314-7.

100. Dodd JM, Jones L, Flenady V, et al. Prenatal administration of progesterone for preventing preterm birth in women considered to be at risk of preterm birth. Cochrane Database Syst Rev 2013;7:CD004947. https://doi.org/10.1002/14651858.CD004947.pub3.

101. Price JT, Vwalika B, Freeman BL, et al. Weekly 17 alpha-hydroxyprogesterone caproate to prevent preterm birth among women living with HIV: a randomised, double-blind, placebo-controlled trial. Lancet HIV 2021;8(10):e605–13. https://doi.org/10.1016/S2352-3018(21)00150-8.

102. Mugo NR, Hong T, Celum C, et al, Partners PrEP Study Team. Pregnancy incidence and outcomes among women receiving preexposure prophylaxis for HIV prevention: a randomized clinical trial - PubMed. Available at: https://pubmed.ncbi.nlm.nih.gov/25038355/. Accessed April 19, 2022.

103. Kinuthia J, Pintye J, Abuna F, et al. PrEP Implementation for Young Women and Adolescents (PrIYA) Program. PrEP uptake among pregnant and postpartum women: Results from a large implementation program within routine maternal child health (MCH) clinics in Kenya. 2018. https://programme.aids2018.org/Abstract/Abstract/7484. [Accessed 19 April 2022]. Accessed.

104. Joseph Davey DL, Baeten JM, Aldrovandi G, et al. Emerging evidence from a systematic review of safety of pre-exposure prophylaxis for pregnant and postpartum women: where are we now and where are we heading? J Int AIDS Soc 2020;23(1):e25426. https://doi.org/10.1002/jia2.25426.

105. Ibekwe E, Haigh C, Duncan F, et al. Clinical outcomes of routine opt-out antenatal human immunodeficiency virus screening: a systematic review. J Clin Nurs 2017;26(3–4):341–55. https://doi.org/10.1111/jocn.13475.

106. Killam WP, Tambatamba BC, Chintu N, et al. Antiretroviral therapy in antenatal care to increase treatment initiation in HIV-infected pregnant women: a stepped-wedge evaluation. AIDS 2010;24(1):85–91. https://doi.org/10.1097/QAD.0b013e32833298be.

107. Aliyu MH, Blevins M, Audet CM, et al. Integrated prevention of mother-to-child HIV transmission services, antiretroviral therapy initiation, and maternal and infant retention in care in rural north-central Nigeria: a cluster-randomised controlled trial. Lancet HIV 2016;3(5):e202–11. https://doi.org/10.1016/S2352-3018(16)00018-7.

108. Differentiated service delivery for families - children, adolescents, and pregnant and breastfeeding women: A background review. Available at: https://differentiatedservicedelivery.org/Portals/0/adam/Content/QLbAMeHLEkCeha-XD45xXQ/File/DSD%20Families%20review_28Nov.pdf. Accessed April 16, 2022.

109. Zerbe A, Brittain K, Phillips TK, et al. Community-based adherence clubs for postpartum women on antiretroviral therapy (ART) in Cape Town, South Africa: a pilot study. BMC Health Serv Res 2020;20(1):621. https://doi.org/10.1186/s12913-020-05470-5.

110. Trafford Z, Gomba Y, Colvin CJ, et al. Experiences of HIV-positive postpartum women and health workers involved with community-based antiretroviral therapy adherence clubs in Cape Town, South Africa | BMC Public Health | Full Text. Available at: https://bmcpublichealth.biomedcentral.com/articles/10.1186/s12889-018-5836-4. Accessed April 16, 2022.

111. Ioannidis JP, Abrams EJ, Ammann A, et al. Perinatal transmission of human immunodeficiency virus type 1 by pregnant women with RNA virus loads <1000 copies/ml. J Infect Dis 2001;183(4):539–45. https://doi.org/10.1086/318530.

112. Garcia PM, Kalish LA, Pitt J, et al. Maternal levels of plasma human immunodeficiency virus type 1 RNA and the risk of perinatal transmission. Women and Infants Transmission Study Group. N Engl J Med 1999;341(6):394–402. https://doi.org/10.1056/NEJM199908053410602.

113. Haberer JE, Bangsberg DR, Baeten JM, et al. Defining success with HIV pre-exposure prophylaxis: a prevention-effective adherence paradigm. AIDS 2015;29(11):1277–85. https://doi.org/10.1097/QAD.0000000000000647.

114. Hill LM, Maseko B, Chagomerana M, et al. HIV risk, risk perception, and PrEP interest among adolescent girls and young women in Lilongwe, Malawi: operationalizing the PrEP cascade. J Int AIDS Soc 2020;23(Suppl 3). https://doi.org/10.1002/jia2.25502.

115. Seifert SM, Chen X, Meditz AL, et al. Intracellular Tenofovir and Emtricitabine Anabolites in Genital, Rectal, and Blood Compartments from First Dose to

Steady State. AIDS Res Hum Retroviruses 2016;32(10–11):981–91. https://doi.org/10.1089/AID.2016.0008.

116. Cottrell ML, Yang KH, Prince HMA, et al. A Translational Pharmacology Approach to Predicting Outcomes of Preexposure Prophylaxis Against HIV in Men and Women Using Tenofovir Disoproxil Fumarate With or Without Emtricitabine. J Infect Dis 2016;214(1):55–64. https://doi.org/10.1093/infdis/jiw077.

117. Patterson KB, Prince HA, Kraft E, et al. Penetration of tenofovir and emtricitabine in mucosal tissues: implications for prevention of HIV-1 transmission - PubMed. Available at: https://pubmed.ncbi.nlm.nih.gov/22158861/. Accessed April 19, 2022.

118. Mweemba O, Zimba C, Chi BH, et al. Contextualising men's role and participation in PMTCT programmes in Malawi and Zambia: A hegemonic masculinity perspective. Glob Public Health. Published online August 10, 2021:1-14. doi:10.1080/17441692.2021.1964559.

119. Golub SA. PrEP Stigma: Implicit and Explicit Drivers of Disparity. Curr Hiv/aids Rep 2018;15(2):190–7. https://doi.org/10.1007/s11904-018-0385-0.

120. Barker P, Barron P, Bhardwaj S, et al. The role of quality improvement in achieving effective large-scale prevention of mother-to-child transmission of HIV in South Africa. AIDS 2015;29(Suppl 2):S137–43. https://doi.org/10.1097/QAD.0000000000000718.

121. Bhardwaj S, Barron P, Pillay Y, et al. Elimination of mother-to-child transmission of HIV in South Africa: rapid scale-up using quality improvement. S Afr Med J 2014;104(3 Suppl 1):239–43. https://doi.org/10.7196/samj.7605.

122. Akama E, Mburu M, Mutegi E, et al. Impact of a Rapid Results Initiative Approach on Improving Male Partner Involvement in Prevention of Mother to Child Transmission of HIV in Western Kenya. AIDS Behav 2018;22(9):2956–65. https://doi.org/10.1007/s10461-018-2140-3.

123. Rustagi AS, Gimbel S, Nduati R, et al. Implementation and Operational Research: Impact of a Systems Engineering Intervention on PMTCT Service Delivery in Côte d'Ivoire, Kenya, Mozambique: A Cluster Randomized Trial. J Acquir Immune Defic Syndr 2016;72(3):e68–76. https://doi.org/10.1097/QAI.0000000000001023.

124. UNICEF, UNAIDS WHO. Key considerations for programming and prioritization. Going the 'Last Mile' to EMTCT: A road map for ending the HIV epidemic in children. Available at: http://www.childrenandaids.org/sites/default/files/2020-02/Last-Mile-To-EMTCT_WhitePaper_UNICEF2020.pdf. Accessed April 16, 2022.

125. Abrams EJ, Myer L, Rosenfield A, et al. Prevention of mother-to-child transmission services as a gateway to family-based human immunodeficiency virus care and treatment in resource-limited settings: rationale and international experiences - American Journal of Obstetrics & Gynecology. Available at: https://www.ajog.org/article/S0002-9378%2807%2900434-6/fulltext. Accessed April 16, 2022.

126. Myer L, Abrams EJ, Zhang Y, et al. Family matters: Co-enrollment of family members into care is associated with improved outcomes for HIV-infected women initiating antiretroviral therapy. J Acquir Immune Defic Syndr 2014;67(Suppl 4):S243–9. https://doi.org/10.1097/QAI.0000000000000379.

127. World Health Organization. PMTCT strategic vision 2010-2015 : preventing mother-to-child transmission of HIV to reach the UNGASS and millennium Development Goals : moving towards the elimination of Paediatric HIV, December 2009. World Health Organization; 2010. Available at: https://apps.who.int/iris/handle/10665/44268. Accessed April 17, 2022.

Maternal Mortality in Low and Middle-Income Countries

Emma R. Lawrence, MD, MS[a],*, Thomas J. Klein, MD, MPH[a],
Titus K. Beyuo, BSc, MBChB, MPhil, MGCS, FWACS[b]

KEYWORDS

- Maternal mortality • LMIC • Pregnancy complication • Maternal death
- Postpartum hemorrhage • Preeclampsia • Eclampsia • Maternal sepsis

KEY POINTS

- Despite a 38% decrease in global maternal mortality during the last decade, rates remain unacceptably high with greater than 800 maternal deaths occurring each day.
- There is a significant regional variation among rates and causes of maternal mortality, and the vast majority occurs in low-income and middle-income countries.
- The leading causes of direct maternal mortality are hemorrhage, hypertensive disorders of pregnancy, sepsis, complications of abortion, and thromboembolism.
- Eliminating preventable maternal mortality hinges on improving clinical management of these life-threatening obstetric conditions, as well as addressing the complex social and economic barriers that pregnant women face to access quality care.

INTRODUCTION

Maternal mortality is defined by the World Health Organization (WHO) as a death that occurs during pregnancy or within 42 days of delivery or termination of the pregnancy, from any cause related to or worsened by pregnancy.[1] Direct maternal mortality results from the pregnant state or its management, whereas indirect maternal mortality results from preexisting or new disease worsened by the physiologic changes of pregnancy.[1] Worldwide, approximately 73% of maternal deaths are attributable to direct causes.[2] Maternal deaths are reported as a maternal mortality ratio (MMR), which quantify the number of maternal deaths per 100,000 live births.[1]

Funding sources: None.
[a] Department of Obstetrics and Gynecology, University of Michigan, L400 UH South, 1500 East Medical Center Drive, Ann Arbor, MI 48109, USA; [b] Department of Obstetrics and Gynaecology, University of Ghana Medical School, PO Box 4236, Accra, Ghana
* Corresponding author.
E-mail address: emmarl@med.umich.edu

Despite a 38% decrease in global maternal mortality during the last decade, rates remain unacceptably high with 810 maternal deaths occurring each day.[3] Maternal mortality was affirmed as a priority by the United Nations Millennium Development Goals, calling for a 75% decrease in the MMR between 1990 and 2015, a target that was unfortunately not achieved. As of 2015, the Sustainable Development Goals call for a reduction in the global MMR to less than 70, with each country less than 140, by the year 2030.[1] As of 2021, the WHO estimates the global MMR at 211, with rates as high as 1150 in South Sudan.[3,4] There is significant regional variation among rates and causes of maternal mortality (**Figs. 1** and **2**). Ninety-four percent of maternal deaths occur in low and middle income countries (LMICs), with two-thirds occurring in Sub-Saharan Africa and one-fifth in Southern Asia.[3]

The leading causes of direct maternal mortality are hemorrhage (27.1%), hypertensive disorders of pregnancy (HDP; 14.0%), sepsis (10.7%), complications of abortion (7.9%), and thromboembolism (3.2%).[2] The following article reviews each of these causes of maternal mortality within the context of LMICs, with a focus on clinical diagnosis and management during the intrapartum period. Importantly, most maternal mortalities are avoidable. Eliminating preventable maternal mortality (**Fig. 3**)[4] hinges on improving clinical management of these life-threatening obstetric conditions, as well as addressing the complex social and economic barriers that pregnant women face to access quality care.

Postpartum Hemorrhage

Postpartum hemorrhage (PPH) has been recently redefined as a total blood loss of 1000 mL or greater, or blood loss associated with signs of hypovolemia, regardless of mode of delivery.[5,6] PPH is the leading cause of global maternal mortality, accounting for 8% in high-income countries and 20% in LMICs.[7]

Risk factors for PPH include prolonged labor, chorioamnionitis, and cesarean delivery (**Table 1**).[5] PPH often occurs in uncomplicated pregnancies so all obstetric facilities should be adequately prepared for management.[9] Prevention of PPH begins during antenatal care (**Fig. 4**).[7,9,10]

Diagnosis of PPH includes recognizing abnormally high blood loss and identifying the cause of hemorrhage. Although quantification of blood loss (QBL) has been

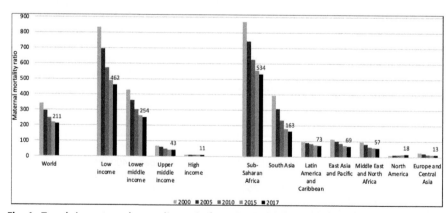

Fig. 1. Trends in maternal mortality ratio from 2000 to 2017 across World Bank-defined regions and income groups. (*Data from* World Health Organization. Trends in maternal mortality 2000 to 2017: estimates by WHO, UNICEF, UNFPA, World Bank Group and the United Nations Population Division. 2019;CC BY-NC-SA 3.0 IGO.)

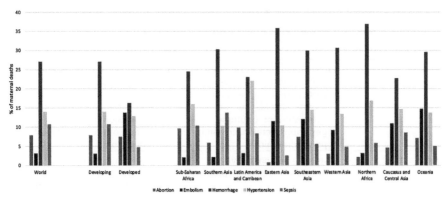

Fig. 2. Leading causes of direct maternal mortality by United Nations-defined region. (*Data from* Say L, Chou D, Gemmill A, et al. Global causes of maternal death: a WHO systematic analysis. Lancet Glob Health. 2014;2(6):e323-e333.)

determined to be more accurate than subjective assessment, QBL is not conclusively linked to improved outcomes.[11] Signs and symptoms of hypovolemia (hypotension, tachycardia, presyncope) typically develop when blood loss exceeds 1500 mL (~25% of total blood volume).[12] Uterine atony is the most common cause of PPH, accounting for nearly 70% of cases. Other leading causes include obstetric lacerations (20%) and retained placenta (10%).[7] Rarer, but serious, causes include coagulopathy, uterine inversion, and uterine rupture. Diagnosis should include assessment of uterine tone, examination of the vagina, vulva, perineum, and cervix for lacerations or hematomas, and examination of the placenta. If retained placenta is suspected, pelvic ultrasound is diagnostically helpful.[7]

Maternal morbidity and mortality associated with PPH is improved with prompt intervention, use of standardized protocols, and implementation of a team-based multidisciplinary approach.[5] An ongoing assessment of blood loss and resuscitation status is essential (**Fig. 5**). Management should be tailored to the specific cause (see **Table 1**). Complications of PPH can include severe anemia, hypoperfusion with resultant acute kidney injury and multisystem failure, and disseminated intravascular coagulopathy (DIC).[5]

Preparation for blood transfusion should begin when blood loss approaches 1500 mL with ongoing bleeding, or with signs of hemodynamic instability.[5] All obstetric facilities should have a supply of type O, Rh-negative blood, particularly those without

❖90% pregnant women attend 4 or more antenatal care visits (towards 8 visits by 2030)
❖90% births attended by skilled health personnel
❖80% women have access postnatal care within 2 d of delivery
❖60% of population has access to emergency obstetric care within 2 h of travel time
❖65% of women able to make informed and empowered decisions regarding sexual relations, contraceptive use, and their reproductive health

Fig. 3. Ending Preventable Maternal Mortality targets for 2025.

Table 1
Cause, risk factors, and management of postpartum hemorrhage

Cause	Risk Factors[7]	Management[8]
Uterine atony	Chorioamnionitis, prolonged labor, precipitous delivery, labor induction or augmentation, uterine fibroids, uterine overdistention (multiple gestations, fetal macrosomia, polyhydramnios)[7]	1. Bimanual uterine massage 2. Uterotonic medications[a] 3. Mechanical compression with balloon tamponade or uterine compression sutures[b] 4. Ligation of uterine arteries[c] 5. Hysterectomy
Genital tract trauma	Operative vaginal delivery, precipitous delivery, episiotomy	• Laceration: repair • Hematoma: compression and close observation; rarely, open hematoma for suture ligation and packing
Retained placenta	Succenturiate placenta, prior uterine surgery, placenta accreta spectrum	• Evacuation of placenta tissue with manual removal, suction curettage, or sharp curettage. Consider ultrasound-guidance • If placenta accreta spectrum suspected, prepare for hysterectomy
Uterine rupture	Prior uterine surgery, obstructed labor	Surgical repair if feasible, prepare for hysterectomy
Coagulopathy	Preeclampsia, intrauterine fetal death, placental abruption, amniotic fluid embolism, inherited or acquired coagulation disorder	Resuscitation with appropriate fluid replacement, consideration of transfusion focused on correction of coagulopathy

[a] Oxytocin (IM 10 units or IV 10–40 units in 500–1000 mL as a continuous infusion), methylergonovine (IM 0.2 mg every 2–4 h), 15-methyl prostaglandin F2α (IM 0.25 mg every 15–90 min), misoprostol (buccal or vaginal or rectal 600–1000 mcg). Oxytocin is typically administered first. A second agent is needed in 3% to 25% of cases.[5]
[b] If balloon tamponade device is not available, consider packing the uterus with gauze.
[c] Internal iliac artery ligation is uncommonly performed due to level of surgical skill required.

a blood bank.[9] Settings with a blood bank should adopt a massive transfusion protocol (**Fig. 6**), which typically involves administration of packed red blood cells, fresh-frozen plasma, and platelets in ratios of 1:1:1, 6:4:1, or 4:4:1.[7] If available, cryoprecipitate should be considered in patients with low fibrinogen or suspected DIC. Administration of 1 g tranexamic acid, intravenously, reduces mortality from obstetric hemorrhage, without affecting thrombosis risk.[13]

Antepartum Hemorrhage

Antepartum hemorrhage (APH), which occurs in 3% to 5% of all pregnancies,[14] is defined as significant bleeding from the genital tract before the onset of labor.[15] APH is, most commonly due to placental abruption, defined as detachment of the placenta before delivery, or placenta previa, defined as the placenta partially or totally covering the internal cervical os.[15] The most serious cause of APH is placenta accreta spectrum disorder, which is an abnormal invasion of placental tissue into or through the myometrium or surrounding organs, resulting in the failure of placental separation during the third stage of labor.[14] In LMICs, rates of APH are rising primarily due to an increase in cesarean deliveries.[14]

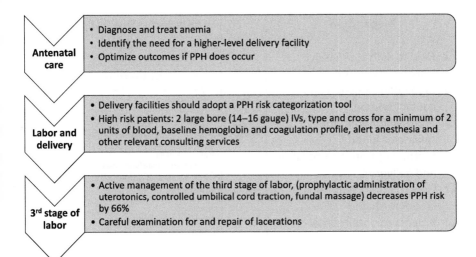

Fig. 4. Prevention of PPH.

Risk factors for placental abruption include preeclampsia, abdominal trauma, smoking, and drug use. History of prior abruption is most predictive, with recurrence rates of 4.4% after one affected pregnancy and 19% to 25% after two.[16] Risk factors for placenta previa include advanced maternal age, multiple gestation, smoking, and prior uterine surgery. The most important risk factors for placenta accreta are placenta previa together with prior cesarean delivery (**Table 2**).[17] Diagnosis of APH is based on history, clinical presentation, and ultrasound imaging (**Fig. 7, Table 3**). Painless vaginal bleeding is associated with placenta previa, whereas nonepisodic pain and a tense abdomen is suggestive of placental abruption.[15]

Management of APH depends on cause, blood loss and maternal hemodynamic status, and gestational age. If placental location is unknown, a speculum examination should assess the degree of bleeding and cervical dilation. Digital cervical examination should be avoided until placenta previa is ruled out. All life-threatening bleeding should prompt delivery, regardless of gestational age. The Kleihauer-Betke test should be performed to determine the appropriate dose of anti-D immunoglobulin (Rhogam) to administer to Rh-negative women to prevent isoimmunization.[15]

❖Accurate assessment of blood loss
❖Monitor vital signs and urine output
❖Intravenous access
❖Fluid resuscitation
❖Consider blood transfusion
❖Identify etiology(s) of bleeding
❖Optimize facility and personnel

Fig. 5. Core management of PPH.

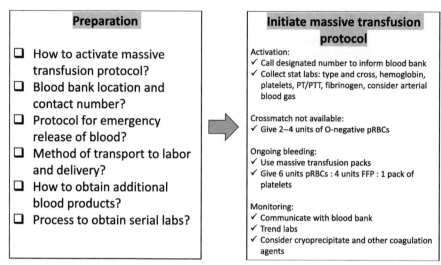

Fig. 6. Example obstetrics transfusion protocol. Concepts from Safe Mother Initiative PPH bundle.

- *Previa*: Uncomplicated placenta previa should be delivered via cesarean delivery between 36 + 0 and 37 + 0 weeks.[22] Surgical planning should minimize placental transection, including consideration of a vertical skin and/or uterine incision, particularly with an anterior previa, transverse fetal lie, and preterm gestation. Placenta previa increases the risk of massive hemorrhage and need for hysterectomy, so delivery should be performed at a facility with a skilled obstetric surgeon and access to blood products.[15]
- *Abruption*: Significant placental abruption is an indication for delivery. Abruption is often associated with rapid onset of labor, and vaginal delivery is preferred if maternal and fetus status are reassuring. The development of DIC should be monitored with laboratory and clinical assessment of blood clotting.[15]
- *Accreta*: In a stable patient with an antepartum diagnosis of suspected placenta accreta spectrum disorder, cesarean delivery should be performed between 34 + 0 and 36 + 6 weeks, with a very low threshold for cesarean hysterectomy.[18] Delivery personnel should be prepared for massive hemorrhage because such deliveries have a median blood loss of 2000 to 7800 mL and median blood

Table 2
Risk of placenta accreta

C-section Number	Placenta Previa	
	No	Yes
First	0.2%	3%
Second	0.3%	11%
Third	0.6%	40%
Fourth	2.1%	61%
Fifth	2.3%	67%

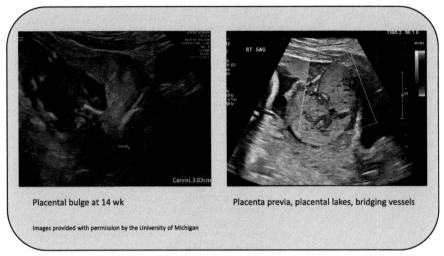

Placental bulge at 14 wk   Placenta previa, placental lakes, bridging vessels

Images provided with permission by the University of Michigan

Fig. 7. Ultrasound images of placenta previa and accreta.

transfusion of 5 units.[23] If suspected accreta is first encountered at the time of vaginal delivery, the patient should be moved to the operating room for a bimanual examination under anesthesia to assess for a partially or totally adherent placenta. Preparation should be made for hysterectomy, including notification of available consulting services such as urology and general surgery. In the setting of a small focal accreta and stable bleeding, leaving the placenta in situ and waiting for resorption can be considered in a well-counseled patient with a strong desire for future fertility or with delivery at a facility without surgical capacity. However, uterine-conserving management is associated with risks of emergency hysterectomy (40%), major morbidity (42%), and recurrence in subsequent pregnancies (20%).[24]

Hypertensive Disorders of Pregnancy

HDP, which include gestational hypertension, preeclampsia, and eclampsia, complicate 10% of pregnancies globally. As management of PPH improves and risk factors for HDP increase, HDP is expected to become the leading cause of maternal mortality in LMICs.[25]

Risk factors for the development of HDP include nulliparity, multiple gestation, HDP in a prior pregnancy, and cardiovascular risk factors such as advanced maternal age, obesity, diabetes, and chronic hypertension.[26,27] In pregnancies with significant or multiple risk factors, low-dose aspirin should be started before 16 weeks gestation, which reduces the risk of severe preeclampsia by 53%.[28] Calcium supplementation may reduce the risk of preeclampsia among women in LMICs with calcium-deficient diets.[29]

Assessment of HDP should include serial blood pressure measurements, laboratory studies (complete blood count with platelet count, creatinine, aspartate transaminase (AST), alanine transaminase (ALT), urine protein), and evaluation of symptoms (right upper quadrant pain, headache, visual disturbances). Hypertension and proteinuria are classic features of preeclampsia; however, newer diagnostic criteria de-emphasize the necessity of proteinuria (**Fig. 8**).[26,27]

Table 3
Ultrasound evaluation of placental abruption, placenta previa, and placenta accreta

Placental Condition	Screening	Ultrasound Findings	Accuracy
Previa	Routine second trimester anatomy ultrasound should assess placental location[a]	Placenta partially or completely covering internal cervical os[19]	Excellent accuracy (PPV 93.3%, NPV 97.6%). Transvaginal superior to transabdominal[19]
Abruption	n/a	Retroplacental clot[20,21]	Sensitivity is poor (24%), however visualizing retroplacental clot is highly specific (96%)[20]
Accreta	n/a	Loss of hypoechoic retroplacental line or bladder-uterine interface, lacunae, hypervascularity extending to/into the bladder[18]	Very good sensitivity (90.7%) and specificity (96.9%) when performed by skilled operators, in pregnancies at risk of accreta[18]

[a] Placenta previa diagnosed on second trimester ultrasound resolves before term in 90% of cases. Detection of a placenta previa or low lying placenta (<20 mm from internal cervical os) and should be reevaluated at 32 wk[19].

Complications of preeclampsia include placental abruption with the development of DIC, acute kidney injury, pulmonary edema, and stroke. Eclampsia can lead to maternal hypoxia, traumatic injury, and aspiration pneumonia.[30] The management of HDP centers on (1) delivery, (2) prevention of seizures, and (3) control of elevated blood pressures.

- *Delivery*: The only definitive treatment of HDP is delivery. Although the decision to deliver term gestations is clear, decision-making for preterm and periviable gestations can be difficult, particularly in LMIC settings where preterm neonatal survival is poor. All cases of HELLP and eclampsia should be stabilized and immediately delivered, regardless of gestational age. Women with preeclampsia with severe features are typically delivered immediately, although cautious inpatient expectant management can be considered for select patients less than 34 weeks gestation with stabilized blood pressures and without signs of end organ damage. Induction of labor and vaginal delivery is a reasonable option, unless evidence of fetal compromise or other contraindications to vaginal delivery. However, success is decreased with lower gestational ages.[26]
- *Prevention of seizures:* Magnesium sulfate is an evidence-proven medication of choice for seizure prophylaxis among patients with preeclampsia with severe features, HELLP, and eclampsia.[31,32] Magnesium sulfate, which can be administered intravenously or intramuscularly, is given as a loading dose followed by maintenance doses. Regimens vary and the ideal dose and duration is unknown[33]; the commonly used Pritchard regimen consists of a 10 mg IM loading dose (5 mg in each buttock) followed by 5 g IM every 4 hours. Adverse effects of magnesium sulfate include respiratory depression and cardiac arrest, with decreased clearance in the setting of AKI. Prevention of magnesium toxicity includes strict monitoring of inputs and outputs, assessment of deep tendon reflexes and vital signs, and consideration of laboratory magnesium levels where

available.[34] Concern for cardiorespiratory compromise should prompt administration of calcium gluconate and consideration of endotracheal intubation. Eclamptic seizures are usually self-limited. The initial management includes placing the patient into the lateral decubitus position, minimizing risk of injury and aspiration, and monitoring vital signs and oxygen saturation levels. Magnesium sulfate should be promptly administered.

- *Control of elevated blood pressures:* Severe hypertension, defined as a systolic blood pressure of 160 mm Hg or higher and/or a diastolic blood pressure of 110 mm Hg or higher persisting more than 15 minutes, should be promptly treated with short-acting antihypertensives. Treatment of severe hypertension in pregnancy can help prevent heart failure, myocardial infarction, acute kidney injury, and stroke. Commonly used short-acting antihypertensives include IV hydralazine, IV labetalol, and oral nifedipine. There are no reported significant differences in efficacy among these medications,[35] and every obstetric facility should adopt a protocol for dose escalation and sequential administration.

INFECTION AND SEPSIS

Maternal sepsis is defined as organ dysfunction resulting from infection during pregnancy, delivery, postabortion, or postpartum period.[36,37] More specifically, puerperal sepsis is an infection of the genital tract occurring between onset of labor or rupture of membranes and 6 weeks postpartum, and includes chorioamnionitis and postpartum endometritis (PPE).[38] Maternal mortality can also result from infections acquired before or during pregnancy, including human immunodeficiency virus (HIV), tuberculosis (TB), and malaria.[39]

Chorioamnionitis and Endometritis

Chorioamnionitis, defined as an infection of the chorion or amnion, is the most common intrapartum infection.[2] More recent terminology includes Intraamniotic Infection and Triple I (Intrauterine Infection and/or Inflammation), with strict diagnostic criteria (**Fig. 9**).[40] PPE is an infection of the decidua by ascending organisms from the vagina.

Gestational hypertension:
- Elevated BP: Systolic ≥140 mm Hg or diastolic ≥90 mm Hg, on 2 occasions at least 4 h apart, after 20 wk, with previously normal BPs

Preeclampsia:
- Elevated BP: Systolic ≥140 mm Hg or diastolic ≥90 mm Hg, on 2 occasions at least 4 h apart, after 20 wk, with previously normal BPs; AND
- Proteinuria: ≥300 mg per 24–h urine collection or ≥ 0.3 mg/dL protein:creatinine ratio or ≥1+ dipstick reading; OR any severe feature below

  Severe Features:
  - Systolic ≥160 mm Hg or diastolic ≥110 mm Hg
  - Platelet count <100,000 3 109/L
  - Serum creatinine >1.1 mg/dL or a doubling of baseline
  - Elevated serum liver transaminases to twice normal, or persistent right upper quadrant pain
  - Pulmonary edema
  - New-onset persistent headache or visual disturbance

Hemolysis Elevated Liver Enzymes and Low Platelets (HELLP):
- Elevated serum liver transaminases to twice normal; AND Platelet count <100,000 3 109/L

Eclampsia:
- New-onset tonic-clonic, focal, or multifocal seizures in pregnancy or postpartum, without another cause

Fig. 8. Diagnostic criteria for hypertensive disorders of pregnancy.

Suspected Triple I
❖ Fever: ≥39.0°C once; or 38.0–39.0°C on ≥2 measurements 30 min apart without another clear source
    PLUS, at least 1 of the following:
❖ Fetal heart rate baseline >160
❖ Maternal white cell count >15,000 (in absence of corticosteroids)
❖ Purulent fluid from cervical os

Confirmed Triple I
❖ All criteria above
    PLUS, at least 1 of the following:
❖ Amniotic fluid with positive gram stain or culture, low glucose, or high white cell count
❖ Infection and/or inflammation on histopathology of placenta, fetal membranes, or umbilical cord

Endometritis
❖ Fever: ≥39.0°C once; or 38.0–39.0°C on ≥2 measurements 30 min apart without another clear source
    PLUS, at least 1 of the following:
❖ Uterine tenderness
❖ Abnormal vaginal discharge or odor
❖ Subinvolution of uterus

Fig. 9. Diagnostic criteria for peripartum infections.

Cesarean delivery is the single most important risk factor for PPE, with an incidence of 1% to 3% following vaginal delivery and up to 27% following cesarean delivery.[41] Additional risk factors include prolonged rupture of membranes, obesity, malnutrition, unclean delivery conditions, and low socioeconomic status. The diagnosis of PPE is made clinically based on maternal fever with signs of endometrial infection (see **Fig. 8**).[42] PPE may be complicated by peritonitis, intra-abdominal abscess formation, and sepsis.[42] Prompt administration of broad-spectrum antibiotics is the main pillar of management of chorioamnionitis and endometritis.[43] Antibiotic choice should be guided by local sensitivity data and guidelines (**Table 4**).[43,44] Especially in situations of delayed diagnosis of endometritis or a lack of clinical improvement after administration of appropriate antibiotics, retained products of conception should be suspected as a nidus of infection. Ultrasound should be used to evaluate for retained products of conception, and if present, prompt removal with dilation and curettage is indicated.

Malaria

Malaria is caused by infection with the mosquito-borne plasmodium parasite, among which *Plasmodium falciparum* is the most endemic in LMICs. The prevalence of malaria and progression to severe malaria is higher in pregnancy.[45] Malaria is also a significant cause of anemia in pregnancy, with the plasmodium parasite causing hemolysis of both parasitized and nonparasitized red blood cells and cytoadherence. Maternal mortality can occur secondary to cerebral malaria, severe anemia, and/or multiorgan failure.[46]

Prevention of malaria hinges on the use of insecticide-treated nets and preventive drug therapy for pregnant women in endemic areas (**Fig. 10**).[45] Despite evidence for efficacy, uptake is suboptimal. The WHO estimates that only 33% of pregnant women in sub-Saharan Africa receive complete preventive drug therapy and 60% use insecticide-treated mosquito nets.[46]

Symptoms of malaria are nonspecific and include fever, headache, myalgias, gastrointestinal issues, and jaundice. Severe malaria may present with neurologic changes and hypoglycemia. The diagnosis of malaria is the same as in nonpregnant populations (**Fig. 11**). Treatment of malaria involves prompt administration of

Table 4
Management of peripartum infections

Clinical Condition	Common Antibiotic Regimen[43,44]	Antibiotic Timing
Chorioamnionitis Suspected Triple I Confirmed Triple I	Ampicillin (2g q6 h) and Gentamicin (5 mg/kg q24 h or 2 mg/kg followed by 1.5 mg/kg q8 h)	Start at time of diagnosis. Continue until delivery If undergoing cesarean delivery, add clindamycin 900 mg
Endometritis	Clindamycin (900 mg q8 h) plus Gentamicin (5 mg/kg q24 h or 1.5 mg/kg q8 h)	Start at time of diagnosis. Continue until 24–28 h of clinical improvement

antimalarial agents and supportive management. Selection of antimalarials depends on severity of the infection, local drug-resistance patterns (chloroquine-resistant vs sensitive), and regional trends in the predominant *Plasmodium* species.[46] Importantly, *P falciparum* can sequester within the placenta, making it more difficult to treat and causing recurrent maternal infection. Placental malaria is associated with maternal anemia, poor neonatal outcomes including preterm delivery, low birthweight, and stillbirth, and transplacental crossing of the malaria parasite leading to congenital malaria. Intravenous artesunate is the medication of choice for the treatment of severe malaria.[47]

Tuberculosis

Worldwide, active TB infection complicates more than 200,000 pregnancies annually, often in conjunction with HIV, and most commonly in Africa and Southeast Asia.[48] In recent years, TB resistant to first-line and second-line medicines have been on the increase and present major challenges to TB management; drug-resistant TB may occur in pregnancy and should be considered in appropriate clinical situations and based on local epidemiology and surveillance data.

TB infections are classified as latent (inactive, asymptomatic, not contagious) versus active (often symptomatic, infectious). Latent TB bacilli may reactivate and cause active TB during pregnancy.[49] Individuals with HIV-coinfection and untreated latent TB are much more likely to develop active TB than those without HIV. Screening for 4 symptoms (cough, fever, weight loss [or poor weight gain pregnancy] or night sweats) is very useful for ruling out active TB in areas with high TB burden and especially in the setting of HIV infection. If a woman screens positive for any of these symptoms, she should be evaluated for active TB. Those with latent TB only should receive TB preventive treatment according to national or WHO guidelines (World Health Organization. WHO consolidated guidelines on tuberculosis. 2020 https://www.who.int/publications/i/item/9789240001503) Symptoms of active TB include fever, cough, weight loss, night sweats, and malaise; however, symptoms may be more difficult to recognize in pregnancy.[49] The approach to diagnosis and treatment is similar to nonpregnant populations (**Figs. 12** and **13**). TB in pregnancy is associated with an increased risk of pneumonia, acute respiratory distress syndrome, need for mechanical ventilation, and mortality.[50,51] Recommendations for TB preventive treatment in household contacts of individuals with active TB is based on national and local epidemiology but is strongly recommended for child contacts aged younger than 5 years, once active TB has been ruled out, because they are at greatest risk of severe and disseminated disease, associated with high morbidity and mortality (World Health Organization. WHO consolidated guidelines on tuberculosis. 2020).

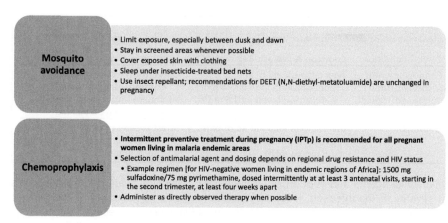

Fig. 10. Prevention of malaria infection in pregnancy.

Human Immunodeficiency Virus

Pregnant women infected with HIV have an 8-fold risk of maternal mortality[52] due in part to immunocompromise with increased risk of severe puerperal and abortion-related sepsis. Indirect causes of maternal mortality in HIV-positive women include higher rates of TB and more severe malaria coinfection, especially with more severe immunosuppression; furthermore, HIV and related immunosuppression may be associated with reduced effectiveness of and/or drug–drug interactions with standard medication regimens, increasing the risk of complications and death.[53] In settings with high TB transmission pregnant women living with HIV who have an unknown or positive test for latent TB and are unlikely to have active TB should receive TB preventive treatment with at least 36 months of daily isoniazid preventive treatment. Baseline liver function testing (LFT) is encouraged when feasible but routine LFT is not indicated in pregnancy in the absence of other risk factors for liver toxicity; vitamin B6 supplementation should be considered. (WHO. WHO consolidated guidelines on tuberculosis. 2020) Maternal outcomes can be improved through antenatal screening for HIV, prevention and treatment of coinfections, and antiretroviral treatment (ART).[52] Although approaches to HIV treatment are beyond the scope of this article, prompt initiation and sustained use of ART throughout pregnancy reduces mortality (see Friday Saidi and Benjamin H. Chi's article, "HIV Treatment and Prevention for

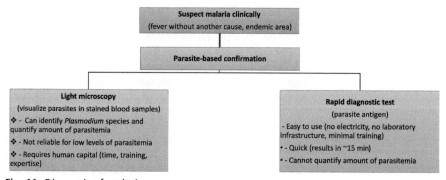

Fig. 11. Diagnosis of malaria.

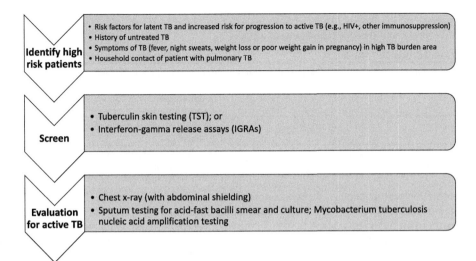

Fig. 12. Screening and diagnosis of TB.

Pregnant and Postpartum Women in Global Settings," in this issue).[54] Global guide-lines for the treatment and prevention of HIV, as well as significant coinfections (eg, TB, malaria) are developed and regularly updated by the World Health Organization (who.int).

Complications of Abortion

Abortion, both spontaneous and elective, represents a major cause of maternal morbidity and mortality.[55] Spontaneous abortion occurs in 10% to 15% of pregnancies.[56] Globally, there were approximately 120 million unintended pregnancies yearly between 2015 and 2019, with 61% (73 million) ending in elective abortion.[57] Unintended pregnancy rates are highest in countries with more restricted access to abortion and contraception,[57] leading to unsafe abortion and associated complications.[55] The rate of serious complications increases with increasing gestational age, described in **Table 5**.[58] The risk of cervical laceration and uterine perforation is reduced with adequate cervical preparation and cervical dilation by highly trained clinicians.

Abortion-related hemorrhage should be managed with uterotonic agents and intracervical vasopressin. If uterotonics are unavailable or unsuccessful, internal compression with a Foley catheter or uterine "Bakri" balloon can tamponade bleeding. Cervical lacerations should be fully visualized and repaired. In a stable patient, fundal perforation with a blunt instrument (dilator or sound) can be managed with close postoperative observation.

> ❖Start treatment immediately
> ❖Benefits outweigh risks in pregnancy
> ❖Consider drug availability and local resistance patterns
> ❖Multi-drug regimen for 6–9 mo with drug-sensitive TB
> ❖Manage drug-resistant TB and/or TB with HIV coinfection
>   in consultation with expert/infectious disease specialist
> ❖Administer as directly observed therapy if possible
> ❖Monitor for drug side effects (increased risk of isoniazid-
>   induced hepatotoxicity in pregnancy)

Fig. 13. Principles of management of active TB.

Table 5
Classification of abortion complications

Classification	Timing	Clinical Problem
Immediate	During, <3 h postabortion	Hemorrhage, tissue trauma (cervical laceration, uterine perforation), hematometra, complication of anesthesia
Delayed	>3 h, up to 28 d	Retained products of conception; infection
Late	>28 d	Rh sensitization; Asherman syndrome with infertility

Perforation with suction or forceps necessitates surgical exploration to evaluate and manage bleeding or organ injury. Septic abortion should be managed with broad-spectrum intravenous antibiotics with anerobic coverage, evaluation for retained products of conception, and evacuation with dilation and curretage if present.[58,59]

Venous Thromboembolism

The risk of venous thromboembolism (VTE) is 10-fold higher in pregnancy than in nonpregnant individuals.[60] Although VTE represents a smaller proportion of maternal mortality in LMICs, the global incidence is increasing because of increasing rates of obesity, diabetes, cardiovascular disease, and cesarean delivery.[61] Nonmodifiable risk factors include inherited thrombophilias and antiphospholipid syndrome.[60] The risk of VTE can be reduced through the consideration of prophylactic anticoagulation in patients with significant risk factors.[60]

Diagnosis of deep venous thrombosis and pulmonary embolism (PE) is based on clinical presentation and confirmatory imaging (**Fig. 14**).[62,60,63] Treatment of acute VTE in pregnancy requires anticoagulation therapy, continued for a minimum of 6 weeks postpartum. Warfarin is teratogenic, and therefore anticoagulation with weight-based dosing of unfractionated heparin or low molecular weight heparin is recommended. In patients with massive PE and associated cardiovascular compromise or those at risk of hemorrhage, intravenous unfractionated heparin is preferred. Management should be done with consultation of hematology, pharmacy, and anesthesia; ICU-level care is often needed. Hospital protocols for the treatment of VTE should account for local availability of anticoagulants.[62,63]

Ectopic Pregnancy

Ectopic pregnancy, defined as an extrauterine gestation, occurs most commonly in the fallopian tube (95%–97%).[64] Approximately 2% to 4% of ectopic pregnancies

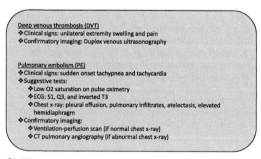

Fig. 14. Diagnosis of VTE.

Delay 1: Seeking care	Delay 2: Reaching care	Delay 3: Receiving adequate care
❖ Poverty; cost of care ❖ Poor health literacy; lack of knowledge of warning signs ❖ Negative prior experience with health care system ❖ Agency to make healthcare decisions	❖ Long distance to health facilities ❖ Low availability or high cost of transportation ❖ Poor roads and infrastructure	❖ Poor referral systems ❖ Lack of medical equipment, medications, blood ❖ Inadequate training and availability of healthcare workers ❖ Capacity for surgical and anesthesia care

Fig. 15. Three delays contributing to preventable maternal mortality.

are interstitial and 1% is ovarian, abdominal, and cervical. Risk factors include a history of pelvic inflammatory disease, tubal surgery, assisted reproductive technologies, and prior ectopic pregnancy.[56] Prevention of ectopic pregnancy is focused on prevention, screening, and treatment of pelvic infections, primarily chlamydia.[65]

Ectopic pregnancy should be suspected in cases of pregnancy with abdominopelvic pain or bleeding, if intrauterine pregnancy has not been confirmed.[56] Ultrasonography is the mainstay of diagnosis, demonstrating the absence of an intrauterine gestational sac and the presence of an adnexal mass consistent with an extrauterine gestation, with or without pelvic free fluid. Typically, transvaginal pelvic ultrasound can detect a gestational sac at approximately 5 weeks gestation, a yolk sac by 5.5 weeks and an embryo with cardiac activity by 6 weeks.[66] If ultrasound is not available or the clinical picture is unclear, dilation and curettage with evaluation for the presence of intrauterine chorionic villi can be both diagnostic and therapeutic.[64]

In LMICs, ectopic pregnancies often present ruptured and require urgent surgical management. Most commonly, treatment is laparotomy with salpingectomy or salpingoophorectomy.[67,68] Laparoscopy is possible in some LMIC settings and depends on availability, surgeon skill set, and patient stability. In situations where ectopic pregnancy is diagnosed in a stable patient, medical decision-making should consider the clinical scenario and patient desires.[64] Options include methotrexate in appropriately counseled patients who have the ability for close monitoring and follow-up, or surgical management with salpingectomy versus salpingostomy.[56]

DISCUSSION

Eliminating preventable maternal mortality depends not only on prevention and clinical management of the life-threatening obstetric conditions outlined in this article but also on overall strengthening of health systems and health-care infrastructure. A push toward facility delivery has been an important focus of improving maternity care; however, facility delivery alone is not sufficient.[69] Reduction of maternal mortality relies on high quality of care, including availability of emergency and surgical services, antibiotics, blood, and the ability to safely and quickly refer to a higher level facility if needed.[70] For women living in more remote settings, maternity waiting homes are one strategy to minimize delays to care and have been associated with improved maternal outcomes.[71] Strategies such as service delivery redesign, which recommend that the majority of care is provided at higher-level facilities,[72] must be balanced with challenges of overcrowding and equitable geographic access for women in rural settings.

The availability of trained health-care providers, with the ability to recognize and manage complications, is an essential component of quality reproductive health care. The largest increase in skilled birth attendants at delivery has occurred in sub-Saharan Africa and Southern Asia; however, major inequities persist. As of 2020, skilled attendance at birth is estimated at 83% globally, nearly 100% in high-income countries but only 64% in sub-Saharan Africa, with higher rates in urban areas and among wealthier women.[73] Brain drain places a large burden on LMIC human resource capacity, and motivation to work in remote areas is often low.[74] Notably, systems that build specialized obstetric capacity locally and provide local opportunities for subspecialization and professional accreditation promote retention.[75]

For pregnant women, there exists multiple challenges to receiving prompt, quality medical care. This is often conceptualized by the Three Delays Model (**Fig. 15**). Cultural beliefs about childbirth, traditional birth practices, and trust in the health-care system all play critical roles. In addition, data availability remains a challenge, contributing to underreporting of maternal mortality in the most affected areas. Thus, meeting targets to reduce maternal mortality involves not only improvements in quality and access to medical care but also better systems for data collection and management, and building capacity of LMIC researchers. The way forward involves a focus on strengthening human resources and health-care infrastructure, driven by global priority-setting to support LMIC-led solutions.

CLINICS CARE POINTS

- Antenatal care is a key opportunity for screening, prevention, and risk-stratification
- Patients with low-risk pregnancies may still develop serious obstetric complications; all delivery facilities should be prepared to manage obstetric emergencies and facilitate expeditious referrals to higher level facilities
- Outcomes are improved with the use of standardized emergency protocols and engagement of multidisciplinary teams
- Multilevel delays in pregnant women accessing quality care contribute to preventable maternal morbidity and mortality

DISCLOSURE

None of the authors has any commercial or financial conflicts of interest.

REFERENCES

1. World Health Organization. Trends in maternal mortality 2000 to 2017: estimates by WHO, UNICEF, UNFPA, World Bank Group and the United Nations Population Division. 2019;CC BY-NC-SA 3.0 IGO.
2. Say L, Chou D, Gemmill A, et al. Global causes of maternal death: a WHO systematic analysis. Lancet Glob Health 2014;2(6):e323–33.
3. Maternal mortality. Available at: https://www.who.int/news-room/fact-sheets/detail/maternal-mortality. Accessed March 13, 2022.
4. New global targets to prevent maternal deaths. Available at: https://www.who.int/news/item/05-10-2021-new-global-targets-to-prevent-maternal-deaths. Accessed March 13, 2022.

5. American College of Obstetricians and Gynecologists. Postpartum hemorrhage. Practice Bulletin No. 183. Obstet Gynecol 2017;130:168–86.
6. Borovac-Pinheiro A, Pacagnella RC, Cecatti JG, et al. Postpartum hemorrhage: new insights for definition and diagnosis. Am J Obstet Gynecol 2018;219(2): 162–8.
7. Bienstock JL, Eke AC, Hueppchen NA. Postpartum Hemorrhage. N Engl J Med 2021;384(17):1635–45.
8. Lalonde A. International Federation of Gynecology and Obstetrics. Prevention and treatment of postpartum hemorrhage in low-resource settings. Int J Gynaecol Obstet 2012;117(2):108–18.
9. Prevention and Management of Postpartum Haemorrhage: Green-top Guideline No. 52. BJOG. 2017;124(5):e106–e149.Pubmed Partial Author stitle Page
10. Begley CM, Gyte GM, Devane D, et al. Active versus expectant management for women in the third stage of labour. Cochrane Database Syst Rev 2019;2: CD007412.
11. Diaz V, Abalos E, Carroli G. Methods for blood loss estimation after vaginal birth. Cochrane Database Syst Rev 2018;9:CD010980.
12. Pacagnella RC, Souza JP, Durocher J, et al. A systematic review of the relation-ship between blood loss and clinical signs. PLoS One 2013;8(3):e57594.
13. Shakur H, Roberts I, Fawole B, et al. Effect of early tranexamic acid administration on mortality, hysterectomy, and other morbidities in women with post-partum hae-morrhage (WOMAN): an international, randomised, double-blind, placebo-controlled trial. Lancet 2017;389(10084):2105–16.
14. Jauniaux E, Ayres-de-Campos D. FIGO Placenta Accreta Diagnosis and Man-agement Expert Consensus Panel. FIGO consensus guidelines on placenta ac-creta spectrum disorders: Introduction. Int J Gynaecol Obstet 2018;140(3): 261–4.
15. Royal College of Obstetricians and Gynaecologists. Antepartum Haemorrhage: Green–top Guideline No. 63. Green–top Guideline. UK: Royal College of Obste-tricians and Gynaecologists; 2011.
16. Qin J, Liu X, Sheng X, et al, Assisted reproductive technology and the risk of pregnancy-related complications and adverse pregnancy outcomes in singleton pregnancies: a meta-analysis of cohort studies. Fertil Steril 2016;105(1):73–85, e1-e6.
17. Silver RM, Landon MB, Rouse DJ, et al. Maternal morbidity associated with mul-tiple repeat cesarean deliveries. Obstet Gynecol 2006;107(6):1226–32.
18. Jauniaux E, Alfirevic Z, Bhide AG, et al. Placenta Praevia and Placenta Accreta: Diagnosis and Management: Green-top Guideline No. 27a. BJOG 2019;126(1): e1–48.
19. Heller HT, Mullen KM, Gordon RW, et al. Outcomes of pregnancies with a low-lying placenta diagnosed on second-trimester sonography. J Ultrasound Med 2014;33(4):691–6.
20. Shinde GR, Vaswani BP, Patange RP, et al. Diagnostic Performance of Ultraso-nography for Detection of Abruption and Its Clinical Correlation and Maternal and Foetal Outcome. J Clin Diagn Res 2016;(8):10. QC04-QC07.
21. ACOG. Massive Transfusion Protocol (MTP). Safe Mother Initiative. 2019. Avail-able at: https://www.acog.org/-/media/project/acog/acogorg/files/forms/districts/smi-ob-hemorrhage-bundle-poster-massive-transfusion-protocol.pdf.
22. American College of Obstetricians and Gynecologists' Committee on Obstetric Practice. Society for Maternal-Fetal Medicine. Medically Indicated Late-Preterm

and Early-Term Deliveries: ACOG Committee Opinion, Number 831. Obstet Gynecol 2021;138(1):e35–9.

23. Wright JD, Pri-Paz S, Herzog TJ, et al. Predictors of massive blood loss in women with placenta accreta. Am J Obstet Gynecol 2011;205(1):38.e1-6.

24. Pather S, Strockyj S, Richards A, et al. Maternal outcome after conservative management of placenta percreta at caesarean section: a report of three cases and a review of the literature. Aust N Z J Obstet Gynaecol 2014;54(1):84–7.

25. Abalos E, Cuesta C, Grosso AL, et al. Global and regional estimates of pre-eclampsia and eclampsia: a systematic review. Eur J Obstet Gynecol Reprod Biol 2013;170(1):1–7.

26. American College of Obstetricians and Gynecologists' Committee on Practice Bulletins-Obstetrics. Gestational hypertension and preeclampsia: ACOG Practice Bulletin, number 222. Obstet Gynecol 2020;135(6):e237–60.

27. National Institute for Health and Care Guidance. Overview | Hypertension in pregnancy: diagnosis and management. NICE guideline [NG133]. 2019. Available at: https://www.nice.org.uk/guidance/ng133. Accessed March 23, 2022.

28. Roberge S, Nicolaides K, Demers S, et al. The role of aspirin dose on the prevention of preeclampsia and fetal growth restriction: systematic review and meta-analysis. Am J Obstet Gynecol 2017;216(2):110–20.e6.

29. Justus Hofmeyr G, Lawrie TA, Atallah ÁN, et al. Calcium supplementation during pregnancy for preventing hypertensive disorders and related problems. Cochrane Database Syst Rev 2018;(10).

30. ACOG. Gestational Hypertension and Preeclampsia. Practice Bulletin 222. 2020. Available at: https://www.acog.org/clinical/clinical-guidance/practice-bulletin/articles/2020/06/gestational-hypertension-and-preeclampsia. Accessed March 28, 2021.

31. Altman D, Carroli G, Duley L, et al. Do women with pre-eclampsia, and their babies, benefit from magnesium sulphate? The Magpie Trial: a randomised placebo-controlled trial. Lancet 2002;359(9321):1877–90.

32. The Eclampsia Trial Collaborative Group. Which anticonvulsant for women with eclampsia? Evidence from the Collaborative Eclampsia Trial. Lancet 1995; 345(8963):1455–63.

33. Long Q, Oladapo OT, Leathersich S, et al. Clinical practice patterns on the use of magnesium sulphate for treatment of pre-eclampsia and eclampsia: a multi-country survey. BJOG 2017;124(12):1883–90.

34. Smith JM, Lowe RF, Fullerton J, et al. An integrative review of the side effects related to the use of magnesium sulfate for pre-eclampsia and eclampsia management. BMC Pregnancy Childbirth 2013;13:34.

35. Duley L, Meher S, Jones L. Drugs for treatment of very high blood pressure during pregnancy. Cochrane Database Syst Rev 2013;(7):CD001449.

36. Woodd SL, Montoya A, Barreix M, et al. Incidence of maternal peripartum infection: A systematic review and meta-analysis. Plos Med 2019;16(12):e1002984.

37. Bonet M, Nogueira Pileggi V, Rijken MJ, et al. Towards a consensus definition of maternal sepsis: results of a systematic review and expert consultation. Reprod Health 2017;14(1):67.

38. Hussein J, Walker L. Puerperal sepsis in low- and middle-income settings: past, present and future. In: Kehoe S, Neilson J, Norman J, editors. Maternal and infant deaths: Chasing Millennium development Goals 4 and 5. Cambridge University Press; 2014. p. 131–48.

39. The Diagnosis and Treatment of Malaria in Pregnancy (Green-top Guideline No. 54b). RCOG. Available at: https://www.rcog.org.uk/guidance/browse-all-

guidance/green-top-guidelines/the-diagnosis-and-treatment-of-malaria-in-pregnancy-green-top-guideline-no-54b/. Accessed March 19, 2022.

40. Higgins RD, Saade G, Polin RA, et al. Evaluation and Management of Women and Newborns With a Maternal Diagnosis of Chorioamnionitis: Summary of a Workshop. Obstet Gynecol 2016;127(3):426–36.

41. Heitkamp A, Meulenbroek A, van Roosmalen J, et al. Maternal mortality: near-miss events in middle-income countries, a systematic review. Bull World Health Organ 2021;99(10):693–707F.

42. Rouse CE, Eckert LO, Muñoz FM, et al. Postpartum endometritis and infection following incomplete or complete abortion: Case definition & guidelines for data collection, analysis, and presentation of maternal immunization safety data. Vaccine 2019;37(52):7585–95.

43. Intrapartum Management of Intraamniotic Infection. Available at: https://www.acog.org/clinical/clinical-guidance/committee-opinion/articles/2017/08/intrapartum-management-of-intraamniotic-infection. Accessed March 19, 2022.

44. Conde-Agudelo A, Romero R, Jung EJ. Garcia Sánchez ÁJ. Management of clinical chorioamnionitis: an evidence-based approach. Am J Obstet Gynecol 2020; 223(6):848–69.

45. Desai M, Hill J, Fernandes S, et al. Prevention of malaria in pregnancy. Lancet Infect Dis 2018;18(4):e119–32.

46. World malaria report. 2020. Available at: https://www.who.int/publications-detail-redirect/9789240015791. Accessed March 31, 2022.

47. World Health Organization. WHO Guidelines for Malaria. 2021. Available at: https://app.magicapp.org/#/guideline/5438.

48. Sugarman J, Colvin C, Moran AC, et al. Tuberculosis in pregnancy: an estimate of the global burden of disease. Lancet Glob Health 2014;2(12):e710–6.

49. Programme GT. WHO Consolidated Guidelines on Tuberculosis, Module 4: Treatment - Drug-Resistant Tuberculosis Treatment. 2020. https://www.who.int/publications/i/item/9789240007048. Accessed March 30, 2022.

50. Sobhy S, Babiker Z, Zamora J, et al. Maternal and perinatal mortality and morbidity associated with tuberculosis during pregnancy and the postpartum period: a systematic review and meta-analysis. BJOG 2017;124(5):727–33.

51. El-Messidi A, Czuzoj-Shulman N, Spence AR, et al. Medical and obstetric outcomes among pregnant women with tuberculosis: a population-based study of 7.8 million births. Am J Obstet Gynecol 2016;215(6):797, e1-e797.e6.

52. Calvert C, Ronsmans C. The contribution of HIV to pregnancy-related mortality: a systematic review and meta-analysis. AIDS 2013;27(10):1631–9.

53. Lathrop E, Jamieson DJ, Danel I. HIV and maternal mortality. Int J Gynaecol Obstet 2014;127(2):213–5.

54. Hodgson I, Plummer ML, Konopka SN, et al. A systematic review of individual and contextual factors affecting ART initiation, adherence, and retention for HIV-infected pregnant and postpartum women. PLoS One 2014;9(11):e111421.

55. Bearak J, Popinchalk A, Ganatra B, et al. Unintended pregnancy and abortion by income, region, and the legal status of abortion: estimates from a comprehensive model for 1990–2019. Lancet Glob Health 2020;8(9):e1152–61.

56. Jones, W. H, Rock, A. J. Te Linde's Operative Gynecology.; 2015.

57. Unintended Pregnancy and Abortion Worldwide. Guttmacher Institute. 2020. Available at: https://www.guttmacher.org/fact-sheet/induced-abortion-worldwide. Accessed March 19, 2022.

58. WHO | Clinical management of abortion complications: a practical guide. 2014. Available at: https://www.who.int/reproductivehealth/publications/unsafe_abortion/MSM_94_1/en/. Accessed March 19, 2022.

59. American College of Obstetricians and Gynecologists' Committee on Practice Bulletins—Gynecology. ACOG Practice Bulletin No. 200: Early Pregnancy Loss. Obstet Gynecol 2018;132(5):e197–207.

60. Mark Landon, Henry Galan, Eric Jauniaux, Deborah Driscoll, Vincenzo Berghella, William Grobman, Sarah Kilpatrick, Alison Cahill. Gabbe's Obstetrics: Normal and Problem Pregnancies. (Elsevier, ed.).; 2020.

61. Friedman AM, Ananth CV. Obstetrical venous thromboembolism: Epidemiology and strategies for prophylaxis. Semin Perinatol 2016;40(2):81–6.

62. American College of Obstetricians and Gynecologists' Committee on Practice Bulletins—Obstetrics. ACOG Practice Bulletin No. 196: Thromboembolism in Pregnancy. Obstet Gynecol 2018;132(1):e1–17.

63. Thrombosis and Embolism during Pregnancy and the Puerperium. Acute Management (Green-top Guideline No. 37b). RCOG. Available at: https://www.rcog.org.uk/guidance/browse-all-guidance/green-top-guidelines/thrombosis-and-embolism-during-pregnancy-and-the-puerperium-acute-management-green-top-guideline-no-37b/. Accessed March 23, 2022.

64. Overview | Ectopic pregnancy and miscarriage. diagnosis and initial management | Guidance | NICE. Available at: https://www.nice.org.uk/guidance/ng126. Accessed March 19, 2022.

65. Tang W, Mao J, Li KT, et al. Pregnancy and fertility-related adverse outcomes associated with Chlamydia trachomatis infection: a global systematic review and meta-analysis. Sex Transm Infect 2020;96(5):322–9.

66. Ultrasound in pregnancy. Practice bulletin No. 175. American College of Obstetricians and Gynecologists. Obstet Gynecol 2016;128:e241–56.

67. Berhe ET, Kiros K, Hagos MG, et al. Ectopic Pregnancy in Tigray, Ethiopia: A Cross-Sectional Survey of Prevalence, Management Outcomes, and Associated Factors. J Pregnancy 2021;2021:4443117.

68. Hamura NN, Bolnga JW, Wangnapi R, et al. The impact of tubal ectopic pregnancy in Papua New Guinea–a retrospective case review. BMC Pregnancy Childbirth 2013;13:86.

69. Gabrysch S, Nesbitt RC, Schoeps A, et al. Does facility birth reduce maternal and perinatal mortality in Brong Ahafo, Ghana? A secondary analysis using data on 119 244 pregnancies from two cluster-randomised controlled trials. Lancet Glob Health 2019;7(8):e1074–87.

70. Gage AD, Carnes F, Blossom J, et al. In Low- And Middle-Income Countries, Is Delivery In High-Quality Obstetric Facilities Geographically Feasible? Health Aff 2019;38(9):1576–84.

71. Powell S. Maternity waiting homes and the impact on maternal mortality in developing countries : a rapid evidence. UNICEF Global Development Commons. 2019. Available at: https://gdc.unicef.org/resource/maternity-waiting-homes-and-impact-maternal-mortality-developing-countries-rapid-evidence.

72. Kruk ME, Gage AD, Arsenault C, et al. High-quality health systems in the Sustainable Development Goals era: time for a revolution. Lancet Glob Health 2018; 6(11):e1196–252.

73. UNICEF. Delivery care: Millions of births occur annually without any assistance from a skilled attendant despite recent progress. UNICEF DATA 2018. Available at: https://data.unicef.org/topic/maternal-health/delivery-care/. Accessed March 14, 2022.

74. Anderson FWJ, Mutchnick I, Kwawukume EY, et al. Who will be there when women deliver? Assuring retention of obstetric providers. Obstet Gynecol 2007;110(5):1012–6.
75. Kekulawala M, Samba A, Braunschweig Y, et al. Obstetric Capacity Strengthening in Ghana Results in Wide Geographic Distribution and Retention of Certified Obstetrician-Gynecologists: A Quantitative Analysis. BJOG 2022. https://doi.org/10.1111/1471-0528.17121.

Pelvic Floor Disorders/ Obstetric Fistula

Saifuddin T. Mama, MD, MPH[a],*, Mohan Chandra Regmi, MBBS, MD[b]

KEYWORDS

- Obstetric fistula • Obstructed labor • Pelvic floor disorder • Pelvic organ prolapse
- Urinary incontinence • Urge incontinence • Stress incontinence • Fecal incontinence

KEY POINTS

- Pelvic floor disorder and obstetric fistula remain a significant problem across the world. There is a high cost to society economically and culturally from this chronic disease burden.
- Focused research on risk factors, outcomes, and management for pelvic floor disorders and obstetric fistula remains a key priority.
- Emphasis on primary prevention strategies centered around patient education and empowerment are essential for reducing the burden of disease.

PELVIC FLOOR DISORDER
Epidemiology

Pelvic floor disorders (PFDs) include disorders with dysfunction of structures of the pelvic floor. It includes structures located within the bony pelvis, that is, urogenital and anorectal viscera, pelvic floor musculature and connective tissues, nerves, and blood vessels.[1–5]

Though common, the actual magnitude of PFD might be quite different from published literature. Most epidemiological surveys for PFD are questionnaire based and not based on clinical examination. A cross-sectional study conducted in the United States reported that 25% of women over the age of 20 were suffering from at least one of the three PFDs: urinary incontinence (UI), pelvic organ prolapse (POP), or fecal incontinence (FI).[6] Studies from low- and middle-income countries (LMIC) suggest the prevalence of PFD at 20% to 41% but many of these studies do not use validated questionnaires. The contribution to literature and research from LMIC has been

Disclosures: past speaker for AbbVie on endometriosis.
Disclosures: no conflict of interest.
[a] Cooper Medical School of Rowan, University, Cooper University Health Care, 101 Haddon Avenue, 5th Floor Suite 503-A, Camden, NJ 08103, USA; [b] BP Koirala Institute of Health Sciences, Dharan, Nepal
* Corresponding author.
E-mail address: mama-saifuddin@cooperhealth.edu

Obstet Gynecol Clin N Am 49 (2022) 735–749
https://doi.org/10.1016/j.ogc.2022.08.001

limited. Islam and colleagues[7-11] reviewed cross-sectional studies between 2010 and 2018. Of 49 studies, 31 studies (63%) were from upper-middle-income countries, 15 (30.6%) were from LMIC and 3 (7.5%) were from low-income countries.[7,12,13]

UI is defined as involuntary loss of urine in the International Continence Society/International Urogynecologic Association (ICS/IUGA) report on the terminology of pelvic floor dysfunction, categorized as a symptom rather than a sign.[14] The stigma of UI is deeply rooted in social and cultural contexts and the definitions used in various studies may vary influencing estimations of the magnitude of this condition in various populations.[15] Women tend to hide these symptoms; the real magnitude of these conditions might be quite different than what has been reported.

UI is generally divided into stress incontinence (SUI, involuntary loss of urine on physical exertion or effort), overactive bladder (OAB) (a broader term that includes urinary urgency and/or frequency with or without incontinence and nocturia (waking at night to void)), urge urinary incontinence (UUI, involuntary loss of urine associated with urgency) and mixed incontinence (a combination of stress and urge incontinence in varying degrees). UI is the most common PFD. In the United States, a cross-sectional study reported UI prevalence at 15.7%.[6] Data from LMIC suggest the prevalence of UI from 15.7% to 30%.[7,13,16] The Sixth International Consultation on Incontinence committee reviewed epidemiological studies on UI and quoted prevalence rates of 5% to 69%. The widespread variation is likely due to the use of different case definitions in different populations with varying age ranges as well as a lack of consistent use of validated questionnaires. Among subtypes, isolated SUI comprises about half of all UI followed by mixed incontinence and UUI. The exact distribution differs depending on the age of the population studied. In the older population, UUI is more common than SUI.[17] Each subtype has different modalities of treatment so validated questionnaires focusing on subtype detection using bother symptoms should be emphasized.

FI with involuntary loss of liquid or solid stool affects one in eight adults with 9% of adult women reporting FI at least monthly.[18] It increases with age and is more common in the elderly and in patients with chronic bowel dysfunction, diabetes, neurological disease, obesity, UI, and prior anal sphincter injury.[18,19] FI of liquid stool is more common than solid stool. FI severely impacts both quality of life and mental health. Less is known about the impact of FI in LMIC but in developed countries, FI increases the risk for nursing home placement.[18] The prevalence of FI in nursing home approaches 50%.[20] Patients with FI experience shame, guilt, depression, and social isolation with only 30% of affected patients seeking care.

POP is defined as a protrusion or herniation of the pelvic organs (uterus, bladder, small bowel, and rectum) into the vaginal walls due to loss of support. ICS defines POP as the descent of one or more of the anterior vaginal wall, posterior vaginal wall, and or vaginal apex which may include the uterus (cervix) or the vaginal cuff scar (post-hysterectomy). These signs on the clinical examination have to be correlated with relevant POP symptoms (eg, feeling a vaginal bulge).[14] POP can cause significant suffering for adult women as they age and result in socioeconomic consequences but may be unacknowledged and a hidden public health issue in many more traditional societies.[21,22]

Most epidemiologic studies on POP are from higher resource settings with fewer reports in Asian and African populations.[7] These studies vary in quality; studies that combine screening questionnaires and clinical examinations usually show higher prevalence. Prevalence estimates using the sensation of mass bulging into the vagina as POP definition range from 5% to 31% globally and in LMIC range up to 61%. Specifically, in some studies, the prevalence of POP is 40% to 50% with a mean age of

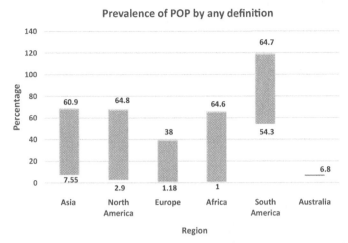

Fig. 1. Pelvic organ prolapse is a public health problem around the globe. (*Data from* Brown HW, Hegde A, Huebner M, et al. International urogynecology consultation chapter 1 committee 2: Epidemiology of pelvic organ prolapse: prevalence, incidence, natural history, and service needs. Int Urogynecol J. 2022; 33(2):173-187. doi:10.1007/s00192-021-05018-z).

presentation as early as 28 years with a symptom duration of 7 years.[23,24] POP is most common in the anterior and apical component followed by the posterior compartment (**Fig. 1**).[17,22,25]

Risk Factors

There are many epidemiologic studies on pelvic floor changes during pregnancy and after different forms of delivery. The mechanism is likely multifactorial including mechanical and neurovascular injury to the pelvic floor muscles and ligaments. PFDs are more common in parous compared with nulliparous women of the same age. As increasing age is also an important risk factor for PFD, the effect of parity is more pronounced in younger women.[4,13,17,21,26] Parity is also an especially important risk factor in LMIC due to the higher average parity, greater numbers of vaginal deliveries with unskilled birth attendants and a greater proportion of women having to undertake heavy manual work before, during, and after pregnancy.[27] Increased prevalence of PFD has been noted in women who had a vaginal delivery (VD) versus women who delivered by cesarean section (CS) in the immediate postpartum period; however, after several years postpartum, the prevalence is comparable (**Fig. 2**). Parous women with VD have a higher chance of surgery for PFD than women who delivered by CS. Women who delivered by CS without labor did not experience any additional risk for POP and FI as compared with nulliparous women. Other childbirth-related factors increasing the risk of PFD include instrument delivery (ID), prolonged second stage of labor, fetal macrosomia, and perineal lacerations.[28–36] It has been estimated that 9 CS would be necessary to prevent 1 UI and 12 CS to prevent 1 POP.[37] However, CS is not risk free having a higher morbidity and mortality rate in comparison to VD. Increasing cesarean births must be weighed against the association with increased risks for future pregnancy and long-term outcomes.[38]

Genetic factors have been associated with UI and POP,[17] but not described for FI. Studies show high concordance of continence status between sister pairs for postmenopausal women suggesting familial factors play a role in the development of UI.[26,39] Women with a family history of POP were more likely to have POP compared

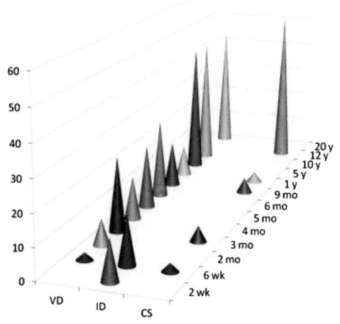

Fig. 2. Higher incidence of urinary incontinence after vaginal delivery than cesarean section in immediate postpartum period but similar incidence 20 years after cesarean section indicating the effect of age. (*Data from Refs*[26,88–93]). X axis: mode of delivery; Y axis: percentage; VD: vaginal delivery; ID: instrument delivery; CS: cesarean section

with women without a family history. Women with a history of surgical correction for POP and reporting a family history of POP were on average 1.4 times more likely to have recurrence after POP surgery than women with surgical correction for POP without a family history.[40]

Obesity is associated with an increased risk of SUI, UUI, and FI. Its influence on POP is less clear.[3,17] Obesity appears to also be associated with poor outcomes for PFD surgery. Bariatric surgery has a benefit on PFD for obese women overall with improvement in UI and POP symptoms but not FI.[41]

Chronic lifting of heavy weights (**Fig. 3**) has been found to be associated with POP in both developed countries and LMIC.[23,42,43] Pelvic surgery including previous POP surgery and hysterectomy are found to be associated with recurrent POP and UI whereas rectal and anal surgery is risk factors for FI.[44–46] Other less well-established risk factors include bowel dysfunction particularly constipation with subsequent straining which may be associated with POP and FI.[47–49] The literature associating joint hypermobility and POP is mixed.[50–52]

Assessment

With improved awareness, more women are reporting symptoms of PFD. Proper assessment is fundamental for quality care and better outcomes in PFD treatment. Insufficient history taking and clinical assessment and poor medical and surgical approaches have no place in patient management. The evaluation of PFD is subjective (patient history and information from questionnaires), semi-objective (eg, voiding diaries and pad tests), and objective (eg, physical examination). Usage of standard

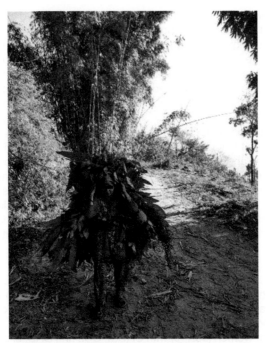

Fig. 3. Women in rural Nepal are subjected to chronic lifting of heavy back loads including carrying feed for livestock/domestic animals.

terminology provided by the ICS/IUGA document on the terminology of pelvic floor dysfunction is advisable to characterize patient signs and symptoms.[14] As the symptoms of PFD may be underreported, leading questions (eg, Do you feel like urinating more than normal during the day or night or both? Do you leak when you cough, laugh, exercise, or only when trying to get to the toilet?) might be helpful to elicit these symptoms. As PFD often coexists, leading questions should be asked for POP and anorectal dysfunction as well (eg, Do you feel a bulge, or pressure in the vagina? Do you have difficulty in defecation including inability to control feces, flatus or both?). Information can be obtained from the patient using a previously validated, self-administered questionnaire ideally completed before the index consultation. The approach should be holistic (type, frequency, severity, precipitating factors, social impact, effect on hygiene and quality of life}, directed to three primary areas, that is, the lower urinary tract, the genital system including sexual function, and the bowel, and individualized based on patient wishes and availability of resources.[17,53–55]

Physical examination should include abdominal examination, vaginal speculum, and bimanual examination, neurologic evaluation of the perineal region as well as assessment of pelvic floor reflexes and muscle tone. Further assessment depends on patient symptoms. A standardized vaginal examination using a prolapse grading system (Pelvic Organ Prolapse Quantification, POP-Q) is used for staging POP.[56] For UI, cough stress test as well as determination of urethral hypermobility and post-void residual volume may guide treatment. Bladder diary documenting frequency of voids, amount voided, fluid intake, and leakage episodes as well as provocation prompting the leakage (eg, stress provocation, urgency sensation) is an integral part of the initial assessment.

Most lab tests and imaging studies are not necessary for assessing PFD. Tests commonly performed for UI are urine analysis and culture to rule out infection.

Although urodynamic studies are commonly used in developed countries to assess lower urinary tract function, it has not been shown to impact treatment outcomes. If needed in LMIC settings, simple office cytometry involving the insertion of a catheter attached to a syringe into the bladder while filling the bladder through the syringe can give information on bladder capacity and detrusor contraction (observation of oscillation of the water column in the attached syringe during bladder filling).[55,57,58] The catheter and syringe can then be removed, and the patient asked to cough to see if there is leakage of urine (SUI).

Evaluating stool consistency with the Bristol stool scale is helpful in the initial evaluation of FI. Passive FI is associated with neurologic dysfunction. FI with urgency is related to stool type and transit. A detailed history should include bowel habits, consistency, FI triggers, underlying medical issues, and prior trauma including obstetric history. Physical examination should assess for hemorrhoids, masses, prolapse, fistula along with an assessment of pelvic floor strength, and evaluation of resting and active anal sphincter tone. Ancillary testing with endoanal ultrasound, defecography, dynamic MRI, and anorectal manometry is usually not required but can be used for complex cases.

Treatment

Conservative management of PFD involves nonsurgical and non-pharmacological approaches. These comprise lifestyle modifications (eg, weight loss, cessation of smoking) and pelvic floor muscle training (PFMT).

More than half of women (53.1%) with UI (SUI, UUI, and OAB) experience improvement with conservative treatment.[17,59–62] In addition to PFMT and lifestyle modifications, other conservative management for OAB and UUI include a scheduled voiding regimen as well as avoidance of food or liquids containing bladder irritants such as caffeinated beverages, carbonated drinks, and diets with high oxalates. Advice on intake of fluids and voiding pattern should be based on the bladder diary completed as part of the patient assessment. Common medical conditions and medications that contribute to urinary issues should be addressed. Postmenopausal women presenting with UI amenable to a trial of vaginal estrogen may report improvement in symptoms. Pharmacological agents (eg, antimuscarinics and beta 3 receptor agonists) are adjuvant to conservative management. Other treatment modalities (eg, OnabotulinumtoxinA intravesical injections, posterior tibial nerve stimulation, and sacral neuromodulation) can be considered if these measures fail but access may be limited in LMIC.[63]

Conservative treatments for SUI include PFMT, lifestyle modifications, and anti-incontinence pessaries. If these unsuccessful, the gold standard surgical treatment is the midurethral sling using type I polypropylene mesh with an efficacy of more than 80%. In LMIC, due to the limited availability of midurethral slings, a pubovaginal sling with autologous rectus fascia or fascia lata as well as a Burch colposuspension (urethropexy) procedure are also evidence-based surgical treatment options for SUI.[54]

Symptomatic POP should be treated with PFMT and lifestyle modifications including weight loss, correction of constipation with habitual straining as well as limiting chronic heavy lifting if possible. Vaginal pessaries can also be used. Women who refuse or are unresponsive to pessary use are offered surgical treatment. Surgical treatment depends on the availability of resources, the expertise of the surgeon, anatomical defects, general health of the patient, concomitant need of anti-incontinence procedure and history of prior pelvic surgery. POP repair can be performed vaginally (vaginal reconstructive procedures or vaginal obliterative procedures) or abdominally (open, laparoscopic or robotic with or without mesh or graft augmentation). Although open, laparoscopic or robotic abdominal sacrocolpopexy is the gold standard procedure for apical POP with attachment of type I polypropylene mesh to the anterior and posterior vagina while suspending the tail of the mesh to the sacrum, vaginal reconstructive procedures with or without a hysterectomy (eg, hysterectomy with a uterosacral ligament suspension, sacrospinous ligament hysteropexy) are almost as effective, do not use mesh, and require very little resources.[64] For patients who do not desire vaginal coital capability, vaginal obliterative procedures should also be considered as these procedures have high rates of success with low rates of complications. In LMIC, vaginal reconstructive procedures or vaginal obliterative procedures are the most commonly performed prolapse surgeries.

For FI, PFMT with or without biofeedback and food diary are mainstay treatments.[65] Increasing fluid intake and fiber to control constipation as well as the use of fiber supplements and antimotility medications such as loperamide for loose stools and diarrhea to optimize stool consistency is crucial. Perianal skin care is recommended with nonirritating cleansers and moisturizing skin barriers. In reproductive age women with FI from obstetric causes with evidence of anal sphincter disruption, anal sphincteroplasty has success rates of 65% to 87% but up to 40% of women may experience ongoing fecal urgency despite successful repair. Other options which may not be readily accessible in LMIC include anal plugs, tibial or sacral neuromodulation, and colonic diversion in recalcitrant cases.

OBSTETRIC FISTULA
Epidemiology

Pelvic fistula is defined as an abnormal communication between two organs of the pelvis (eg, urethra, bladder, ureter, uterus, cervix, ureter, and rectum) and includes vesicovaginal fistula (VVF), urethrovaginal fistula, vesicocervical fistula, vesicouterine fistula, ureterovaginal fistula and rectovaginal fistula (RVF).[3] Pelvic fistula in higher and lower resource settings may result from obstetric complications, surgery, radiation, trauma, infection, malignancy, and congenital malformations. In LMIC, most pelvic fistulas (97%) are obstetric fistula (OF) that result from obstetric complications specifically obstructed labor with labor ranging from 2.5 to 4 days. The compression of the fetal head within the maternal pelvis if unrelieved will lead to tissue compression and compromised blood supply resulting in hypoxia and ischemia with eventual pressure necrosis and fistula development. Most infants are stillborn.[66] As the access to emergency obstetric care improves, OF can also be associated with CS; however, it remains unclear if most of these fistulas are the result of unrecognized iatrogenic injury to the bladder during the CS or if the fistulas are the result of obstetric labor which lead to the CS. Most OF involves the lower urinary tract with concomitant VVF and RVF occurring in 10% to 15% of patients.[67,68] In any setting but particularly in conflict zones, postcoital injury due to rape and trauma can also result in fistula formation.[69]

The exact global prevalence and incidence of are unknown. World Health Organization estimates 2 million cases worldwide. Several articles in aggregate estimate the prevalence of LMIC of between 10 and 150 per 100,000 women[70–72] with some pooled prevalence data from population-based studies suggesting 29 per 100,000 women.[67] This highlights the need for population-level demographic data collection using validated screening questionnaires.

Risk Factors

Zhang and colleagues[66] in a systematic review with 33 articles meeting criteria for OF in LMIC noted multiple risk factors including younger age at first pregnancy, low health literacy, low socioeconomic status, and financial constraints. Women with OF suffer from malnutrition with short stature. They live in settings with no access to prenatal or emergency care including access to safe CS, lack of transportation even after obstructed labor is determined, and may live in settings where harmful childbirth practices involving random cuts in the vagina during labor are routine ("Gishiri cutting"). In addition, even if these women are able to reach a health facility with emergency obstetric services such as CS, they may be at risk of iatrogenic injury during the CS.[73,74] The exact location may vary depending on the mechanism with most distal fistulas, those that involve the vagina and distal bladder and urethra, resulting from obstructed labor, whereas the more proximal fistulas, those that involve the upper vagina and or cervix and bladder, resulting from iatrogenic injury during CS.[75]

Assessment

Thorough history should include onset, duration, characteristics of leakage, obstetric history, risk factors, and social history including social/psychologic support systems. Detailed physical and pelvic examination evaluates vaginal depth, caliber, mobility, stricture, and scarring as well as identification of the fistula track by organs involved, location especially relative to key structures such as the ureters, size, number, and level of scarring. Bladder dye test involves retrograde fill with saline and methylene blue or blue food dye with a tampon or gauze placed in the vagina can be performed to confirm VVF. If the bladder dye test is negative (gauze in the vagina is not blue) and there is suspicion of a ureterovaginal fistula, phenazopyridine can be given orally and a tampon or gauze placed in the vagina to assess for proximal orange staining. Patient with vesicouterine fistula may present with Youssef's syndrome with cyclic hematuria, UI and amenorrhea.[76] Most OF do not require imaging and most relevant imaging modalities such as CT urogram and MRI may not be readily available in LMIC; however, intravenous pyelogram, which may be available, even in rural settings, may help identify ureteral involvement or if the OF is not seen clinically.

In addition to the presentation of continual incontinence, OF patients can also present with bladder calculi (2%) (**Fig. 4**), cervical stenosis leading to hematometra, severe vaginal and perineal scarring such as loss of labia minora, and perineal dermatitis with secondary ulceration from chronic urine exposure. In addition, due to the wide extent of pressure and ischemic injury from the obstructed labor, patients may also have extensive pelvic floor and pelvic and lower extremity nerve compromise with loss of anal reflex on examination, motor weakness primarily of the L5 nerve root with leg drop, and limb contractures from immobility.

There is no standardized diagnosis and staging system for OF. Several classifications have been suggested including one by Waaldijk for VVF mainly focused on whether the closing mechanism of the urethra is involved and if the fistula is circumferential (the entire proximal bladder is detached from the distal urethra).[74] Another classification system is by Goh focused on distance of fistula from urethral meatus, size of fistula, and level of the surrounding fibrosis.[77] For RVF, a classification by Tsang[78] focused on simple versus complex, proximal versus distal location, and size and etiology of the fistula has been used.

Before embarking on surgical management, the patient should be optimized regarding nutrition and hydration as well as the treatment of concomitant parasitic diseases. Preoperative planning includes evaluating for possible ureteral involvement, deciding if intraoperative ureteral stent placement is needed, whether a hysterectomy is necessary, and the route of surgery.

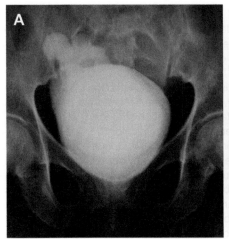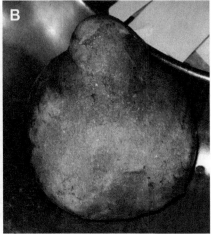

Fig. 4. (*A*) Plain film showing large calcification within the bladder. (*B*) Bladder calculi.

Treatment

Although most OF will require surgical management, conservative treatment with a pro-longed bladder catheter placed immediately after obstetric injury (for 1–2 months) can lead to closure of small VVF (<1 cm). OFs that involve the bladder and rectum can usually be surgically managed vaginally whereas those that involve the ureters and or uterus may need to be addressed abdominally. Prognostic indicators for successful OF repair include length of urethra, size and number of fistulas, location of fistula, size of the bladder, and the degree of scarring.[73,74,79] Successful repair is aimed at closing the fistula and restoring normal anatomy if there is significant vaginal and perineal scarring and involves adequate exposure, wide mobilization to result in tension-free closure, correct identification of the fistula tract with a stent or pediatric Foley catheter if needed, avoiding injury to relevant structures such as the ureters and anal sphincter if not already involved, and possible excision of the tract depending on the degree of scarring. OF are typically closed in at least two layers. For VVF, retrograde filling of the bladder after the first layer closure is performed to confirm watertight closure. Bladder catheter can be placed after closure for continuous bladder drainage for 1–2 weeks.[73,74,80–82] There appears to be no benefit to postoperative antibiotic use during this time.[83] A Martius or omental J flap can be used to introduce vascularity to the fistula closure on a case-by-case basis. Although a CT cys-togram can be used before bladder catheter removal to confirm successful closure, as this is not feasible in LMIC a retrograde bladder dye test can be done. Sexual abstinence is recommended for 6-12 weeks post repair with some patients reporting improved sex-ual function after repair.[84] Success rates of closure after the first attempt is in the 80% to 95% range with decreased rates of success (60% to 90%) for subsequent attempts at repair. Even after successful OF closure, UI and FI remain a significant problem, in up to 15% to 25% of patients along with persistent vaginal stricture, dyspareunia, and infer-tility.[85] In one study, the success rate of pregnancy after uterine preserving surgery for VVF was 31%.[86] Furthermore, women with OF may be socially isolated, marginalized, ostracized, are often economically dependent on others, and have low literacy. There is a high rate of mental health dysfunction with persistent depression. These women are more likely to be divorced or abandoned.[66] These psychosocial issues may also impact reintegration into the community even after a successful repair. This underscores the need for improved patient education and health systems to increase access to care.

Prevention

PFD and OF represent a serious worldwide public health problem for women and the focus should be on primary prevention. Identification of risk factors for PFD is complicated by the long duration between the occurrence of the putative risk factor (eg, childbirth) and the clinical manifestation of PFD, such as POP. PFD have a long latency period and may go through periods of remission. In addition, although CS seems to be protective of PFD compared with VD or ID, given the potential maternal and fetal risks of CS, especially in LMIC, this is not an effective prevention strategy. A strategy of offering CS to women at substantially higher than average risk for PFD may be appropriate but this requires a clear delineation of accurate risk factors which presently have not been identified clearly. Nevertheless, increasing awareness of PFD should be incorporated into clinical practice including discussions on prevention strategies targeting modifiable risk factors such as obesity.[87] For OF, identification of risk factors and appropriate counseling during pregnancy and labor is essential for prevention but is challenging in LMIC due to multiple factors including overcrowded hospitals, lack of trained staff, level of patient literacy, and limited resources including shortages in medications, supplies, and equipment. In addition to health care infrastructure limitations, many parts of the world also lack other essential public services to empower women and potentially prevent the development of these conditions including education and transportation services. For now, identifying women with and at risk for these conditions remains a key element in health resource allocation.

SUMMARY

PFD and OF are common conditions afflicting women globally and in LMIC but further work, particularly in risk factor identification and development of prevention strategies, is needed particularly in LMIC. Development of effective prevention and treatment programs in these settings must consider all aspects of public services including education to improve patient and public literacy and awareness of these conditions as well as transportation to readily access care and health care infrastructure with adequate resources including medication and equipment as well as trained personal.

CLINICS CARE POINTS

- Detailed history taking with elucidation of risk factors along with careful pelvic exam for pelvic floor disorders and obstetric fistula remains crucial for accurate diagnosis.
- Awareness of psychosocial and cultural factors that impact both prevention and treatment of pelvic floor disorders can help mitigate their occurrence.
- Diligence and perseverance in the care of patients focused on individualizing the treatment whether medical or surgical embedded within the existing cultural and social norms is essential.

REFERENCES

1. Bump RC, Norton PA. Epidemiology and natural history of pelvic floor dysfunction. Obstet Gynecol Clin North Am 1998;25(4):723–46.
2. Goh J, Romanzi L, Elneil S, et al. An International Continence Society (ICS) report on the terminology for female pelvic floor fistulas. Neurourol Urodyn 2020;39(8): 2040–71.

3. Pomian A, Lisik W, Kosieradzki M, et al. Obesity and pelvic floor disorders: a review of the literature. Med Sci Monit 2016;22:1880–6.
4. Shrestha LB. Population aging in developing countries. Health Aff (Millwood) 2000;19(3):204–12.
5. Bo K, Frawley HC, Haylen BT, et al. An International Urogynecological Association (IUGA)/International Continence Society (ICS) joint report on the terminology for the conservative and nonpharmacological management of female pelvic floor dysfunction. Int Urogynecol J 2017;28:191–213.
6. Nygaard I, Barber MD, Burgio KL, et al. Prevalence of symptomatic pelvic floor disorders in US women. JAMA 2008;300(11):1311–6.
7. Islam RM, Oldroyd J, Rana J, et al. Prevalence of symptomatic pelvic floor disorders in community-dwelling women in low and middle-income countries: a systematic review and meta-analysis. Int Urogynecol J 2019;30(12):2001–11.
8. Hartigan SM, Smith AL. Disparities in Female Pelvic Floor Disorders. Curr Urol Rep 2018;19(2):16.
9. Mishra GD, Cooper R, Kuh D. A life course approach to reproductive health: theory and methods. Maturitas 2010;65(2):92–7.
10. Delancey JO, Kane Low L, Miller JM, et al. Graphic integration of causal factors of pelvic floor disorders: an integrated life span model. Am J Obstet Gynecol 2008; 199(6):610.e1–6105.
11. Hallock JL, Handa VL. The epidemiology of pelvic floor disorders and childbirth: an update. Obstet Gynecol Clin North Am 2016;43(1):1–13.
12. Dheresa M, Worku A, Oljira L, et al. Factors associated with pelvic floor disorders in Kersa District, eastern Ethiopia: a community-based study. Int Urogynecol J 2019;30(9):1559–64.
13. Beketie ED, Tafese WT, Assefa ZM, et al. Symptomatic pelvic floor disorders and its associated factors in South-Central Ethiopia. PLoS One 2021;16(7):e0254050.
14. Haylen BT, de Ridder D, Freeman RM, et al. An International Urogynecological Association (IUGA)/International Continence Society (ICS) joint report on the terminology for female pelvic floor dysfunction. Int Urogynecol J 2010;21(1):5–26.
15. Elstad EA, Taubenberger SP, Botelho EM, et al. Beyond incontinence: the stigma of other urinary symptoms. J Adv Nurs 2010;66(11):2460–70.
16. Zuchelo LTS, Santos EFS, Dos Santos Figueiredo FW, et al. Pelvic floor disorders in postpartum adolescents in the Western Amazon: a cross-sectional study. Int J Womens Health 2018;10:477–86.
17. Abrams P, Andersson KE, Apostolidis A, et al. 6th International Consultation on Incontinence. Recommendations of the International Scientific Committee: Evaluation and treatment of urinary incontinence, pelvic organ prolapse and fecal incontinence. Neurourol Urodyn 2018;37(7):2271–2.
18. Kheng-Seong N, Sivakumaran Y, Nassar N, et al. Fecal incontinence: community prevalence and associated factors– a systematic review. Dis Colon Rectum 2015; 58:1194–209.
19. Brown HW, Dyer KY, Rogers RG. Management of fecal incontinence. Obstet Gynecol 2020;136(4):811–21.
20. Nelson RL. Epidemiology of fecal incontinence. Gastroenterology 2004;126:S3–7.
21. Walker GJ, Gunasekera P. Pelvic organ prolapse and incontinence in developing countries: review of prevalence and risk factors. Int Urogynecol J 2011;22(2): 127–35.
22. Lien YS, Chen GD, Ng SC. Prevalence of and risk factors for pelvic organ prolapse and lower urinary tract symptoms among women in rural Nepal. Int J Gynaecol Obstet 2012;119(2):185–8.

23. Joshi D, Jha N, Sharma Paudel I, et al. Factors associated with pelvic organ prolapse in eastern region of nepal: a case control study. J Nepal Health Res Counc 2020;18(3):416–21.

24. Ministry of Health and Population, Nepal. Nepal demographic and health survey 2006. Kathamandu. Ministry of health (MoH). New Era: Macro International Inc; 2007.

25. Brown HW, Hegde A, Huebner M, et al. International urogynecology consultation chapter 1 committee 2: epidemiology of pelvic organ prolapse: prevalence, incidence, natural history, and service needs. Int Urogynecol J 2022;33(2):173–87.

26. Rortveit G, Daltveit AK, Hannestad YS, et al, Norwegian EPINCONT Study. Urinary incontinence after vaginal delivery or cesarean section. N Engl J Med 2003;348(10):900–7.

27. López-López AI, Sanz-Valero J, Gómez-Pérez L, et al. Pelvic floor: vaginal or caesarean delivery? A review of systematic reviews. Int Urogynecol J 2021; 32(7):1663–73.

28. Hansen BB, Svare J, Viktrup L, et al. Urinary incontinence during pregnancy and 1 year after delivery in primiparous women compared with a control group of nulliparous women. Neurourol Urodyn 2012;31(4):475–80.

29. Memon HU, Handa VL. Vaginal childbirth and pelvic floor disorders. Womens Health (Lond) 2013;9(3):265–77.

30. Boyles SH, Li H, Mori T, et al. Effect of mode of delivery on the incidence of urinary incontinence in primiparous women. Obstet Gynecol 2009;113(1):134–41.

31. Leijonhufvud A, Lundholm C, Cnattingius S, et al. Risks of stress urinary incontinence and pelvic organ prolapse surgery in relation to mode of childbirth. Am J Obstet Gynecol 2011;204(1):70.e1–707.

32. Handa VL, Blomquist JL, Roem J, et al. Longitudinal study of quantitative changes in pelvic organ support among parous women. Am J Obstet Gynecol 2018;218(3):320.e1–7.

33. Cattani L, Decoene J, Page AS, et al. Pregnancy, labour and delivery as risk factors for pelvic organ prolapse: a systematic review. Int Urogynecol J 2021;32(7): 1623–31.

34. Pretlove SJ, Thompson PJ, Toozs-Hobson PM, et al. Does the mode of delivery predispose women to anal incontinence in the first year postpartum? A comparative systematic review. BJOG 2008;115(4):421–34, published correction appears in BJOG. 2010 Sep;117(10):1307-1308.

35. Blomquist JL, Muñoz A, Carroll M, et al. Association of delivery mode with pelvic floor disorders after childbirth. JAMA 2018;320(23):2438–47.

36. Schwarzman P, Paz Levy D, Walfisch A, et al. Pelvic floor disorders following different delivery modes-a population-based cohort analysis. Int Urogynecol J 2020;31(3):505–11.

37. Gyhagen M, Bullarbo M, Nielsen TF, et al. The prevalence of urinary incontinence 20 years after childbirth: a national cohort study in singleton primiparae after vaginal or caesarean delivery. BJOG 2013;120(2):144–51.

38. Keag OE, Norman JE, Stock SJ. Long-term risks and benefits associated with cesarean delivery for mother, baby, and subsequent pregnancies: Systematic review and meta-analysis. PLoS Med 2018;15(1):e1002494.

39. Buchsbaum GM, Duecy EE, Kerr LA, et al. Urinary incontinence in nulliparous women and their parous sisters. Obstet Gynecol 2005;106(6):1253–8.

40. Samimi P, Jones SH, Giri A. Family history and pelvic organ prolapse: a systematic review and meta-analysis. Int Urogynecol J 2021;32(4):759–74.

41. Lian W, Zheng Y, Huang H, et al. Effects of bariatric surgery on pelvic floor disorders in obese women: a meta-analysis. Arch Gynecol Obstet 2017;296(2):181–9.
42. Bodner-Adler B, Shrivastava C, Bodner K. Risk factors for uterine prolapse in Nepal. Int Urogynecol J Pelvic Floor Dysfunct 2007;18(11):1343–6.
43. Jørgensen S, Hein HO, Gyntelberg F. Heavy lifting at work and risk of genital prolapse and herniated lumbar disc in assistant nurses. Occup Med (Lond) 1994; 44(1):47–9.
44. Hsieh CH, Chang WC, Lin TY, et al. Long-term effect of hysterectomy on urinary incontinence in Taiwan. Taiwan J Obstet Gynecol 2011;50(3):326–30.
45. Altman D, Falconer C, Cnattingius S, et al. Pelvic organ prolapse surgery following hysterectomy on benign indications. Am J Obstet Gynecol 2008; 198(5):572.e1–5726.
46. Pernikoff BJ, Eisenstat TE, Rubin RJ, et al. Reappraisal of partial lateral internal sphincterotomy. Dis Colon Rectum 1994;37(12):1291–5.
47. Jelovsek JE, Barber MD, Paraiso MF, et al. Functional bowel and anorectal disorders in patients with pelvic organ prolapse and incontinence. Am J Obstet Gynecol 2005;193(6):2105–11.
48. Morgan DM, DeLancey JO, Guire KE, et al. Symptoms of anal incontinence and difficult defecation among women with prolapse and a matched control cohort. Am J Obstet Gynecol 2007;197(5):509.e1–5096.
49. Sharma A, Marshall RJ, Macmillan AK, et al. Determining levels of fecal incontinence in the community: a New Zealand cross-sectional study. Dis Colon Rectum 2011;54(11):1381–7.
50. Marshman D, Percy J, Fielding I, et al. Rectal prolapse: relationship with joint mobility. Aust N Z J Surg 1987;57(11):827–9.
51. Norton PA, Baker JE, Sharp HC, et al. Genitourinary prolapse and joint hypermobility in women. Obstet Gynecol 1995;85(2):225–8.
52. Knoepp LR, McDermott KC, Muñoz A, et al. Joint hypermobility, obstetrical outcomes, and pelvic floor disorders. Int Urogynecol J 2013;24(5):735–40.
53. Smith CA, Witherow RO. The assessment of female pelvic floor dysfunction. BJU Int 2000;85(5):579–87.
54. Good MM, Solomon ER. Pelvic floor disorders. Obstet Gynecol Clin North Am 2019;46(3):527–40.
55. Holroyd-Leduc JM, Tannenbaum C, Thorpe KE, et al. What type of urinary incontinence does this woman have? JAMA 2008;299(12):1446–56.
56. Bump RC, Mattiasson A, Bø K, et al. The standardization of terminology of female pelvic organ prolapse and pelvic floor dysfunction. Am J Obstet Gynecol 1996; 175(1):10–7.
57. Grigoriadis T, Athanasiou S. Investigation of pelvic floor disorders. Climacteric 2019;22(3):223–8.
58. Nager CW, Brubaker L, Litman HJ, et al. A randomized trial of urodynamic testing before stress-incontinence surgery. N Engl J Med 2012;366(21):1987–97.
59. Bascur-Castillo C, Carrasco-Portiño M, Valenzuela-Peters V, et al. Effect of conservative treatment of pelvic floor dysfunctions in women: an umbrella review. Int J Gynecol Obstet 2022;00:1–20.
60. Dumoulin C, Cacciari LP, Hay-Smith EJC. Pelvic floor muscle training versus no treatment, or inactive control treatments, for urinary incontinence in women. Cochrane Database Syst Rev 2018;10(10):CD005654.
61. Ladi-Seyedian SS, Sharifi-Rad L, Nabavizadeh B, et al. Traditional biofeedback vs. pelvic floor physical therapy-is one clearly superior? Curr Urol Rep 2019; 20(7):38.

62. Rahn DD, Ward RM, Sanses TV, et al. Vaginal estrogen use in postmenopausal women with pelvic floor disorders: systematic review and practice guidelines. Int Urogynecol J 2015;26(1):3–13.
63. Helfand BT, Evans RM, McVary KT. A comparison of the frequencies of medical therapies for overactive bladder in men and women: analysis of more than 7.2 million aging patients. Eur Urol 2010;57(4):586–91.
64. Maher C, Feiner B, Baessler K, et al. Surgery for women with apical vaginal prolapse. Cochrane Database Syst Rev 2016;10(10):CD012376.
65. Bols EMJ, Hendriks EJM, Berghmans BCM, et al. A systematic review of etiological factors for postpartum fecal incontinence. Acta Ob et Gyn 2010;89:302–14.
66. Zheng AX, Anderson FWJ. Obstetric fistula in low income countries. IJOG 2009; 104(2):85–9.
67. Adler AJ, Ronsmans C, Calvert C, et al. Estimating the presence of obstetric fistula: a systematic review and meta-analysis BMC. Pregnancy Childbirth 2013; 13:246.
68. Bodner-Adler B, Hanzal E, Pablik E, et al. Management of vesicovaginal fistulas in women following benign gynecologic surgery: A systematic review and meta-analysis. PLoS One 2017;12(2):e0171554.
69. Muleta M, Williams G. Postcoital injuries treated at the Addis Ababa Fistula Hospital, 1991–97. Lancet 1999;354(9195):2051–2.
70. Prual A, Bouvier-Colle MH, de Bernis L, et al. Severe maternal morbidity from direct obstetric causes in West Africa: incidence and case fatality rates. Bull World Health Organ 2000;78(5):593–7.
71. Vangeenderhuysen C, Prual A, Ould el Joud D. Obstetric fistulae: incidence estimates for sub-Saharan Africa. Int J Gynecol Obstet 2001;73(1):65–6.
72. Muleta M, Fantahun M, Tafesse B, et al. Obstetric fistula in rural Ethiopia. East Afr Med J 2007;84(11):525–33.
73. Hancock B. Practical obstetric fistula surgery. London: Royal Society of Medicine Press; 2009.
74. Waaldijk K. Step-by-step surgery of vesicovaginal fistulas. Edinburgh: Campion Press; 1994.
75. Washington BB, Raker CA, Kabeja GA, et al. Demographic and delivery characteristics associated with obstetric fistula in Kigali, Rwanda. Int J Ob Gynec 2015; 129:34–7.
76. Battacharjee S, Kohli UA, Sood A, et al. Vesicouterine fistula: Youssef's syndrome. Med J Armed Forces India 2015;71(Suppl 1):S175–7.
77. Goh JTW. A new classification for female genital tract fistula. Aust New Zealand J. Ob Gyne 2004;44:502–4.
78. Tsang CBS. Rothenberger DA Rectovaginal fistulas therapeutic options. Surg Clin North America 1997;77(1):95–114.
79. Nardos R, Browning A, Chen CC. Risk factors that predict failure after vaginal repair of obstetric vesicovaginal fistulae. Am J Obstet Gynecol 2009;200(5): 578.e1–4.
80. Randazzo M, Lengauer L, Rochat CH, et al. Best practices in robotic assisted repair of vesicovaginal fistula: a consensus report from the European Association of urology robotic urology section scientific working group for reconstructive urology. Eur Urol 2020;78:432–42.
81. Miklos JR, Moore RD, Chinthakanan O. Laparoscopic and robotic assisted vesicovaginal fistula repair: a systematic review of the literature. JMIG 2015;22(5): 727–36.

82. Barone MA, Widmer M, Arrowsmith S, et al. Breakdown of simple female genital fistula repair after 7 day versus 14 day postoperative bladder catherisation: a randomized, controlled, open label, non-inferiority trial. Lancet 2015;386(9988): 56–62.

83. Tomlinson AJ. Thornton JG a randomized controlled trial of antibiotic prophylaxis for vesicovaginal fistula repair. BJOG 2005;105(4):397–9.

84. Mohr S, Brandner S, Mueller MD, et al. Kuhn A Sexual function after vaginal and abdominal fistula repair. Am J Obstet Gynecol 2014;211(1):74.e1–6.

85. Bengtson AM, Kopp D, Tang JH, et al. Identifying patients with vesicovaginal fistula at high risk of urinary incontinence after surgery. Obstet Gynecol 2016; 128(5):945–53.

86. Porcaro AB, Zicari M, Antoniolli SZ, et al. Vesicouterine fistula following cesarean section. Int Urol Nephrol 2002;34:335–44.

87. Bazi T, Takahashi S, Ismail S, et al. Prevention of pelvic floor disorders: international urogynecological association research and development committee opinion. Int Urogynecol J 2016;27(12):1785–95.

88. Foldspang A, Hvidman L, Mommsen S, et al. Risk of postpartum urinary incontinence associated with pregnancy and mode of delivery. Acta Obstet Gynecol Scand 2004;83(10):923–7.

89. Lukacz ES, Lawrence JM, Contreras R, et al. Parity, mode of delivery, and pelvic floor disorders. Obstet Gynecol 2006;107(6):1253–60.

90. Wesnes SL, Hunskaar S, Bo K, et al. The effect of urinary incontinence status during pregnancy and delivery mode on incontinence postpartum. A cohort study. BJOG 2009;116(5):700–7.

91. Ekström A, Altman D, Wiklund I, et al. Planned cesarean section versus planned vaginal delivery: comparison of lower urinary tract symptoms. Int Urogynecol J Pelvic Floor Dysfunct 2008;19(4):459–65.

92. Farrell SA, Allen VM, Baskett TF. Parturition and urinary incontinence in primiparas. Obstet Gynecol 2001;97(3):350–6.

93. Dolan LM, Hilton P. Obstetric risk factors and pelvic floor dysfunction 20 years after first delivery. Int Urogynecol J 2010;21(5):535–44.

Genital Tract Infections in Women, Pregnancy and Neonates

Alphonse N. Ngalame, MD, DES O&G, MPH[a],
Mwangelwa Mubiana-Mbewe, BSc, MBChB, MMed, MBA[b],
Jodie A. Dionne, MD, MSPH[c],*

KEYWORDS

- Chlamydia • Genital tract infections • Gonorrhea • Herpes simplex virus
- Infection in pregnancy • Sexually transmitted infections • Syphilis • Trichomoniasis

KEY POINTS

- The global burden of STI is highest among reproductive-age women who reside in LMIC.
- Unfortunately, the diagnosis and treatment of genital tract infections has been limited in LMIC settings by poor access to sensitive diagnostic testing and a reliance on syndromic management of sexually transmitted infections (STIs).
- As most STIs in women are asymptomatic, routine and affordable screening is needed to identify infections and prevent short- and long-term adverse health outcomes.

INTRODUCTION

Genital tract infections in women are highly prevalent and most are asymptomatic. Genital tract infections during pregnancy occur in up to 40-50% of women.[1] Rates of sexually transmitted infections (STIs) are highest in certain low- and middle-income countries (LMIC) regions, specifically sub-Saharan Africa, Latin America, and the Caribbean.[2] Genital tract infections are caused by a wide variety of pathogens. The main causative organisms discussed in this article include bacteria (*Chlamydia trachomatis*, *Neisseria gonorrhoeae*, *Treponema pallidum*), parasites (*Trichomonas vaginalis*), yeast (*Candida albicans*), and viruses (herpes simplex virus [HSV]).[3] Ulcerative and nonulcerative STIs facilitate the acquisition and transmission

[a] Department of Obstetrics and Gynecology, Faculty of Health Sciences, University of Buea, PO Box 12, Buea, Cameroon; [b] Centre for Infectious Diseases Research, PO Box 34681, Plot 34620 Corner Lukasu/Danny Pule Road, Lusaka, Zambia; [c] Department of Medicine, Division of Infectious Diseases, University of Alabama at Birmingham, 703 19th Street South, Birmingham, AL 35294, USA
* Corresponding author.
E-mail address: jdionne@uabmc.edu

Obstet Gynecol Clin N Am 49 (2022) 751–769
https://doi.org/10.1016/j.ogc.2022.07.004
0889-8545/22/© 2022 Elsevier Inc. All rights reserved.

obgyn.theclinics.com

of HIV in women to their infants and sexual partners.[4] HIV infection in women and pregnancy is discussed in a separate article.

STIs can lead to adverse maternal, fetal, and neonatal outcomes in women and during and after pregnancy. These outcomes include pelvic inflammatory disease (PID), tubal infertility, ectopic pregnancy, premature rupture of membranes, miscarriages, preterm birth, fetal growth restriction as well as neonatal morbidities such as skin lesions, conjunctivitis, pneumonia, sepsis, meningitis, encephalitis, organ dysfunction, and perinatal mortality.[3] In this article, each infection will be divided into sections focused on the impact on women, pregnancy, and exposed neonates with a focused discussion of epidemiology, clinical outcome, and diagnostic details with relevance to LMIC settings. A summary of adverse infection outcomes is found in **Table 1** with diagnostic options in **Table 2**, and recommended treatment for genital tract infections in **Table 3**.

The most common STIs can be divided into 2 syndromes: ulcerative conditions (syphilis and HSV) and nonulcerative conditions (chlamydia, gonorrhea, and trichomoniasis). Vaginitis is a common nonulcerative condition in pregnancy that is often caused by candidiasis, which is not considered an STI, or bacterial vaginosis (BV), a dysbiosis in the vaginal flora that can be transmitted between partners.

The epidemiology of neonatal infection is dependent on the timing of infection in pregnancy and acquired immunity in the mother. Case detection and effective management relies on the availability of antenatal and neonatal STI screening programs and timely treatment. Although some perinatal STIs such as syphilis and HIV have well-established screening programs in ANC clinics, implementation in LMIC settings

Table 1
Summary of genital tract infections and adverse outcomes

Infection (Organism)	Outcomes in Women	Pregnancy Outcomes	Fetal/Neonatal Outcomes
Chlamydia (*Chlamydia trachomatis*)	Cervicitis PID Ectopic pregnancy Tubal infertility	Ectopic pregnancy PROM Preterm delivery low birth weight	Fetal loss, preterm delivery, low birth weight Conjunctivitis, pneumonia
Gonorrhea (*Neisseria gonorrhoeae*)	Cervicitis PID Ectopic pregnancy Tubal infertility DGI	Ectopic pregnancy PROM Fetal growth restriction Low birth weight	Low birth weight, preterm delivery, ophthalmia neonatorum, DGI
Syphilis (*Treponema pallidum*)	Genital ulcer disease Uveitis Alopecia Meningovascular disease Cardiovascular disease (aortitis)	Fetal loss stillbirth Preterm delivery Low birth weight congenital syphilis	Fetal loss stillbirth Preterm delivery Low birth weight Congenital syphilis
Herpes Simplex (HSV Type 1 + 2)	Recurrent genital ulcer disease Viral hepatitis Keratitis Meningitis/ Encephalitis	Spontaneous abortion Preterm delivery Stillbirth	Preterm delivery, low birth weight, encephalitis, disseminated disease, skin, eye, and mouth disease

Abbreviations: DGI, disseminated gonococcal infection; PROM, premature rupture of membranes.

Table 2
Diagnostic options for genital tract infections in women and newborns in LMIC

	Gold Standard Testing (Often Unavailable in LMIC)	Testing in LMIC Settings	Rapid or Point of Care Test	Self-collection Option	Newborn Testing
Syphilis	Serologic screening with confirmatory test	Serologic screening with or without confirmation	Rapid treponemal test with 75–99% sensitivity. Dual syphilis/HIV available	Pilot studies in HIC	VDRL/RPR
HSV 1 + 2	HSV culture HSV PCR of active lesion	Serology	Available in HIC or research study	Pilot studies in HIC	Clinical; culture of lesions; PCR
CT/NG	CT/NG culture or RNA/DNA NAAT	CT serology	N/A	Option per WHO	CT/NG: Culture of conjunctival swab
TV	NAAT	Direct microscopy (wet mount)	Available in HIC or research only	Option per WHO	Not available
BV	Nugent Score on Gram stain vaginal fluid smear	Amsel score	Under investigation	Option per WHO	Not available
Candidiasis	culture	Microscopy	Available in HIC or research only	Option per WHO	Not available
Pelvic Inflammatory Disease	Laparoscopic examination, endometrial biopsy or pelvic imaging studies	None. Clinical diagnosis.	CT/NG/MG NAAT in HIC or research study	HIC only	Not applicable

Abbreviations: HIC, high-income countries; MG, *Mycoplasma genitalium*; NAAT, nucleic acid amplification test; RPR, rapid plasmin regain; VDRL, Venereal Disease Research Laboratory.

Table 3
Treatment of common genital tract infections in women, pregnancy, and neonates according to 2021 guidelines from the WHO and US CDC

	Women	Pregnancy	Neonates
Syphilis	Early: Benzathine penicillin G 2.4 MU intramuscularly in a single dose Late or latent[a]: Benzathine penicillin G 2.4 MU intramuscularly weekly x 3 doses (same for WHO and CDC)	Early: Benzathine penicillin G 2.4 MU intramuscularly in a single dose Late or latent WHO[a]: erythromycin 500 mg orally 4 times a day for 14 days Late or latent CDC[a]: Benzathine penicillin G 2.4 MU intramuscularly weekly x 3 doses	WHO: Aqueous benzyl penicillin 50 000 U/kg/12 hrs intravenously for 10–15 days OR Procaine penicillin 50 000 U/kg/day single dose intramuscularly for 10–15 days CDC: Aqueous crystalline penicillin G 50,000 U IV/kg/12 hrs × 7 days then every 8 hours × 3 days to complete 10 day regimen OR Procaine penicillin G 50,000 U IM/kg/day x 10 days
HSV (same for WHO and CDC)	Primary infection: Acyclovir 400 mg orally daily 3 times a day for 10 days. Recurrent infection: Acyclovir 400 mg orally daily 3 times a day for 5 days.	Primary infection: Acyclovir 400 mg orally daily 3 times a day for 10 days. Recurrent infection: Acyclovir 400 mg orally daily 3 times a day for 5 days.	Acyclovir 60 mg/kg/day in divided doses 8 hourly for 21 days if disseminated or CNS disease OR 14 days if not
CT/NG (uncomplicated) (CT treatment same for WHO and CDC)	CT: doxycycline 100 mg orally twice daily for 7 days NG WHO: ceftriaxone 250 mg IM, single dose + azithromycin 1 gram orally, single dose NG CDC: ceftriaxone 500 mg IM, single dose alone if CT has been ruled out)	CT: Azithromycin 1 gram orally, single dose OR Erythromycin 500 mg orally, 4 times a day for 7 days NG WHO: ceftriaxone 250 mg IM, single dose + azithromycin 1 gram orally, single dose NG CDC: ceftriaxone 500 mg IM, single dose alone if CT has been ruled out)	CT: Azithromycin 20 mg/Kg orally for 3 days OR Erythromycin 50 mg/Kg/ per day in 4 divided doses for 14 days NG: ophthalmia Ceftriaxone 50 mg/Kg IM single dose DGI: Ceftriaxone 25–50 mg/Kg/day once IV/IM for 10–14 days (Cefotaxime 50 mg/Kg 12 hourly)
PID	PID WHO outpatient mgmt: ceftriaxone 250 mg IM, single dose + azithromycin 1gm PO, single dose + doxycycline 100 mg PO twice daily x 14 days + metronidazole 400 or 500 mg PO twice daily x 14 days PID CDC: Ceftriaxone 1g Q24 hrs + Doxycycline 100 mg PO/IV q 12 hrs + Metronidazole 500 mg PO/IV q12 hrs	PID CDC: Consult with ID Expert Consider Ceftriaxone 1g Q24 hrs + Azithromycin 500 mg PO/IV q 24 hrs + Metronidazole 500 mg PO/IV q12 hrs (no PID regimen in pregnancy specified by WHO)	N/A

MG (same for WHO and CDC)	Azithromycin 500 mg orally D1, then 250 mg orally on D2-5.	Azithromycin 500 mg orally D1, then 250 mg orally on D2-5.	Guidance not established
TV (same for WHO and CDC)	Metronidazole 2 grams orally in a single dose	Metronidazole 200 mg or 250 mg orally three times a day for 7 days (avoid 1st trimester use, if possible)	Guidance not established
BV (same for WHO and CDC)	Metronidazole 400 mg or 500 mg orally twice daily for 7 days	Metronidazole 200 mg or 250 mg orally three times a day for 7 days (avoid 1st trimester use) Alternative: clindamycin 300 mg orally twice daily for 7 days)	Routine treatment not indicated for exposure
Candidiasis (C albicans) (same for WHO and CDC)	Miconazole vaginal suppository 200 mg at night for 3 nights	Miconazole vaginal suppository 200 mg at night for 3 nights	Routine treatment not indicated for exposure

Abbreviations: BV, bacterial vaginosis; CDC, Centers for Disease Control and Prevention; CT, *Chlamydia trachomatis*; MG, *Mycoplasma genitalium*; NG, *Neisseria gonorrhoeae*; TV, *Trichomonas vaginalis*; WHO, World Health Organization.

[a] Late or latent syphilis defined by WHO as syphilis acquired >2 years ago; late/latent syphilis defined by CDC as syphilis acquired >1 year ago.

Data from Centers for Disease Control and Prevention. Sexually Transmitted Disease Surveillance 2019. Atlanta: U.S. Department of Health and Human Services; 2021. Available at https://www.cdc.gov/std/statistics/2019/default.htm; and World Health Organization (WHO). Guidelines for the management of symptomatic sexually transmitted infections. Available at https://www.who.int/publications/i/item/9789240024168. Published 2021.

is variable. Screening for other STIs is limited to symptomatic patients and access to highly sensitive diagnostic testing is poor.

TRANSMISSION OF GENITAL TRACT INFECTIONS

The most common mode of STI transmission to women is through sexual contact from an infected partner with pathogen transfer between mucous membranes, intact skin, and/or infected seminal secretions or cervicovaginal fluid. The increased vulnerability to STI acquisition among women is multifactorial and can be attributed to anatomic, biologic, immunologic, and social and/or behavioral factors. Younger women, pregnant women, and women living with HIV are at higher risk of STIs compared to other populations.[5] The timing of STI vertical transmission varies. Maternal genital infections can be transmitted to the infant in-utero, during delivery or after delivery, although transmission at the time of vaginal delivery during exposure to infected maternal tissues, cervicovaginal fluid, and/or blood is most common.

ULCERATIVE GENITAL TRACT INFECTIONS
Syphilis

Epidemiology
Syphilis is a curable STI caused by the bacterium *T pallidum*. Global age-standardized incidence rates for syphilis have been increasing among young adults since 2010.[2] Syphilis prevalence among women in Africa averaged 1.6% in 2016.[6] Among pregnant women, syphilis prevalence averaged 1.5%, compared to 0.7% globally.[3,7] The estimated congenital syphilis case rate in Africa in 2016 was 1119 cases per 100,000 live births (a decrease from 1377 cases per 100,000 in 2012).[7] More than 6 in 10 cases of congenital syphilis globally occurred in the World Health Organization (WHO) Africa region with the second highest rate in the Mediterranean region with 635 cases per 100,000 live births. These numbers are likely to underestimate true congenital syphilis case rates because most newborns are asymptomatic and infection is challenging to diagnose.

T pallidum readily crosses the placenta and fetal infection can occur at any stage of pregnancy. Vertical transmission occurs most frequently during the early infectious stages of syphilis—primary, secondary, and early latent infection—within the first year following maternal acquisition of infection. In the absence of treatment, 52% of pregnant women with syphilis will experience an adverse birth outcome. A study in Uganda at a referral hospital found syphilis prevalence of 4.1% among women who had delivered and 3.8% among their exposed newborns.[8] Most of the women had not been treated for syphilis during pregnancy.

Clinical outcomes
Untreated primary and secondary syphilis in pregnancy is highly transmissible in up to 80% of cases while untreated late syphilis is transmitted via the placenta in up to 20-25% of cases.[9] Syphilis is the second largest cause of preventable stillbirths globally, after malaria.[7] Outcomes of vertical transmission include early fetal death or stillbirth (21%), clinical disease in infancy (16%), neonatal death (9%), and low birth weight or preterm delivery (6%).[7]

In the exposed infant, congenital syphilis has a wide variety of clinical presentations involving multiple systems. Early congenital syphilis presents in the first two years of life. Clinical features include hepatosplenomegaly, hepatitis, maculopapular rash with desquamation of palms and soles, and syphilitic rhinitis (snuffles).[10] Long bone involvement includes osteochondritis and periostitis[10] and congenital syphilis may also cause sensorineural deafness and chorioretinitis.[11]

Diagnosis

All pregnant women should be screened for syphilis during pregnancy to prevent complications. Universal screening should be performed at the time of initial presentation for prenatal care, ideally during the first trimester. In some locations, repeat screening is performed during the third trimester and at the time of delivery. Follow-up testing is necessary to detect incident infection during pregnancy. It is critical for facilities to ensure universal syphilis screening among women who present late for prenatal care or receive care at different facilities as screening and treatment may be inconsistent and poorly documented. In the traditional diagnostic algorithm for syphilis, serologic screening detects nontreponemal antibodies: rapid plasmin reagin (RPR) or VDRL (Venereal Disease Research Laboratory). When the screening test is positive, a more specific confirmatory treponemal antibody test is performed. These include TPPA (*T pallidum* particle agglutination), TPHA (*T pallidum* hemagglutination assay), FTA (fluorescent treponemal antibody assay), and enzyme immunoassay antibody testing (EIA or CIA). In some cases, the reverse screening algorithm is used which begins with a treponemal screening test. Fortunately, rapid point of care syphilis testing is also increasingly available in LMIC settings. Most rapid test kits use treponemal antibody testing and some of these tests have lower sensitivity compared to laboratory-based testing. Interpretation of treponemal results can be challenging as antibodies persist lifelong, irrespective of appropriate antibiotic therapy and treatment response. In these cases, RPR/VDRL testing with a comparison of current titers and past titers is useful to look for evidence of active or recently acquired infection. A two-dilution increase in the titer of the nontreponemal test indicates reinfection and a two-dilution decrease in the titer indicates appropriate response to therapy. A one-dilution increase in RPR/VDRL titer is considered equivocal and warrants repeat testing later on. In general, RPR/VDRL titers are repeated every 3 months to assess for response because it takes time for antibody levels to fall after antibiotic therapy. False-positive syphilis testing in pregnancy can occur for EIA/CIA and RPR/VDRL tests but fortunately, the specificity of treponemal antibody tests (TPHA, TPPA, FTA-Abs) is excellent. Any positive syphilis test in a pregnant woman warrants consideration as a true positive result with early treatment indicated if infection cannot be ruled out. Routine culture of *T pallidum* is not possible and PCR testing for syphilis is only currently available in the research setting. Unlike other systemic infections, the period of spirochetemia during early syphilis is brief. This limits the utility of molecular testing of the peripheral blood.

In exposed infants, syphilis diagnostic testing is based on clinical suspicion and 65% of infants with syphilis have a normal examination at birth. Index of suspicion is raised by uncertain or inadequate maternal treatment (poor documentation or nonpenicillin regimen); maternal treatment less than 30 days before delivery; or less than 4-fold decrease in maternal RPR/VDRL titers after treatment.[11] RPR or VDRL are the initial diagnostic tests in exposed infants. If positive, confirmation with treponemal testing is indicated.[9] Passively acquired antibodies in the neonate should be < 4 times lower than maternal antibody titers and can persist for 3–6 months. Neurosyphilis can be confirmed with a positive CSF VDRL, increased protein, and pleocytosis. Long bone radiography may show periostitis and osteochondritis. Infants also need a full blood count, and benefit from ophthalmological examination and auditory brainstem response testing.

Herpes Simplex Virus

Epidemiology

Genital herpes is caused by HSV type 1 or 2.[12] HSV-1 seroprevalence among women in the general population in Africa is 94% and HSV-2 seroprevalence is 43%, with significantly higher rates of HSV-2 among women living with HIV and sex workers.[13,14] Among pregnant women in Tanzania, HSV-2 seroprevalence was 34%.[3] Global prevalence of neonatal HSV infection is 10 cases per 100,000 live births or 14,000 cases per year.[11,15] Most congenital herpes simplex infection in Africa is caused by HSV2, whereas HSV-1 is the predominant cause in the Americas, Europe, and the Western Pacific. The risk of HSV transmission is much higher in primary maternal infection (30–50%) compared to recurrent HSV infection in a person with chronic reactivation illness (<2%).[11]

Clinical outcomes

Although many HSV infections are asymptomatic, typical lesions are multiple shallow painful vesicles or ulcers of the perianal and genital area. Primary infection is often more severe than reactivation illness and malaise, myalgia, headache, and lymphadenopathy may occur. Symptomatic HSV episodes disappear within 3 weeks and the frequency of recurrent episodes varies widely from person to person. As HSV infection is lifelong with variable reactivation from the dorsal root ganglion, viral shedding and asymptomatic transmission can occur in the presence or absence of visible lesions. Primary HSV infection in pregnant women can lead to miscarriage, premature delivery, low birth weight, and neonatal herpes. Most cases of neonatal herpes occur through direct contact with maternal secretions at birth, although postnatal infection can also occur through contact with oral HSV. Transplacental transmission is rare, accounting for 5% of cases.[16] Vertical transmission is highest after primary infection during pregnancy (50%). Current strategies with proven efficacy for preventing neonatal herpes are cesarean delivery and suppressive therapy with acyclovir. Women with a primary or nonprimary first-episode outbreak in pregnancy, as well as women with a clinical history of genital herpes, should be offered suppressive therapy with acyclovir beginning at 36 weeks of gestation.[17]

Cesarean section performed before rupture of the membranes is estimated to reduce the risk of transmission by approximately 60% and is recommended in the setting of active genital lesions or prodromal symptoms (eg, vulvar pain or burning) at the time of labor.[17,18] The majority of women with recurrent infection have a very low risk of delivering a baby with neonatal herpes and vaginal delivery is recommended in the absence of active lesions or prodromal symptoms.

Severe HSV pregnancy outcomes include spontaneous abortion, stillbirth, and congenital anomalies. Most neonates with herpes virus infection have skin vesicles and the mortality rate without treatment is 60%. [16]Presentation can be a multiorgan disseminated disease, central nervous system disease, or skin, eyes, and/or mouth (SEM) disease.[19] Infants with SEM disease may progress to encephalitis if untreated. Infants with intrauterine infection can present with microcephaly or hydranencephaly, chorioretinitis, and keratoconjunctivitis[20]

Diagnosis

Routine HSV screening is not recommended for asymptomatic women nor during pregnancy. Pregnant women with symptoms should undergo serological testing (IgG) and identification by culture, PCR, or direct antibody fluorescence to identify the subtype of HSV infection. In LMIC settings, the diagnosis of HSV is often based on clinical suspicion in a woman with genital ulcer disease without laboratory evidence of active syphilis infection.

Diagnosis of congenital herpes infection relies on a high index of suspicion in an infant with skin vesicles. Confirmatory diagnosis is by culture of suspicious lesions, eye and mouth swabs, and cerebrospinal fluid PCR.[20]

NONULCERATIVE GENITAL TRACT INFECTIONS
Chlamydia

Epidemiology
C trachomatis is an obligate intracellular parasite that infects cervical cells in women and the urethra in men. It can also infect extragenital pharyngeal and rectal sites. Chlamydia prevalence among women averages 3.8% globally and 5% in Africa.[6] The highest infection rates consistently occur in adolescents and young women ages 15-24 years. In recent studies of pregnant women, chlamydia prevalence was 5.4% in Cameroon, 7.4% in the southeastern United States, and 16.8% in the Aboriginal population in Australia.[21,22]

Clinical outcomes
Although 85% of women with chlamydia are asymptomatic, some may present with postcoital bleeding, abnormal vaginal discharge, spotting, dysuria, lower abdominal pain, dysmenorrhea, and dyspareunia.[23] Productive cervical infection leads to cervicitis with inflammation. In some cases, *C trachomatis* ascends into the upper genital tract to cause PID, salpingitis, and tubo-ovarian abscess. Long-term sequelae of PID include tubal infertility in 10%, chronic pelvic pain, and ectopic pregnancy. Chlamydia is the most common cause of tubal infertility in women. The risk of vertical transmission of chlamydia during pregnancy is 60%. The neonate usually acquires infection during delivery through an infected cervix, although infection after delivery by cesarean section has been reported.[24] Untreated maternal chlamydia infection can result in preterm labor, premature rupture of membranes, and low birth weight. Timely treatment during pregnancy prevents these adverse outcomes.[25–28]

Among infants born to mothers with chlamydia, 20-50% develop conjunctivitis and up to 20% can develop pneumonia.[25] Chlamydia conjunctivitis presents at 5-12 days of life and, unlike gonorrhea, erythromycin ointment does not prevent ocular chlamydial infection. Infants with pneumonia present at 1-3 months of age as a subacute illness with repetitive staccato cough and tachypnoea. Some develop long-term abnormal pulmonary function.[25]

Diagnosis
The existing diagnostic gold standard of chlamydia culture (with HeLa 229 or McCoy cells) is expensive and limited to specialized laboratories. Most laboratories in high-income countries (HIC) and their national testing guidelines recommend the use of highly sensitive molecular testing (nucleic acid amplification testing [NAAT]) to detect *C trachomatis*. Genital NAAT testing in women and in pregnancy can be performed on a self-collected vaginal swab, a provider-collected cervical or vaginal swab, or on urine. Specialized equipment needed for molecular diagnostic testing is not yet widely available in LMIC settings. Some providers perform serologic antibody testing for *C trachomatis* but this has limited performance in diagnosing active infection. Syndromic management is used for women with vaginitis or dysuria who may have *C trachomatis* but the utility of this WHO-recommended algorithm is limited because most women with chlamydia are asymptomatic.[29] Diagnosis of neonatal Chlamydia conjunctivitis is typically culture of specimen obtained by a conjunctival swab. Fluorescent antibody tests are another useful diagnostic test that may not be routinely available in LMIC settings.

Infants suspected to have chlamydia pneumonia are diagnosed based on clinical presentation, typical radiologic findings of hyperinflation with bilateral diffuse infiltrates and accompanying peripheral eosinophilia. CT NAAT or direct fluorescent antibody testing can be performed on a nasopharyngeal swab.

Gonorrhea

Epidemiology

N gonorrhoeae is an intracellular, gram-negative diplococcus that infects the endocervix in women and the urethra in men as well as extragenital sites (rectum, pharynx, and conjunctiva). The global prevalence of gonorrhea in women in 2016 was 0.9% and 1.9% in the African region.[6] Among pregnant women, the prevalence in Tanzania was 0.5% and 1.3% in Cameroon.[3,30] In a Kenyan study, the incidence of gonococcal and chlamydial ophthalmia were 3.6 and 8.1 per 100 live births, respectively.[31] Transmission of gonococcal infection was higher in pregnant women with chlamydia coinfection.[31] In Iran, neonatal ophthalmia prevalence rates were much higher for women with chlamydia compared to gonorrhea (11.7% vs 0.4%).[32]

Clinical outcomes

Gonococcal infection is asymptomatic in most women. Typical symptoms include purulent vaginal discharge and dysuria, with inflamed cervix and purulent leukorrhea noted on examination. Gonococcal cervicitis can lead to PID in 10-20% of cases and in recent studies, 20% of PID was associated with gonorrhea infection.[33,34] Pregnancy complications include premature delivery, chorioamnionitis, spontaneous miscarriage, and premature rupture of membranes.[35] Neonatal transmission occurs in 30-50% of cases, with the main presentation of gonococcal ophthalmia neonatorum which can lead to perforation of the globe and blindness. To prevent ocular infection, prophylactic erythromycin eye ointment is prescribed at birth for all infants, regardless of the mode of delivery or maternal infection status.[36] Severe infection can present as disseminated gonococcal infection (DGI) or sepsis with or without meningitis and/or arthritis. Other presentations include rhinitis, vaginitis, and urethritis.

Diagnosis

Confirmatory diagnosis is based on the detection of gonococci by Gram stain microscopy, culture, or NAAT testing performed on genital fluids, blood, and joint fluids. In LMIC, Gram stain and culture are the main methods of diagnosis. Where these are not available, diagnosis is purely clinical. Syndromic management of vaginitis is recommended by WHO but diagnostic accuracy for the detection of gonorrhea in women is limited. Fortunately, the role of improved molecular diagnostic options for gonorrhea among women in LMIC is under investigation.[30] Diagnosing gonococcal infection in the newborn is guided by clinical presentation and culture. Cultures can be performed on samples collected from conjunctival discharge or from the blood in the setting of DGI.

Trichomonas

Epidemiology

T vaginalis (TV) is one of the most common nonviral STIs. Global TV prevalence in 2016 was 5.3% among women and 12% among women in Africa.[6] In a recent meta-analysis, the prevalence of trichomoniasis among pregnant women in Africa was 14%.[37] Trichomonas infection can involve the vagina, urethra, and paraurethral glands.

Clinical outcomes

T vaginalis infection is usually mild and 85% of infected women are asymptomatic.[38] The symptomatic forms are manifested by pruritus, dysuria, dyspareunia, frothy green or yellow purulent discharge, vulvovaginitis, pelvic pain, or vulvar ulcerations. Maternal TV infection has been associated with preterm delivery and low birth weight.[39] Reports of respiratory infection in exposed infants have been documented.[40,41]

Diagnosis

In women, diagnosis is made by microscopic examination of vaginal secretions, dipstick tests, or nucleic acid amplification tests. No routine testing is available for neonatal TV.

Bacterial Vaginosis

Epidemiology

BV is a sexually associated infection and the most common cause of abnormal vaginal discharge in women with global prevalence ranging from 23-29%.[42,43] Prevalence in pregnancy was 7% in Vietnam and ranged from 29% to 52% in sub-Saharan Africa.[37,44] BV is associated with sexual activity in women who have sex with women and/or men, it rarely occurs in patients before sexual debut. BV is currently understood to be a dysbiosis that results from an imbalance of vaginal ecosystem with insufficient numbers of healthy lactobacillus species and a predominance of several other bacteria, including *Gardnerella vaginalis*. BV pathogenesis is complex and factors associated with transmission and persistence (such as antibiotic exposure and biofilm formation) are under investigation.[45]

Clinical outcomes

More than 50% of BV is asymptomatic.[46] Clinical symptoms often include the presence of a thin, white, malodorous vaginal discharge, itching, and vaginal or vulvar pain or burning. BV is associated with PID, postpartum endometritis, and postprocedural gynecologic infections. The impact of BV on birth outcomes remains unclear. Although some data suggest that BV in pregnancy may be associated with spontaneous preterm delivery, others show an association with premature rupture of membranes, low birth weight, and NICU admission in full-term newborns.[47-51] Additional studies focused on BV and birth outcomes are needed.

Diagnosis

Routine screening for BV in women and pregnancy is not recommended.[52-54] The clinical diagnosis of BV is based on the Amsel score, which is positive if at least 3 parameters are present: (1) grayish-white, fluid leucorrhea, that is homogeneous and adherent to the vaginal mucosa, (2) foul-smelling discharge, either spontaneously or after adding a drop of 10% potassium hydroxide to the vaginal secretions (Sniff-test), (3) vaginal pH greater than 4.5, or (4) presence of clue cells on direct examination of the vaginal secretions. The complementary examination for a more precise diagnosis of BV in the research setting is the Nugent Gram stain criteria, which is based on microscopic examination of a smear of vaginal secretions on a slide. Newer molecular tests for BV are available in HIC settings.[55]

Routine treatment of women who have asymptomatic BV is not generally recommended; exceptions include women who are to undergo gynecologic surgery and in pregnancy treatment may be considered in women with prior preterm birth. Both pregnant and nonpregnant women with symptomatic BV should be treated.

Candidiasis

Epidemiology

Vulvovaginal candidiasis (VVC) affects approximately 75% of women during their lifetime and 138 million women globally suffer from recurrent vaginal candidiasis, defined as 4 or more episodes a year.[56-59] *C albicans* is the cause of VVC in 85% of cases and *Candida glabrata* is the second most common cause. *C glabrata* is more likely to be resistant to first-line azole therapy. VVC rates during pregnancy are twice that of nonpregnant women.[60,61] In Ghana, the prevalence of VVC in pregnant women was

37%. This is attributed to physiological changes such as elevated hormone levels, decreased cellular immunity, reduced vaginal pH, and increased vaginal glycogen concentration,[62] which facilitate the proliferation of candida species. Other risk factors for VVC in women include antibiotic therapy, immunosuppression, diabetes, and corticosteroid use.[63]

Clinical outcomes

VVC is a mycotic infection characterized by vulvar pruritus and whitish, curdled leucorrhea. Vaginal candidiasis has not been associated with low birth weight or preterm delivery in most studies.[61,64] Some studies have suggested an association between fetal anomalies and exposure to oral fluconazole treatment during the first trimester of pregnancy.[65,66] Newborns are often colonized with the same candida species as their mother.[67]

Diagnosis

In the setting of typical symptoms, the diagnosis of VVC is confirmed in clinic by microscopic examination of vaginal secretions with the presence of pseudohyphae. Samples can also be sent for culture and identification, though presumptive treatment is routinely practiced.

Pelvic inflammatory disease. PID is an upper genital tract infection with polymicrobial etiology. About half of diagnosed PID cases are caused by an STI such as chlamydia, gonorrhea, or *Mycoplasma genitalium* infection.[68,69] Organisms associated with BV have also been linked to PID. Women with PID often have subtle or nonspecific symptoms (eg, abnormal bleeding, dyspareunia, vaginal discharge) or are asymptomatic. Laparoscopic examination, endometrial biopsy, or pelvic imaging studies are considered the gold standard for diagnosing PID but are not practical for routine diagnosis, especially in LMIC. Therefore, diagnosis is generally based on clinical assessment. No single historical, physical, or laboratory finding is both sensitive and specific for the diagnosis of acute PID. However, even women with mild or asymptomatic PID may be at risk for long-term complications from PID, including infertility, ectopic pregnancy, and chronic pelvic pain.[70,71] Therefore, health care providers should maintain a low threshold for the clinical diagnosis of PID. Presumptive treatment for PID should be initiated for sexually active young women and other women at risk for STIs if they are experiencing pelvic or lower abdominal pain, if no cause for the illness other than PID can be identified, or if one or more of the following 3 minimum clinical criteria are present on pelvic examination: cervical motion tenderness, uterine tenderness, or adnexal tenderness. This approach maximizes sensitivity. One or more of the following additional criteria can be used to enhance the specificity of the minimum clinical criteria and support a PID diagnosis:[72]

- Oral temperature >38.3°C (>101°F)
- Abnormal cervical mucopurulent discharge or cervical friability
- Presence of abundant numbers of WBCs on saline microscopy of vaginal fluid
- Elevated erythrocyte sedimentation rate
- Elevated C-reactive protein
- Laboratory documentation of cervical infection with *N gonorrhoeae* or *C trachomatis*

PID treatment regimens should provide empiric, broad-spectrum coverage of likely pathogens (see **Table 3**), including GC and chlamydia and anaerobic organisms. If an IUD user receives a diagnosis of PID, treatment can be instituted with the IUD remaining in place.[73] Women should demonstrate clinical improvement <3 days after therapy initiation. Sexual partners should be presumptively treated for GC and chlamydia. Hospitalization should be seriously considered under the following circumstances:[72,74]

(1) the diagnosis is uncertain; (2) surgical emergencies, such as appendicitis and ectopic pregnancy cannot be ruled out; (3) a pelvic abscess is suspected; (4) severe illness precludes management on an outpatient basis; (5) the person is pregnant; (6) the person is unable to follow or tolerate an outpatient regimen; or (7) the person has failed to respond to outpatient therapy.

For sexually active women with symptom of lower abdominal pain, WHO suggests assessing for PID and treating syndromically (**Fig. 1**).

Future research to improve outcomes of genital tract infection in women. An effective public health response to STI in women relies on a system that ensures access to testing and treatment in all adolescents and sexually active adults to reduce community transmission rates. Syndromic management of STI leads to many missed opportunities for diagnosis and treatment in symptomatic and asymptomatic women. These missed opportunities to diagnose and treat STIs in women can lead to long-term complications including tubal infertility, ectopic pregnancy, and chronic pelvic pain.[75] Advocacy for routine screening of women and pregnant women in LMIC settings for treatable genital

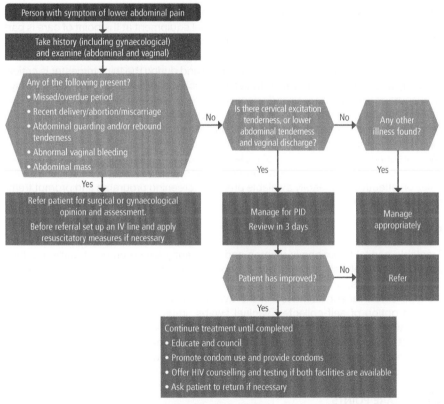

Fig. 1. Current WHO syndromic management guidelines for lower abdominal pain. (*From* World Health Organization (WHO). Guidelines for the management of symptomatic sexually transmitted infections. Available at https://www.who.int/publications/i/item/9789240024168. Published 2021.)

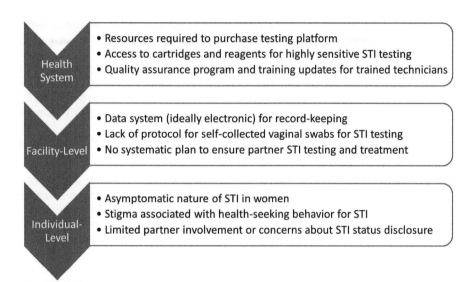

Fig. 2. Barriers to genital tract STI testing among women in LMIC settings.

infection should be supported. The development of novel, affordable, high-quality diagnostic testing that can be performed with minimal equipment at the point of care is part of the solution.[76,77] Barriers to quality diagnostic testing at the system level, facility level, and individual level are highlighted in **Fig. 2**. Programs to ensure universal access to syphilis screening in pregnancy at entry to care and during the third trimester is critical including addressing barriers in LMIC settings such as reagent stock-outs. Novel ways to encourage and ensure safe and effective partner STI treatment to reduce reinfection rates in pregnancy are also needed. Alternative options for the treatment of syphilis in pregnancy are also needed as persistent shortages of benzathine penicillin are common. Studies focused on the natural history and outcomes of *M genitalium*, TV, and BV in pregnancy, and the impact of maternal infection on fetal and neonatal outcomes is also needed. Prevention of neonatal infection acquired from the maternal genital tract relies on effective and readily available prenatal screening programs and prompt treatment of identified infection.

SUMMARY

Treatable genital infections in women and pregnancy are common globally and they pose a significant risk to the health of women and infants in LMIC settings. Timely testing, diagnosis, and treatment of STI are critical, but access is limited for many women. Given recent advances in the availability of high-quality diagnostic testing and the option of self-collected vaginal swabs, improved health outcomes are expected when international guidelines and clinical practice shift from syndromic management of symptomatic persons to routine, universal screening for chlamydia, gonorrhea, and syphilis in women and during pregnancy. Urgent change in practice is needed to meet the WHO's strategy of global STI elimination by 2030.

CLINICS CARE POINTS

- Most bacterial STI in women and pregnancy are asymptomatic.

- Untreated STI in pregnancy leads to adverse birth outcomes including preterm delivery, low birthweight and congenital syphilis.
- Review of maternal health information and treatment history is highly relevant to the assessment of infants with in-utero STI exposure.
- Molecular diagnostic STI testing is highy sensitive but not yet widely available in low and middle-income countries.

DISCLOSURE

Authors have no disclosures or financial conflicts of interest.

REFERENCES

1. Marai W. Lower genital tract infections among pregnant women: a review. East Afr Med J 2001;78(11):581–5.
2. Zheng Y, Yu Q, Lin Y, et al. Global burden and trends of sexually transmitted infections from 1990 to 2019: an observational trend study. Lancet Infect Dis 2021. https://doi.org/10.1016/s1473-3099(21)00448-5.
3. Msuya SE, Uriyo J, Hussain A, et al. Prevalence of sexually transmitted infections among pregnant women with known HIV status in northern Tanzania. Reprod Health 2009;6:4.
4. Cohen MS, Council OD, Chen JS. Sexually transmitted infections and HIV in the era of antiretroviral treatment and prevention: the biologic basis for epidemiologic synergy. J Int AIDS Soc 2019;22(Suppl Suppl 6):e25355.
5. Control UCfD. Sexually Transmitted Disease Surveillance Report 2018. 2019. https://www.cdc.gov/std/stats18/default.htm. [Accessed 1 July 2022].
6. Rowley J, Vander Hoorn S, Korenromp E, et al. Chlamydia, gonorrhoea, trichomoniasis and syphilis: global prevalence and incidence estimates, 2016. Bull World Health Organ 2019;97(8):548–562p.
7. Korenromp EL, Rowley J, Alonso M, et al. Global burden of maternal and congenital syphilis and associated adverse birth outcomes-Estimates for 2016 and progress since 2012. PLoS One 2019;14(2):e0211720.
8. Oloya S, Lyczkowski D, Orikiriza P, et al. Prevalence, associated factors and clinical features of congenital syphilis among newborns in Mbarara hospital, Uganda. BMC Pregnancy Childbirth 2020;20(1):1–7.
9. Arnold SR, Ford-Jones EL. Congenital syphilis: a guide to diagnosis and management. Paediatrics Child Health 2000;5(8):463–9.
10. Cooper JM, Sánchez PJ. Congenital syphilis. Semin Perinatol 2018;42(3):176–84.
11. Azimi P. Syphilis (Treponema pallidum). In: Kliegman RM, Behrman RE, Hal BJ, editors. Nelson textbook of pediatrics. 18th edition. Philadelphia, PA: Saunders Elsevier Inc; 2007. p. 1263–9.
12. Organization WH. Global health sector strategy on Sexually Transmitted Infections, 2016-2021. 2016. https://www.who.int/reproductivehealth/publications/rtis/ghss-stis/en/. [Accessed 1 July 2022].
13. Harfouche M, Abu-Hijleh FM, James C, et al. Epidemiology of herpes simplex virus type 2 in sub-Saharan Africa: Systematic review, meta-analyses, and meta-regressions. EClinicalMedicine 2021;35:100876.
14. Harfouche M, Chemaitelly H, Abu-Raddad LJ. Herpes simplex virus type 1 epidemiology in Africa: systematic review, meta-analyses, and meta-regressions. J Infect 2019;79(4):289–99.

15. Looker KJ, Magaret AS, May MT, et al. First estimates of the global and regional incidence of neonatal herpes infection. Lancet Glob Health 2017;5(3):e300–9.
16. Pinninti SG, Kimberlin DW. Preventing herpes simplex virus in the newborn. Clin Perinatol 2014;41(4):945–55.
17. Management of Genital Herpes in Pregnancy: ACOG practice bulletinacog practice bulletin, number 220. Obstet Gynecol 2020;135(5):e193–202.
18. Brown ZA, Wald A, Morrow RA, et al. Effect of serologic status and cesarean delivery on transmission rates of herpes simplex virus from mother to infant. JAMA 2003;289(2):203–9.
19. Fernandes ND, Arya K, Ward R. Congenital Herpes Simplex. StatPearls [Internet]. Treasure Island (FL): StatPearls Publishing; 2022. p. 1360–5.
20. Stanberry LR. Herpes simplex virus. In: Nelson textbook of pediatrics. 18th edition. Saunders Elsevier Inc; 2007.
21. Kiguen AX, Marramá M, Ruiz S, et al. Prevalence, risk factors and molecular characterization of Chlamydia trachomatis in pregnant women from Córdoba, Argentina: a prospective study. PLoS One 2019;14(5):e0217245.
22. Graham S, Smith LW, Fairley CK, et al. Prevalence of chlamydia, gonorrhoea, syphilis and trichomonas in Aboriginal and Torres Strait Islander Australians: a systematic review and meta-analysis. Sex Health 2016;13(2):99–113.
23. Morré SA, Rozendaal L, van Valkengoed IG, et al. Urogenital Chlamydia trachomatis serovars in men and women with a symptomatic or asymptomatic infection: an association with clinical manifestations? J Clin Microbiol 2000;38(6):2292–6.
24. La Scolea LJ JR, Paroski JS, Burzynski L, et al. Chlamydia trachomatis infection in infants delivered by cesarean section. Clin Pediatr 1984;23(2):118–20.
25. Adachi K, Nielsen-Saines K, Klausner JD. Chlamydia trachomatis infection in pregnancy: the global challenge of preventing adverse pregnancy and infant outcomes in Sub-Saharan Africa and Asia. Biomed Res Int 2016;2016:1–21.
26. Ahmadi A, Ramazanzadeh R, Sayehmiri K, et al. Association of Chlamydia trachomatis infections with preterm delivery; a systematic review and meta-analysis. BMC Pregnancy Childbirth 2018;18(1):240.
27. Olson-Chen C, Balaram K, Hackney DN. Chlamydia trachomatis and adverse pregnancy outcomes: meta-analysis of patients with and without infection. Matern Child Health J 2018;22(6):812–21.
28. Reekie J, Roberts C, Preen D, et al. Chlamydia trachomatis and the risk of spontaneous preterm birth, babies who are born small for gestational age, and stillbirth: a population-based cohort study. Lancet Infect Dis 2018. https://doi.org/10.1016/s1473-3099(18)30045-8.
29. Chirenje ZM, Dhibi N, Handsfield HH, et al. The etiology of vaginal discharge syndrome in zimbabwe: results from the zimbabwe STI etiology study. Sex Transm Dis 2018;45(6):422–8.
30. Mbah CE, Jasani A, Aaron KJ, et al. Association between chlamydia trachomatis, neisseria gonorrhea, mycoplasma genitalium, and trichomonas vaginalis and secondary infertility in cameroon: a case-control study. PLoS One 2022;17(2):e0263186.
31. Laga M, Nzanze H, Brunham R, et al. Epidemiology of ophthalmia neonatorum in Kenya. Lancet 1986;328(8516):1145–9.
32. Pourabbas B, Rezaei Z, Mardaneh J, et al. Prevalence of Chlamydia trachomatis and Neisseria gonorrhoeae infections among pregnant women and eye colonization of their neonates at birth time, Shiraz, Southern Iran. BMC Infect Dis 2018;18(1):1–4.

33. Darville T. Pelvic inflammatory disease due to neisseria gonorrhoeae and chlamydia trachomatis: immune evasion mechanisms and pathogenic disease pathways. J Infect Dis 2021;224(12 Suppl 2):S39–46.

34. Tsevat DG, Wiesenfeld HC, Parks C, et al. Sexually transmitted diseases and infertility. Am J Obstet Gynecol 2017;216(1):1–9.

35. Adachi K, Klausner JD, Xu J, et al. Chlamydia trachomatis and Neisseria gonorrhoeae in HIV-infected Pregnant Women and Adverse Infant Outcomes. Pediatr Infect Dis J 2016;35(8):894–900.

36. Bell TA, Grayston JT, Krohn MA, et al. Randomized trial of silver nitrate, erythromycin, and no eye prophylaxis for the prevention of conjunctivitis among newborns not at risk for gonococcal ophthalmitis. Eye Prophylaxis Study Group. Pediatrics 1993;92(6):755–60.

37. Nyemba DC, Haddison EC, Wang C, et al. Prevalence of curable STIs and bacterial vaginosis during pregnancy in sub-Saharan Africa: a systematic review and meta-analysis. Sex Transm Infect 2021. https://doi.org/10.1136/sextrans-2021-055057.

38. Sutton M, Sternberg M, Koumans EH, et al. The prevalence of Trichomonas vaginalis infection among reproductive-age women in the United States, 2001-2004. Clin Infect Dis 2007;45(10):1319–26.

39. Kamal AM, Ahmed AK, Mowafy NME-S, et al. Incidence of antenatal trichomoniasis and evaluation of its role as a cause of preterm birth in pregnant women referring to Minia University Hospital, EGYPT. Iranian J Parasitol 2018;13(1):58.

40. Carter JE, Whithaus KC. Neonatal respiratory tract involvement by Trichomonas vaginalis: a case report and review of the literature. Am J Trop Med Hyg 2008; 78(1):17–9.

41. Bruins MJ, van Straaten IL, Ruijs GJ. Respiratory disease and Trichomonas vaginalis in premature newborn twins. Pediatr Infect Dis J 2013;32(9):1029–30.

42. Peebles K, Velloza J, Balkus JE, et al. High global burden and costs of bacterial vaginosis: a systematic review and meta-analysis. Sex Transm Dis 2019;46(5): 304–11.

43. Kenyon C, Colebunders R, Crucitti T. The global epidemiology of bacterial vaginosis: a systematic review. Am J Obstet Gynecol 2013;209(6):505–23.

44. Goto A, Nguyen QV, Pham NM, et al. Prevalence of and factors associated with reproductive tract infections among pregnant women in ten communes in Nghe An Province, Vietnam. J Epidemiol 2005;15(5):163–72.

45. Muzny CA, Schwebke JR. Pathogenesis of bacterial vaginosis: discussion of current hypotheses. J Infect Dis 2016;214(Suppl 1):S1–5. https://doi.org/10.1093/infdis/jiw121.

46. Klebanoff MA, Schwebke JR, Zhang J, et al. Vulvovaginal symptoms in women with bacterial vaginosis. Obstet Gynecol 2004;104(2):267–72.

47. Laxmi U, Agrawal S, Raghunandan C, et al. Association of bacterial vaginosis with adverse fetomaternal outcome in women with spontaneous preterm labor: a prospective cohort study. J Matern Fetal Neonatal Med 2012;25(1):64–7.

48. Haahr T, Ersbøll AS, Karlsen MA, et al. Treatment of bacterial vaginosis in pregnancy in order to reduce the risk of spontaneous preterm delivery - a clinical recommendation. Acta Obstet Gynecol Scand 2016;95(8):850–60.

49. Juliana NCA, Suiters MJM, Al-Nasiry S, et al. The Association between vaginal microbiota dysbiosis, bacterial vaginosis, and aerobic vaginitis, and adverse pregnancy outcomes of women living in sub-saharan africa: a systematic review. Front Public Health 2020;8:567885.

50. Mulinganya G, De Vulder A, Bisimwa G, et al. Prevalence, risk factors and adverse pregnancy outcomes of second trimester bacterial vaginosis among pregnant women in Bukavu, Democratic Republic of the Congo. PLoS One 2021;16(10):e0257939.

51. Dingens AS, Fairfortune TS, Reed S, et al. Bacterial vaginosis and adverse outcomes among full-term infants: a cohort study. BMC Pregnancy Childbirth 2016;16(1):278.

52. Guise JM, Mahon SM, Aickin M, et al. Screening for bacterial vaginosis in pregnancy. Am J Prev Med 2001;20(3 Suppl):62–72.

53. Owens DK, Davidson KW, Krist AH, et al. Screening for Bacterial Vaginosis in Pregnant Persons to Prevent Preterm Delivery: US Preventive Services Task Force Recommendation Statement. JAMA 2020;323(13):1286–92.

54. Brabant G. [Bacterial vaginosis and spontaneous preterm birth]. J Gynecol Obstet Biol Reprod (Paris) 2016;45(10):1247–60. Vaginose bactérienne et prématurité spontanée.

55. Broache M, Cammarata CL, Stonebraker E, et al. Performance of a vaginal panel assay compared with the clinical diagnosis of vaginitis. Obstet Gynecol 2021; 138(6):853–9.

56. Gonçalves B, Ferreira C, Alves CT, et al. Vulvovaginal candidiasis: epidemiology, microbiology and risk factors. Crit Rev Microbiol 2016;42(6):905–27.

57. Denning DW, Kneale M, Sobel JD, et al. Global burden of recurrent vulvovaginal candidiasis: a systematic review. Lancet Infect Dis 2018;18(11):e339–47.

58. Yano J, Sobel JD, Nyirjesy P, et al. Current patient perspectives of vulvovaginal candidiasis: incidence, symptoms, management and post-treatment outcomes. BMC Womens Health 2019;19(1):48.

59. Boyd Tressler A, Markwei M, Fortin C, et al. Risks for recurrent vulvovaginal candidiasis caused by non-albicans candida versus candida albicans. J Womens Health (Larchmt) 2021;30(11):1588–96.

60. Wenjin Q, Yifu S. Epidemiological study on vaginal Candida glabrata isolated from pregnant women. Scand J Infect Dis 2006;38(1):49–54.

61. Roberts CL, Rickard K, Kotsiou G, et al. Treatment of asymptomatic vaginal candidiasis in pregnancy to prevent preterm birth: an open-label pilot randomized controlled trial. BMC Pregnancy Childbirth 2011;11:18.

62. Konadu DG, Owusu-Ofori A, Yidana Z, et al. Prevalence of vulvovaginal candidiasis, bacterial vaginosis and trichomoniasis in pregnant women attending antenatal clinic in the middle belt of Ghana. BMC Pregnancy Childbirth 2019; 19(1):341.

63. Jafarzadeh L, Ranjbar M, Nazari T, et al. Vulvovaginal candidiasis: an overview of mycological, clinical, and immunological aspects. J Obstet Gynaecol Res 2022. https://doi.org/10.1111/jog.15267.

64. Cotch MF, Hillier SL, Gibbs RS, et al. Epidemiology and outcomes associated with moderate to heavy Candida colonization during pregnancy. Vaginal Infections and Prematurity Study Group. Am J Obstet Gynecol 1998;178(2):374–80.

65. Zhang Z, Zhang X, Zhou YY, et al. The safety of oral fluconazole during the first trimester of pregnancy: a systematic review and meta-analysis. BJOG 2019; 126(13):1546–52.

66. Budani MC, Fensore S, Di Marzio M, et al. Maternal use of fluconazole and congenital malformations in the progeny: a meta-analysis of the literature. Reprod Toxicol 2021;100:42–51.

67. Zisova LG, Chokoeva AA, Amaliev GI, et al. Vulvovaginal candidiasis in pregnant women and its importance for candida colonization of newborns. Folia Med (Plovdiv) 2016;58(2):108–14.
68. Goller JL, De Livera AM, Fairley CK, et al. Population attributable fraction of pelvic inflammatory disease associated with chlamydia and gonorrhoea: a cross-sectional analysis of Australian sexual health clinic data. Sex Transm Infect 2016;92(7):525–31.
69. Sharma H, Tal R, Clark NA, et al. Microbiota and pelvic inflammatory disease. Semin Reprod Med 2014;32(1):43–9.
70. Wiesenfeld HC, Hillier SL, Meyn LA, et al. Subclinical pelvic inflammatory disease and infertility. Obstet Gynecol 2012;120(1):37–43.
71. Trent M, Bass D, Ness RB, et al. Recurrent PID, subsequent STI, and reproductive health outcomes: findings from the PID evaluation and clinical health (PEACH) study. Sex Transm Dis 2011;38(9):879–81.
72. Centers for Disease Control and Prevention. Sexually Transmitted Disease Surveillance 2019. Atlanta: U.S: Department of Health and Human Services; 2021.
73. Chen MJ, Kim CR, Whitehouse KC, et al. Development, updates, and future directions of the World Health Organization Selected Practice Recommendations for Contraceptive Use. Int J Gynaecol Obstet 2017;136(2):113–9.
74. Organization WH. Guidelines for the management of symptomatic sexually transmitted infections. 2021. https://www.who.int/publications/i/item/9789240024168. [Accessed 1 July 2022].
75. Sonkar SC, Wasnik K, Kumar A, et al. Evaluating the utility of syndromic case management for three sexually transmitted infections in women visiting hospitals in Delhi, India. Sci Rep 2017;7(1):1465.
76. Peters R, Klausner JD, de Vos L, et al. Aetiological testing compared with syndromic management for sexually transmitted infections in HIV-infected pregnant women in South Africa: a non-randomised prospective cohort study. BJOG 2021; 128(8):1335–42.
77. Wi TE, Ndowa FJ, Ferreyra C, et al. Diagnosing sexually transmitted infections in resource-constrained settings: challenges and ways forward. J Int AIDS Soc 2019;22(Suppl 6):e25343.

Prevention of Cervical Cancer in Low-Resource African Settings

Masangu Mulongo, MBBCh[a], Carla J. Chibwesha, MD, MSc[a,b,*]

KEYWORDS

- Human papillomavirus • HPV • Cervical cancer screening
- Cervical cancer prevention • Africa • Low- and middle-income countries • LMICs

KEY POINTS

- Cervical cancer is the second most common cancer among women and approximately 85% of the global disease burden occurs in low- and middle-income countries (LMICs).
- Cervical cancer incidence, mortality, and disparities in cancer outcomes are projected to rise exponentially in the coming decades, particularly in LMICs.
- In 2020, the World Health Organization (WHO) renewed its commitment to reducing the burden of cervical cancer through a *Global Strategy to Accelerate the Elimination of Cervical Cancer as a Public Health Problem.*
- In support of the ambitious agenda set out in the WHO strategy, global efforts to eliminate cervical cancer are currently focused on expanding access to human papillomavirus vaccination and cervical cancer screening, as well as improving linkage to treatment for women with preinvasive and invasive cervical disease.

THE BURDEN OF CERVICAL CANCER IN AFRICA

Globally, breast cancer is the most prevalent cancer among women, with cervical cancer ranked fourth overall but surpassing breast cancer in many African countries.[1,2] Among an estimated 604,000 new cases of cervical cancer worldwide in 2020, approximately 85% of cases occurred among women living in Africa, Latin America, and Southeast Asia.[1]

Age-standardized incidence and mortality from cervical cancer are highest in Africa. For example, the age-standardized incidence of cervical cancer is 36 per 100,000 women in Southern Africa, compared with a rate of 6 per 100,000 women in North

[a] Clinical HIV Research Unit, Wits Health Consortium, Themba Lethu Clinic, Helen Joseph Hospital, Perth Road, Auckland Park, Johannesburg 2092, South Africa; [b] Division of Global Women's Health, Department of Obstetrics and Gynecology, University of North Carolina at Chapel Hill, 3009 Old Clinic Building, Campus Box 7577, Chapel Hill, NC, USA
* Corresponding author. Division of Global Women's Health, Department of Obstetrics and Gynecology, University of North Carolina at Chapel Hill, 3009 Old Clinic Building, Campus Box 7577, Chapel Hill, NC 27599-7577.
E-mail address: carla_chibwesha@med.unc.edu

Obstet Gynecol Clin N Am 49 (2022) 771–781
https://doi.org/10.1016/j.ogc.2022.08.008
0889-8545/22/© 2022 Elsevier Inc. All rights reserved.

America and 7 per 100,000 in Western Europe.[3] Differences in mortality from cervical cancer between countries in the Global North and South are equally concerning. The International Agency for Research on Cancer currently estimates that the age-standardized mortality from cervical cancer is 21 per 100,000 women in Southern Africa compared with a rate of 2 per 100,000 women in North America and Western Europe.[3] These disparities are only expected to rise.[4]

Although the broader backdrop of inequality is beyond the scope of this article, the vast disparities in cervical cancer incidence and mortality between low- and middle-income countries (LMICs) and high-income countries can largely be attributed to differences in health care access more broadly, as well as to specific barriers to cervical cancer screening and treatment. These barriers include gaps in policy and public health programming, scarcity of trained clinical and laboratory personnel, under-resourced health facilities, and a lack of awareness that cervical cancer is preventable at the community level that, in turn, leads to low uptake of services.[5,6]

Simply put, too few African girls are vaccinated against human papillomavirus (HPV),[7] and not enough women are screened (or treated) for cervical disease.[8] In addition to the scarcity of HPV vaccination and population-based cervical cancer screening programs,[9] the generalized HIV epidemic in sub-Saharan Africa contributes to the region's high cervical cancer rates.[10] Stigma, lack of knowledge about cancer, lack of awareness of the benefits of screening and early detection, long waiting times at health facilities, and poor linkage between screening and treatment services also play a role.[11–13]

In 2020, the World Health Organization (WHO) launched an ambitious call to action through its *Global Strategy to Accelerate the Elimination of Cervical Cancer as a Public Health Problem*. The strategy outlines the so-called 90 to 70 to 90 targets for 2030, which are intended to put countries on the path to reducing the age-standardized incidence of cervical cancer from 13 per 100,000 to 4 per 100,000 women worldwide. This includes (1) 90% of girls vaccinated against HPV by age 15 years; (2) 70% of women screened for cervical cancer by age 35 and 45 years; and (3) 90% of women with precancer or invasive cancer appropriately treated. WHO's impact modeling projects remarkable benefits from achieving the 90 to 70 to 90 targets in LMICs by 2030. Cervical cancer incidence would fall 42% by 2045% and 97% by 2120, whereas 300,000 cervical cancer deaths would be averted by 2030, over 14 million deaths by 2070, and over 62 million by 2120.[14]

HUMAN PAPILLOMAVIRUS AND THE PATHOGENESIS OF CERVICAL CANCER

High-risk HPV (hrHPV) is the necessary cause of virtually all cervical cancers.[15,16] Following infection of the metaplastic cells of the cervical transformation zone, HPV integrates into the host genome and inactivates the tumor suppressors p53 and retinoblastoma. This leads to uncontrolled cellular proliferation and the accumulation of mutations.[17] The most common cervical lesions are of squamous cell origin, and the precancerous state known as cervical intraepithelial neoplasia (CIN) is graded by the proportion of abnormal epithelium.

Although all sexually active individuals are exposed to HPV over the course of their lifetimes, most infections are cleared by the immune system. Genetic predisposition, hormonal factors, host immune response, and tobacco use all affect susceptibility to persistent HPV infection and progression to cancer.[18] Of more than 100 HPV types, at least 14 are considered "high risk" or oncogenic, with HPV 16 and 18 accounting for approximately 70% of cervical cancers worldwide.[19]

HUMAN IMMUNODEFICIENCY VIRUS AND CERVICAL CANCER

HIV infection markedly increases a woman's lifetime risk of persistent hrHPV infection and cervical disease.[20–23] Women living with HIV are significantly more likely to be diagnosed with precancer and 6 times more likely to be develop invasive cervical cancer.[24–26] Although the introduction of combination antiretroviral therapy (ART) has led to remarkable reductions in the incidence of cancers such as Kaposi's sarcoma and non-Hodgkin lymphoma among individuals living with HIV, the role of ART in reducing the incidence of cervical cancer and its precursor lesions remains unclear.[27]

A 2021 meta-analysis estimating the cervical cancer burden associated with HIV found that although 1 in 20 cervical cancers is attributable to HIV globally, as many as 1 in 5 cervical cancers in sub-Saharan Africa are attributable to HIV.[10] Sub-Saharan Africa is the global epicenter of the HIV pandemic: approximately 21 of the 38 million people currently living with HIV are African and 14 million are African women.[28] As increasing numbers of women initiate ART in sub-Saharan Africa, we anticipate that longer life expectancies for these women will be coupled with a rising burden of chronic diseases, including cervical cancer.[29,30]

HUMAN PAPILLOMAVIRUS VACCINATION: PRIMARY PREVENTION

There are currently three HPV vaccines being marketed in many countries throughout the world: a bivalent, a quadrivalent, and a nonavalent vaccine. All three vaccines are highly effective in preventing infection with HPV 16 and 18 and in preventing precancerous cervical lesions caused by these virus types.[31–33] The nonavalent vaccine provides additional protection against HPV 31, 33, 45, 52, and 58. The safety of all three vaccines has been shown in clinical trial data and post-marketing surveillance conducted on several continents.[18]

Global cost-effectiveness analyses using country-based evidence suggests that vaccinating preadolescent girls is usually cost-effective, particularly in resource-constrained settings where alternative cervical cancer prevention and control measures often have limited coverage.[18] WHO recommends that HPV vaccines should be included in national immunization programs, as part of a coordinated and comprehensive strategy to prevent cervical cancer, with the primary target group girls 9 to 14 years of age, before sexual activity. In April 2022, the WHO Strategic Advisory Group of Experts on Immunization (SAGE) evaluated the evidence on the efficacy of single-dose vaccine schedules and concluded that a single-dose HPV vaccine delivers protection comparable to two-dose schedules.[34] The option for a single dose of the vaccine is less costly, less resource intensive, and easier to administer, allowing for financial and human resources to be redirected to other health priorities. The SAGE committee recommended prioritizing multi-age cohort catch-up of missed and older cohorts of girls and updating dose schedules for HPV as follows:

- One or two-dose (0, 6 months) schedule for the primary target of girls aged 9 to 14
- One or two-dose schedule (0, 6 months) for young women aged 15 to 20
- Two doses with a 6-month interval for women older than 21

Immunocompromised individuals, including those with HIV, should receive at least two doses and three doses if possible.

Table 1
Three approaches to cervical cancer screening and future tests

Molecular	Cytologic	Visual Inspection
Nucleic acid amplification tests (NAAT)[a] • High-risk HVP DNA/NAAT • mRNA DNA methylation[b] Protein biomarkers[b] • HPV antibodies • Oncoproteins	Conventional Pap smear[a] Liquid-based cytology (LBC)[b] Dual staining to identify p16 and Ki-67[a]	Visual inspection with acetic acid or with Lugol's iodine (VIA/VILI)[a] • Naked eye • Magnified by colposcope or camera Automated visual evaluation of digital images[b]

[a] Current tests
[b] Tests under evaluation (future tests)
  From WHO guideline for screening and treatment of cervical pre-cancer lesions for cervical cancer prevention, second edition. Geneva: World Health Organization; 2021. Licence: CC BY-NC-SA 3.0 IGO.

SCREENING FOR CERVICAL CANCER: SECONDARY PREVENTION
Limitations of Cervical Cancer Screening Using Cytology and Visual Methods

Cervical cancer is preventable through vaccination (primary prevention) against HPV and/or screening (secondary prevention) for cervical precancer, known as CIN grade 2/3 (CIN 2/3) or adenocarcinoma in situ (AIS).[35–37] Cytology screening (**Table 1**) (Pap smear) has traditionally been the gold standard for secondary prevention of cervical cancer. Over the past 50 years, cytology screening has significantly impacted cancer prevention and saved lives of millions of women living in high-income countries.[38]

The interval between HPV acquisition and progression to invasive cancer is usually 20 years or longer and CIN2/3 and AIS, the most immediate precursors of invasive disease, progress to invasive cancer over a period of 5 to 10 years,[39] This prolonged natural history offers an extended window to detect the presence of precancerous lesions and prevent progression to invasive cancer. The rationale behind Pap smear screening programs is that women found to have cytologic abnormalities are referred for diagnostic confirmation through colposcopy and cervical biopsy. If CIN2/3, AIS, or invasive cancer is confirmed, women are then treated. Precancer lesions can generally be cured using current surgical approaches (excision or ablation),[40] although cure is often harder to achieve in HIV-infected women.[41] Among women with invasive cancer, survival rates for early-stage cancer are more than 90% in countries with advanced care. However, survival drops substantially when diagnosis occurs at later stages and resources and expertise for management even in early stages is limited geographically.[9,42]

Cytology screening is both logistically complex and costly to implement. It requires multiple visits (for screening and to obtain test results, confirmatory diagnosis, and treatment), resulting in long waiting times and follow-up losses.[43] Cytology programs also rely on expensive laboratory infrastructure and well-trained clinical and laboratory personnel. These requirements all create obstacles to the successful implementation and scale-up of cytology screening in LMIC settings.[38]

To overcome the limitations of cytology, visual inspection with acetic acid (VIA) and Lugol's iodine (VILI) is used in many African health systems.[44] With VIA, for example, cervical lesions develop a white color (called acetowhite lesions) when 5% acetic acid (household vinegar) is applied to the cervical epithelium, whereas healthy cervical tissue remains pink. As the screening results are available in real time, women with acetowhite lesions can be offered same-day treatment.[45,46] VIA programs are also commonly led by nurses and other mid-level clinical providers, making them easier to scale in settings with limited human resources for health. VILI is based on similar principles.[47]

Although VIA is more affordable than cytology and allows for same-day treatment, acetowhitening is not specific for cervical cancer or its precursors. Noncancerous conditions, such as areas of immature squamous metaplasia and cervicitis, also result in the cervical epithelium turning white upon the application of acetic acid. Visual screening is ultimately a subjective method, with high inter-operator variability, resulting in considerable rates of false positives, false negatives, and overtreatment.[48,49] In addition, VIA/VILI should not be relied upon when the whole transformation zone cannot be visualized, which is typical after menopause. A recent systematic review and meta-analysis assessed the diagnostic accuracy of smartphone images of the cervix with VIA/VILI, used to capture and share images in an effort to improve sensitivity and interobserver variability. With CIN2+ as the reference standard, sensitivity was 75%, specificity was 62%, negative predictive value was 94% and positive predictive value was 27%.[50] The authors concluded that this technique may provide additional support to health care providers delivering care in low-resource settings. Although VIA is suitable in certain settings and circumstances, limitations in its accuracy and its subjectivity have resulted in only a modest impact on reducing the cervical disease burden in the most affected areas.[43]

With both cytology and visual screening having relatively low sensitivity for detecting precancer and invasive cervical cancer, repeat screening at short intervals (3 years) is recommended by WHO.[51]

Primary Human Papillomavirus Screening

Screening tests that detect the presence of hrHPV are highly sensitive, identifying nearly all cases of precancer and invasive cervical cancer.[52,53] Numerous cohort studies and randomized trials have shown that HPV testing accurately identifies more cervical disease at the first screening and also leads to a reduction in subsequent cases of precancer and invasive cancer,[51,54–58] including among women living with HIV.[59] In 2021, WHO endorsed HPV testing for cervical cancer screening in its updated clinical guidance on cervical cancer prevention.[60] Other international guidelines also recommended primary HPV screening in both high- and low-resources settings,[61,62] and national guidelines in LMICs are gradually being updated to include plans to transition to primary HPV screening from cytology or visual screening.

There are now more than 10 commercially available HPV DNA and RNA tests suitable for cervical cancer screening.[63] Although pricing for HPV tests has decreased as the market has expanded in recent years, many remain cost prohibitive for African health systems.[53] Assays such as careHPV (QIAGEN, Netherlands),[64] Xpert HPV (Cepheid, USA),[65] and AmpFire HPV (Atila BioSystems, USA)[66] are lower in cost. However, all three tests still require laboratory infrastructure, and their utilization remains constrained by affordability. To make primary HPV screening a reality across resource-limited settings, there is an urgent need to develop more affordable point-of-care and/or near-patient HPV tests.

An added benefit of primary HPV screening is that samples can be self-collected with a sensitivity equivalent to provider-collected sampling.[67] Self-sampling can either be done in clinical settings or in a woman's home and has the potential to increase cervical cancer screening coverage—particularly in underserved areas, where pelvic examinations may not be performed routinely and women may not be actively engaged in care. HPV self-sampling may also reduce the burden on health care

Table 2 Summary recommendations from WHO	
WHO suggests using either of the following strategies for cervical cancer prevention among the general population of women	HPV DNA Detection in a Screen-and-treat Approach Starting at the age of 30 y with Regular screening every 5–10 y. HPV DNA detection in a screen, triage and treat approach starting at the age of 30 y with regular screening every 5–10 y.
WHO suggests using the following strategy for cervical cancer prevention among women living with HIV	HPV DNA detection in a screen, triage and treat approach starting at the age of 25 y with regular screening every 3 to 5 y.

From WHO guideline for screening and treatment of cervical pre-cancer lesions for cervical cancer prevention, second edition. Geneva: World Health Organization; 2021. Licence: CC BY-NC-SA 3.0 IGO.

providers and, in so doing, reduce the health care costs associated with cervical cancer screening.[68,69]

Over 30 randomized trials and observational studies have evaluated self-collected HPV testing. A 2019 meta-analysis found that HPV self-sampling increased the uptake of cervical cancer screening, with the most robust results coming from studies in which HPV tests were either sent directly to women's home or provided through door-to-door outreach campaigns.[70] However, most studies have been conducted in high-income settings, where linkage to diagnostic confirmation and treatment is more readily available. Developing implementation strategies for HPV self-sampling in LMICs is therefore a high priority. Current screening recommendations by WHO prioritize women aged 30 to 49 in the general population and aged 25 to 49 in those with HIV infection. Women who have had prior treatment for confirmed CIN 2+ or AIS or as a result of a positive screening test should receive a follow-up HPV test at 12 months .

To be effective, cervical cancer screening programs must achieve high rates of screening coverage and ensure that women who screen positive are managed correctly, and receiving timely treatment. WHO currently recommends primary HPV screening with or without triage before treatment (**Table 2**).[60] Programs that omit the triage step use a strategy known as HPV "test-and-treat". Modeled after the so-called VIA/VILI "screen-and-treat" method, primary HPV screening is followed by same-day treatment for women who screen positive without further confirmation. Although programs that include a triage step—for diagnostic confirmation of precancer—often do this using colposcopy (and cervical biopsy), this approach carries many of the same limitations of cytology-based screening, including higher cost, scarcity of trained health care personnel for colposcopy and pathology, and inconvenience to women who must return for at least three visits (ie, screening, diagnostic confirmation, and treatment). VIA/VILI may also be used to triage women after a positive HPV test result and in both the "test-and-treat" or the "test, triage, and treat" strategies, and can be used to assess eligibility for ablative treatment.

TREATMENT OF PRECANCEROUS LESIONS

Cervical precancerous lesions can be treated by ablative methods that include the destruction of abnormal tissue by burning or freezing (cryotherapy, thermal ablation) and surgical excision of abnormal tissue (loop electrosurgical excision procedure [LEEP]) or cervical conization. In LMICs the most commonly available treatment is ablation with cryotherapy. Cryotherapy generally uses compressed nitrous oxide or carbon dioxide gas, which can present challenges in due to the high cost and infrastructure required for transport and maintenance. New cryotechnologies (eg, CryoPen and CryoPop) are more portable, less expensive, and have less reliance on infrastructure for electricity or gas. Thermal ablation is a technology that uses a heated probe to destroy abnormal tissue, typically at temperatures 100°C to 120°C and is increasingly being adopted as an alternative to cryotherapy. Both cryotherapy and thermal ablation can be used by mid-level providers and are commonly used in screen-and-treat or test-and-treat programs.[71] However, ablative treatments should not be used in women in whom the transformation zone is not visible, which is typical after menopause.

LEEP uses a wire loop heated with an electric current to excise abnormal tissue and is necessary when the lesion is too large to be treated effectively by ablation. LEEP can be performed under local anesthesia on an outpatient basis. Cervical conization in LMICs is generally reserved for more advanced or recurrent precancerous lesions, especially those involving disease in the endocervical canal, and is done under general or regional anesthesia. Both LEEP and conization require more highly trained providers. Both LEEP and conization also result in a pathologic specimen that can assess severity of disease and confirm complete excision, but this may be of limited value in settings where there is a scarcity of trained pathology personnel and equipment.

SUMMARY

Prevention of cervical cancer and achievement of the targets set by WHO to accelerate the elimination of cervical cancer requires attention to both primary and secondary prevention strategies. Girls and young women require broad access to HPV vaccination for the primary prevention of cervical cancer. Newer recommendations for a single dose HPV vaccine option in most cases will make HPV vaccination less expensive and easier to implement.

Organized cytology screening programs have resulted in marked declines in cervical cancer incidence and mortality across much of the industrialized world. In LMICs, however, implementation of cytology screening has been limited by logistical challenges and high costs. Moreover, visual screening programs are inherently subjective and have not reduced the incidence and mortality from cervical cancer in the highest-burden countries in Africa. For secondary prevention, screening programs need to expand their use of primary HPV screening and, as the availability of HPV (and other molecular) tests expands, new assays must be accurate, affordable, and simple enough to scale up rapidly across underserved regions in Africa. Finally, it is important to build efficient mechanisms for both recall and linkage to high-quality treatment.

FUNDING

Dr C.J. Chibwesha is funded by the United States National Institutes of Health to study implementation barriers to cervical cancer screening in South Africa, HPV self-sampling, and combination treatment approaches for cervical precancer in women living with HIV (R21TW011715, U54CA254564, and R01CA250850). Dr. C.J. Chibwesha is also funded by the South African Medical Research Council to study HPV self-sampling. Trainee support for Dr M. Mulongo was provided by the United States National Institutes of Health (D43TW009340 and U54CA254564).

DISCLOSURE

The authors declare no commercial or other financial conflicts of interest.

REFERENCES

1. Sung H, Ferlay J, Siegel RL, et al. Global Cancer Statistics 2020: GLOBOCAN Estimates of Incidence and Mortality Worldwide for 36 Cancers in 185 Countries. CA Cancer J Clin 2021;71(3):209–49.

2. Bray F, Ren JS, Masuyer E, et al. Global estimates of cancer prevalence for 27 sites in the adult population in 2008. Int J Cancer 2013;132(5):1133–45.

3. International Agency for Research on Cancer. GLOBOCAN: Cancer Today. Available at: https://gco.iarc.fr/today/home. August 2022. Accessed August 12, 2022.

4. International Agency for Research on Cancer. GLOBOCAN: Cancer Tomorrow. Available at: https://gco.iarc.fr/tomorrow/en. Accessed August 12, 2022.

5. Denny L. Control of cancer of the cervix in low- and middle-income countries. Ann Surg Oncol 2015;22(3):728–33.

6. Sankaranarayanan R. Screening for cancer in low- and middle-income countries. Ann Glob Health 2014;80(5):412–7.

7. Oberlin AM, Rahangdale L, Chinula L, et al. Making HPV vaccination available to girls everywhere. Int J Gynaecol Obstet 2018;143(3):267–76.

8. Gakidou E, Nordhagen S, Obermeyer Z. Coverage of cervical cancer screening in 57 countries: low average levels and large inequalities. Plos Med 2008;5(6): e132.

9. International Agency for Research on Cancer. Cervical cancer elimination in Africa: where are we now and where do we need to be?. Available at: https://www.uicc.org/sites/main/files/atoms/files/UICC-Cervical_Cancer_in_Africa_FA_Single.pdf. Accessed August 12, 2022.

10. Stelzle D, Tanaka LF, Lee KK, et al. Estimates of the global burden of cervical cancer associated with HIV. Lancet Glob Health 2021;9(2):e161–9.

11. Francis SA, Nelson J, Liverpool J, et al. Examining attitudes and knowledge about HPV and cervical cancer risk among female clinic attendees in Johannesburg, South Africa. Vaccine 2010;28(50):8026–32.

12. Chirwa S, Mwanahamuntu M, Kapambwe S, et al. Myths and misconceptions about cervical cancer among Zambian women: rapid assessment by peer educators. Glob Health Promot 2010;17(2 Suppl):47–50.

13. Adewumi K, Nishimura H, Oketch SY, et al. Barriers and Facilitators to Cervical Cancer Screening in Western Kenya: a Qualitative Study. J Cancer Educ 2021. https://doi.org/10.1007/s13187-020-01928-6.

14. World Health Organization. Global strategy to accelerate the elimination of cervical cancer as a public health problem. Available at: https://www.who.int/publications/i/item/9789240014107. Accessed August 12, 2022.

15. Bosch FX, Manos MM, Munoz N, et al. Prevalence of human papillomavirus in cervical cancer: a worldwide perspective. International biological study on cervical cancer (IBSCC) Study Group. J Natl Cancer Inst 1995;87(11):796–802.

16. Walboomers JM, Jacobs MV, Manos MM, et al. Human papillomavirus is a necessary cause of invasive cervical cancer worldwide. J Pathol 1999;189(1):12–9.

17. Crosbie EJ, Einstein MH, Franceschi S, et al. Human papillomavirus and cervical cancer. Lancet 2013;382(9895):889–99.

18. World Health Organization. Human papillomavirus vaccines: WHO position paper, May 2017-Recommendations. Vaccine 2017;35(43):5753–5.

19. Castellsague X. Natural history and epidemiology of HPV infection and cervical cancer. Gynecol Oncol 2008;110(3 Suppl 2):S4–7.

20. Denny LA, Franceschi S, de Sanjose S, et al. Human papillomavirus, human immunodeficiency virus and immunosuppression. Vaccine 2012;30(Suppl 5): F168–74.

21. Clifford GM, Goncalves MA, Franceschi S, et al. Human papillomavirus types among women infected with HIV: a meta-analysis. AIDS 2006;20(18):2337–44.

22. Denny L, Boa R, Williamson AL, et al. Human papillomavirus infection and cervical disease in human immunodeficiency virus-1-infected women. Obstet Gynecol 2008;111(6):1380–7.

23. Singh DK, Anastos K, Hoover DR, et al. Human papillomavirus infection and cervical cytology in HIV-infected and HIV-uninfected Rwandan women. J Infect Dis 2009;199(12):1851–61.

24. Chirenje ZM. HIV and cancer of the cervix. Best Pract Res Clin Obstet Gynaecol 2005;19(2):269–76.

25. Einstein MH, Phaeton R. Issues in cervical cancer incidence and treatment in HIV. Curr Opin Oncol 2010;22(5):449–55.

26. Castle PE, Einstein MH, Sahasrabuddhe VV. Cervical cancer prevention and control in women living with human immunodeficiency virus. CA Cancer J Clin 2021; 71(6):505–26.

27. Franceschi S, Jaffe H. Cervical cancer screening of women living with HIV infection: a must in the era of antiretroviral therapy. Clin Infect Dis 2007;45(4):510–3.

28. UNAIDS. Global. HIV Statistics 2022. Available at: https://www.unaids.org/sites/ default/files/media_asset/UNAIDS_FactSheet_en.pdf. Accessed August 12, 2022.

29. Brower V. AIDS-related cancers increase in Africa. J Natl Cancer Inst 2011; 103(12):918–9.

30. Casper C. The increasing burden of HIV-associated malignancies in resource-limited regions. Annu Rev Med 2011;62:157–70.

31. Ault KA, Future IISG. Effect of prophylactic human papillomavirus L1 virus-like-particle vaccine on risk of cervical intraepithelial neoplasia grade 2, grade 3, and adenocarcinoma in situ: a combined analysis of four randomised clinical trials. Lancet 2007;369(9576):1861–8.

32. Lehtinen M, Paavonen J, Wheeler CM, et al. Overall efficacy of HPV-16/18 AS04-adjuvanted vaccine against grade 3 or greater cervical intraepithelial neoplasia: 4-year end-of-study analysis of the randomised, double-blind PATRICIA trial. Lancet Oncol 2012;13(1):89–99.

33. Joura EA, Giuliano AR, Iversen OE, et al. A 9-valent HPV vaccine against infection and intraepithelial neoplasia in women. N Engl J Med 2015;372(8):711–23.

34. World Health Organization. One-dose Human Papillomavirus (HPV) vaccine offers solid protection against cervical cancer. Available at: https://www.who.int/ news/item/11-04-2022-one-dose-human-papillomavirus-(hpv)-vaccine-offers-solid-protection-against-cervical-cancer. Accessed August 12, 2022.

35. Jit M, Brisson M. Potential lives saved in 73 countries by adopting multi-cohort vaccination of 9-14-year-old girls against human papillomavirus. Int J Cancer 2018;143(2):317–23.

36. Jit M, Brisson M, Portnoy A, et al. Cost-effectiveness of female human papillomavirus vaccination in 179 countries: a PRIME modelling study. Lancet Glob Health 2014;2(7):e406–14.

37. Gelband H, Sankaranarayanan R, Gauvreau CL, et al. Costs, affordability, and feasibility of an essential package of cancer control interventions in low-income and middle-income countries: key messages from Disease Control Priorities, 3rd edition. Lancet 2016;387(10033):2133–44.

38. Wilailak S, Kengsakul M, Kehoe S. Worldwide initiatives to eliminate cervical cancer. Int J Gynaecol Obstet 2021;155(Suppl 1):102–6.

39. Sawaya GF, Huchko MJ. Cervical Cancer Screening. Med Clin North Am 2017; 101(4):743–53.

40. Saslow D, Solomon D, Lawson HW, et al. American Cancer Society, American Society for Colposcopy and Cervical Pathology, and American Society for Clinical Pathology screening guidelines for the prevention and early detection of cervical cancer. J Low Genit Tract Dis 2012;16(3):175–204.

41. Heard I. Prevention of cervical cancer in women with HIV. Curr Opin HIV AIDS 2009;4(1):68–73.

42. Maranga IO, Hampson L, Oliver AW, et al. Analysis of factors contributing to the low survival of cervical cancer patients undergoing radiotherapy in Kenya. PLoS One 2013;8(10):e78411.

43. Alfaro K, Maza M, Cremer M, et al. Removing global barriers to cervical cancer prevention and moving towards elimination. Nat Rev Cancer 2021;21(10):607–8.

44. Sankaranarayanan R, Anorlu R, Sangwa-Lugoma G, et al. Infrastructure requirements for human papillomavirus vaccination and cervical cancer screening in sub-Saharan Africa. Vaccine 2013;31(Suppl 5):F47–52.

45. Parham GP, Sahasrabuddhe VV, Westfall AO, et al. Implementation of cervical cancer prevention services for HIV-infected women in Zambia: measuring program effectiveness. HIV Ther 2010;4(6):713–22.

46. Parham GP, Mwanahamuntu MH, Kapambwe S, et al. Population-level scale-up of cervical cancer prevention services in a low-resource setting: development, implementation, and evaluation of the cervical cancer prevention program in Zambia. PLoS One 2015;10(4):e0122169.

47. World Health Organization. A practical manual on visual screening for cervical neoplasia. Available at: https://screening.iarc.fr/viavili.php. Accessed August 12, 2022.

48. Sankaranarayanan R, Basu P, Wesley RS, et al. Accuracy of visual screening for cervical neoplasia: Results from an IARC multicentre study in India and Africa. Int J Cancer 2004;110(6):907–13.

49. Arbyn M, Sankaranarayanan R, Muwonge R, et al. Pooled analysis of the accuracy of five cervical cancer screening tests assessed in eleven studies in Africa and India. Int J Cancer 2008;123(1):153–60.

50. Allanson ER, Phoolcharoen N, Salcedo MP, et al. Accuracy of Smartphone Images of the Cervix After Acetic Acid Application for Diagnosing Cervical Intraepithelial Neoplasia Grade 2 or Greater in Women With Positive Cervical Screening: A Systematic Review and Meta-Analysis. JCO Glob Oncol 2021;7:1711–21.

51. Sankaranarayanan R, Nene BM, Dinshaw KA, et al. A cluster randomized controlled trial of visual, cytology and human papillomavirus screening for cancer of the cervix in rural India. Int J Cancer 2005;116(4):617–23.

52. Kuhn L, Denny L. The time is now to implement HPV testing for primary screening in low resource settings. Prev Med 2017;98:42–4.

53. Bosch FX, Robles C, Diaz M, et al. HPV-FASTER: broadening the scope for prevention of HPV-related cancer. Nat Rev Clin Oncol 2016;13(2):119–32.

54. Ronco G, Dillner J, Elfstrom KM, et al. Efficacy of HPV-based screening for prevention of invasive cervical cancer: follow-up of four European randomised controlled trials. Lancet 2014;383(9916):524–32.

55. Zhao Y, Bao H, Ma L, et al. Real-world effectiveness of primary screening with high-risk human papillomavirus testing in the cervical cancer screening

programme in China: a nationwide, population-based study. BMC Med 2021; 19(1):164.

56. Aitken CA, van Agt HME, Siebers AG, et al. Introduction of primary screening using high-risk HPV DNA detection in the Dutch cervical cancer screening programme: a population-based cohort study. BMC Med 2019;17(1):228.

57. Arrossi S, Thouyaret L, Laudi R, et al. Implementation of HPV-testing for cervical cancer screening in programmatic contexts: The Jujuy demonstration project in Argentina. Int J Cancer 2015;137(7):1709–18.

58. Denny L, Kuhn L, De Souza M, et al. Screen-and-treat approaches for cervical cancer prevention in low-resource settings: a randomized controlled trial. JAMA 2005;294(17):2173–81.

59. Kuhn L, Wang C, Tsai WY, et al. Efficacy of human papillomavirus-based screen-and-treat for cervical cancer prevention among HIV-infected women. AIDS 2010; 24(16):2553–61.

60. World Health Organization. WHO guideline for screening and treatment of cervical precancer lesions for cervical cancer prevention. Available at: https://www.who.int/publications/i/item/9789240030824. Accessed August 12, 2022.

61. Jeronimo J, Castle PE, Temin S, et al. Secondary Prevention of Cervical Cancer: ASCO Resource-Stratified Clinical Practice Guideline. J Glob Oncol 2017;3(5): 635–57.

62. U.S. Preventive Services Task Force. Cervical cancer screening. Accessed at: https://www.uspreventiveservicestaskforce.org/uspstf/recommendation/cervical-cancer-screening#fullrecommendationstart. Accessed August 12, 2022.

63. Arbyn M, Simon M, Peeters E, et al. 2020 list of human papillomavirus assays suitable for primary cervical cancer screening. Clin Microbiol Infect 2021;27(8): 1083–95.

64. Jeronimo J, Bansil P, Lim J, et al. A multicountry evaluation of careHPV testing, visual inspection with acetic acid, and papanicolaou testing for the detection of cervical cancer. Int J Gynecol Cancer 2014;24(3):576–85.

65. Einstein MH, Smith KM, Davis TE, et al. Clinical evaluation of the cartridge-based GeneXpert human papillomavirus assay in women referred for colposcopy. J Clin Microbiol 2014;52(6):2089–95.

66. Zhang W, Du H, Huang X, et al. Evaluation of an isothermal amplification HPV detection assay for primary cervical cancer screening. Infect Agent Cancer 2020;15:65.

67. Arbyn M, Smith SB, Temin S, et al. Detecting cervical precancer and reaching underscreened women by using HPV testing on self samples: updated meta-analyses. BMJ 2018;363:k4823.

68. Nelson EJ, Maynard BR, Loux T, et al. The acceptability of self-sampled screening for HPV DNA: a systematic review and meta-analysis. Sex Transm Infect 2017;93(1):56–61.

69. Gupta S, Palmer C, Bik EM, et al. Self-Sampling for Human Papillomavirus Testing: Increased Cervical Cancer Screening Participation and Incorporation in International Screening Programs. Front Public Health 2018;6:77.

70. Yeh PT, Kennedy CE, de Vuyst H, et al. Self-sampling for human papillomavirus (HPV) testing: a systematic review and meta-analysis. BMJ Glob Health 2019; 4(3):e001351.

71. Unitaid. Cervical cancer screening and treatment of precancerous lesions for secondary prevention of cervical cancer: technology landscape. Available at: https://unitaid.org/assets/Cervical_Cancer_Technology-landscape-2019.pdf. Accessed August 12, 2022.

Breast, Ovarian, Uterine, Vaginal, and Vulvar Cancer Care in Low- and Middle-Income Countries
Prevalence, Screening, Treatment, Palliative Care, and Human Resources Training

Achille Van Christ Manirakiza, MD[a],
Krista S. Pfaendler, MD, MPH[b],*

KEYWORDS

- Breast cancer • Ovarian cancer • Uterine cancer • Vaginal cancer • Vulvar cancer
- Palliative care • Cancer training • Resource-limited setting

KEY POINTS

- Women's cancers are on the increase in low- and middle-income countries (LMICs) and contribute to increased cancer mortality in these countries.
- Screening strategies are limited in many LMICs, and sustainable, evidence-based prevention guidelines are lacking.
- LMICs face similar obstacles in reliable availability of all the cancer treatment components and skilled professionals.
- Multiple innovative initiatives in areas of management and training are upcoming, stemming from multilateral collaborations.

BACKGROUND

Breast, ovarian, uterine, vulvar, and vaginal cancer numbers are on the increase worldwide.[1,2] Their distribution has been widely heterogeneous over the years, with a larger proportion of ovarian and uterine cancers in high-income countries (HICs), but a greater share of vulvar and vaginal cancers in low- and middle-income countries (LMICs).[3,4] The

[a] Oncology Service, Department of Medicine, King Faisal Hospital, P.O. Box 2534, Kigali, Rwanda; [b] Division of Gynecologic Oncology, WVU Cancer Institute Mary Babb Randolph Cancer Center, West Virginia University, 1 Medical Center Drive, PO Box 9186, Morgantown, WV 26506-9186, USA
* Corresponding author.
E-mail address: krista.pfaendler@hsc.wvu.edu

Obstet Gynecol Clin N Am 49 (2022) 783–793
https://doi.org/10.1016/j.ogc.2022.08.004
0889-8545/22/© 2022 Elsevier Inc. All rights reserved.

contributing factors to breast and noncervical gynecologic cancer incidence and mortality in LMICs include ongoing changes in individual lifestyles, limited human papillomavirus (HPV) vaccination and breast cancer screening programs, late disease presentations, and inadequate access and availability of treatment resources.

The International Agency for Research on Cancer Global Cancer Observatory (IARC–GLOBOCAN) for the years 2012 and 2020 has shown an increase in occurrence of breast, uterine and ovarian cancers in less developed countries (**Fig. 1**). Vulvar and vaginal cancers were not part of the detailed GLOBOCAN 2012 tables to allow comparisons. Such an increase could be explained by longer life expectancy as a result of other public efforts in curbing communicable diseases,[2] in conjunction with a commendable effort in low-resource settings in introducing and maintaining reliable national cancer registries. In addition, although ovarian and uterine cancer rates have stabilized or declined over the years in HICs due to increased health awareness and early detection and treatment, a different phenomenon fueled by changes in childbearing patterns with less parity has contributed to their increase in LMICs.

Breast cancer in LMICs displays different behavior when compared with ovarian and uterine cancer trends and contributes to close to half of the world disease-specific incidence and early mortality, with more than 400,000 new cases and 200,000 deaths seen in low and middle Human Development Index (HDI) countries in the year 2020,[2] defined as countries with the least human development in terms of health, education, and living conditions. In these countries, mostly younger women are found with aggressive disease, contrasting with an older disease presentation in HICs, with racial and life expectancy factors at play.

Vulvar and vaginal cancers have been historically rare malignancies, with recorded statistics of about 9,000 and 8,000, respectively, in low and middle HDI countries in 2020.[2] The numbers remain increased almost uniformly in less developed countries, with a particular spike in Eastern and Southern Africa, corresponding with HPV hotspots worldwide.

A focused literature review was performed with search criteria including original research articles, reports, and reviews conducted in and for LMICs, according to the World Bank classification. Relevant research done in HICs was reviewed for comparison purposes. General search terms were limited to breast, ovarian, uterine, vulvar, and vaginal cancers. Themes found were summarized and reported under

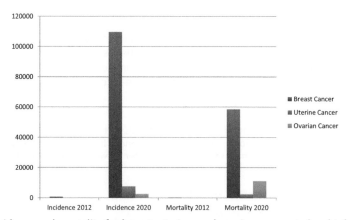

Fig. 1. Incidence and mortality for breast, uterine, and ovarian cancers in low high development index (HDI) countries based on GLOBOCAN data.

general sections of screening, treatment (surgery, chemotherapy, radiation therapy, palliative/end of life care), and physicians' training.

DISCUSSION
Screening

The World Health Organization (WHO) has adopted mammograms as the baseline tools for breast cancer screening.[5] Where available, together with well-defined screening guidelines, they have contributed to improvement in diagnosis and treatment to reduce breast cancer mortality. There are specific frameworks to gain more from mammographic screening, with appropriate age at screening (age 40–75 years), breast cancer history in the family, and availability of machines and skilled operators being the pillars around having organized mammography-based breast cancer screening.

A review of capacity, policies, and practices of breast cancer screening around the world had previously shown inadequate screening resources in LMICs.[5] For example, no country in Latin America, Africa, or a large part of the Central and West Asia regions has an organized breast cancer screening program, and there is a documented over-reliance on nongovernmental organizations in the case of the sub-Saharan African region.[5] Screening policies that exist in a few of those countries show inconsistency in recommended age ranges at screening and whether an addition of clinical breast examination and self-breast examination to mammography is necessary for screening. Social disparities in the access to breast cancer screening services and subsequent treatment in low-resource settings are also an important factor to poor screening practices noted in these regions.[6–8]

With different risk and presenting factors, breast cancer screening has been redefined in LMICs. Despite repetitive efforts to provide mammograms through bilateral partnerships, mammogram-based screening strategies are considered imprudent and unsustainable, given the additional costs that many LMICs cannot afford.[9–11] Mature results of a large randomized controlled study in India have revealed increased early diagnosis and reduced breast cancer mortality rates attributable to clinical breast examination[12] and multiple reports advocate for it as a suitable alternative to mammogram but suggest organized screening programs to fully profit from its gains.[13,14] Although several countries mention self-breast examination as a screening tool, clinical downstaging is an innovative alternative being increasingly tested and stands as a combination of self- and clinical breast examination.[11]

There are no known screening recommendations for vulvar and vaginal cancer screening in general, and detection of these depend on cervical cancer screening programs. Little is known on efforts being made in LMICs regarding their screening and control. HPV is a major cause of vulvar and vaginal cancers. There is a growing body of evidence showing large proportions of vulvar and vaginal cancers are prevented by HPV vaccination programs in high-resource settings, but this success has not been reported in low-resource settings.[15]

The US Preventive Services Task Force recommends against routine screening for ovarian cancer but provides room for both ovarian and uterine cancer screening for high-risk individuals based on family history.[16]

There is a dearth of information related to ovarian and endometrial cancer early detection programs in LMICs, and a number of alternatives have been recommended, spanning from surgical, genetic, and whole-gynecological screening options in single visits.[13,17] For each of these given options, scarcity of materials, inadequate numbers and skills of professionals, and affordability of the suggested tests (genetic tests, for example) are added to a poor health awareness overall and remain problematic to implement in low-resource settings.

Ovarian cancer fatality is increasing in low-resource settings, owing to late stages at presentation. There is a growing interest in mapping the genetics behind carcinogenesis, and ovarian cancers are usually taken together with breast cancers in existing programs. Findings in the few African studies point toward different BRCA-1/2 germline mutations when compared with studies of Caucasian populations, but some similarities have been found in the Latin American populations.[18,19]

Endometrial cancers do not have a standard screening test, but increasing advocacy has been made toward availing health awareness to postmenopausal and at-risk women.[13]

Treatment

Surgery

Surgery is a crucial component of breast and gynecologic cancer care, with roles in prevention (eg, mastectomy or salpingo-oophorectomy high-risk individuals), diagnosis, curative treatment, and palliation. Although 80% of cancer cases require some form of surgical intervention at least once during the disease course,[19] it is estimated that 94% of individuals in LMICs do not have access to safe, timely and affordable surgical and anesthesia care in comparison to 14.9% of individuals in HICs.[20] For breast and noncervical gynecologic cancers, surgical management includes a combination of simple and radical surgical procedures as well as sentinel lymph node mapping and sampling or complete lymph node dissection, with the specific combination of procedures needed for each cancer determined by the stage and distribution of disease as well as histopathology of the tumor. The Lancet Oncology Commission on global cancer surgery identified that many patients do not have access to cancer surgery and that adjuncts to surgery, such as imaging and pathology, are also inadequate.[21] In some countries, there is no local pathology capacity available, requiring specimens to be transported to a large city for processing and evaluation[22]; transport of samples can result in lot samples and/or significant lag times to treatment while awaiting results.

Perioperative care

In some cases, adoption of newer perioperative care programs may be more readily feasible in LMICs than expansion of existing surgical services or may be able to be implemented in conjunction with expansion of surgical services. One of the biggest global advances in perioperative care in the last decade has been demonstration of efficacy of enhanced recovery after surgery (ERAS) programs and implementation of such programs. In a prospective study evaluating impact of ERAS protocol on patients undergoing surgery for advanced ovarian cancer in a low-resource setting from March 2017 to February 2018, Agarwal and colleagues[22] evaluated 45 patients and compared them with 45 historical controls who had received conventional management from January 2016 to December 2016. During their study, they found that compliance with ERAS protocol was 90.6% and occurrence of moderate or severe complications and hospital stay were significantly reduced in the ERAS group with no difference in 30-day readmission rates between groups. The investigators concluded that ERAS programs could be implemented successfully in low-resource settings if the program is modified to meet local needs to avoid increasing health care costs.

Further, an international survey of perioperative practice in gynecologic oncology conducted through social media reported that 37% of 454 respondents in 62 countries reported that ERAS was implemented in their institution.[23] The survey reported greater than 80% adherence to deep vein thrombosis prophylaxis, early removal of urinary catheters after surgery, and early introduction of ambulation but less adherence to use of bowel preparation, carbohydrate loading, use of nasogastric tubes and peritoneal drains, intraoperative temperature monitoring, and early feeding. Among respondents, ERAS protocols in gynecologic cancer surgeries were more widely adopted in Europe (38%) and the Americas (33%) compared with Asia (19%) and Africa (10%). For additional information regarding global ERAS implementation in other disease sites, see article XXX.

Surgical innovation
A surgical innovation in recent years that has shown promise in some ovarian, fallopian tube, and primary peritoneal cancers has been the use of heated intraperitoneal chemotherapy (HIPEC) for peritoneal surface malignancies. Cytoreductive surgery with HIPEC requires a multidisciplinary approach and represents a resource-intensive surgical procedure with significant morbidity and mortality. Deo and colleagues[24] report initiation of a multidisciplinary peritoneal surface malignancy program in 2015 in a high-volume public sector tertiary care center in North India that treated 232 patients with CRS and HIPEC between January 2015 and December 2020 where they achieved optimal cytoreduction in 94.4% of patients, with 28.0% experiencing morbidities including deep vein thrombosis, subacute intestinal obstruction, sepsis, abdominal wound dehiscence, lymphocele, urinoma, acute renal failure, and enterocutaneous fistula and 3.5% treatment-related mortality.

Chemotherapy
Scant literature regarding chemotherapy availability in LMICs for breast and noncervical gynecologic cancers can be identified. In a case report on ovarian cancer management, the investigators from the Democratic Republic of Congo reported no availability of chemotherapy.[25] Availability, cost, and access have been studied in LMICs, and variations have been identified, with a more consistent report of nonavailability of targeted therapy in the case of breast cancer (trastuzumab).

The WHO announced a global action plan for the prevention and control of noncommunicable diseases from 2013 to 2020, which included a global target for 80% availability of basic technologies and essential medicines to treat noncommunicable diseases in both public and private facilities.[26] The WHO 22nd Model List of Essential Medicines published in 2021 includes a long list of immunomodulators and antineoplastics, including basic chemotherapy medications for breast and noncervical gynecological cancers.[27] Because of the WHO focus on increasing access and availability of chemotherapy medications, it is expected that the number of patients and use of chemotherapy will increase substantially. This prompted an online survey investigating chemotherapy handling practices in LMICs, which identified median level of implementation of safe handling practices of 63% in LMICs (32% in low-income countries, 63% in lower-middle-income countries, and 85% in upper-middle-income countries).[28]

Radiation
Although external beam radiotherapy (external radiation) and brachytherapy (internal radiation) are important components of breast, uterine, vaginal, and vulvar cancer treatment, it requires substantial capital investment in equipment, health care infrastructure including ability to maintain equipment, and availability of highly trained health care professionals in several disciplines (radiation oncologists, medical physicists, dosimetrists, or treatment planners) to coordinate treatment.[29] Developing radiotherapy capacity can take multiple years. Even within LMICs, most of the

radiotherapy resources are concentrated in big cities and can be difficult for the rural population to access. More than half of patients in LMICs who require radiotherapy do not have access to treatment and that percentage increases to more than 90% in low-income countries.

Publications regarding radiation oncology infrastructure in LMICs is limited. A systematic review of 49 articles regarding radiotherapy capacity in LMICs published in 2015 revealed significantly limited resources on the African continent and a wide disparity within the African continent, with 60% of all machines concentrated in Egypt and South Africa, whereas 29 countries in Africa lacked any radiation therapy resource.[30] The International Atomic Energy Agency (IAEA) organized the Directory of Radiotherapy Centers (DIRAC), which serves as a central record and quantification of international radiotherapy capacity. The updated DIRAC database reports that there are now 253 radiation therapy centers in the African continent, including 105 brachytherapy units.[30] Even with data updated through 2021, DIRAC data indicate that 53% (133/253) radiation therapy centers in Africa are in Egypt and South Africa. The database demonstrates significant disparities globally, with 8 radiotherapy machines per million people in high-income countries but 0 to 1 per million population in LMICs.[31]

The IAEA held a meeting of experts in November 2018 to review the status of radiotherapy globally and to identify opportunities for outreach, advocacy, and communication, which might support funding global radiotherapy initiatives.[32] The investigators highlight that although the upfront cost of financing equipment is often cited as a barrier, training health care professionals to deliver safe and effective treatment and introducing safe and efficient practices are essential to long-term viability of a radiotherapy program.

Palliative and supportive care

Because breast, ovarian, uterine, vaginal, and vulvar cancer rates are increasing in LMICs, and many patients present with advanced stage disease, symptom management, and provision of palliative care pose urgent needs. There is a widespread recognition of palliative care as a key component of a holistic treatment of patients with cancer, and there has been a growing body of literature demonstrating that early integration of palliative care and supportive care results in improved quality of life, symptom control, patient and caregiver satisfaction, illness understanding, survival, costs of care, and quality of end-of-life care.[33] Early integration of bowel regulation and pain management can improve quality of life early in the cancer trajectory during chemotherapy treatment. Communication is paramount to provision of quality palliative/supportive care to ensure authenticity and autonomy for decision-making with support and guidance from a health care professional.[34]

However, there is a near-universal lack of access to palliative care education in most low-income countries.[35–37] In many settings, palliative care for women's cancers is incorporated only near the end of life. In cases where palliative care is available, pain management is considered as central to sufficient palliative care provision, whereas management of other symptoms and addressing aspects of spirituality and overall quality of life throughout the treatment journey are sometimes left behind. As much as pain has been reported as the main symptom in patients needing palliative care in South Africa and Uganda; sexual health, body image, and psychological problems were reported with similar rates as pain.[38]

In low-resource settings, advanced cancers that are not amenable to treatment are referred from tertiary care to lower level hospitals near the patients' residences for palliative care. Home-based palliative care is an alternative to hospital- or unit-based palliative care.[39–41] Advances in technology have allowed patients to access palliative care in the most remote settings and boosted timely communication and provision of care between health care professionals and patients.[42]

A systematic review of English language studies investigated technology-based interventions of pain, depression, and quality of life in patients with cancer.[43] Most of the studies in their review were conducted in the United States and other HICs. Telehealth interventions effectively evaluated cancer pain outcomes but not depression and quality of life outcomes. Because these were telephone-based interventions utilizing professional interventionists (nurses, psychologists, or counselors) or peer counselors who are cancer survivors, it is possible that these strategies could be applied in LMICs. A team in Tanzania evaluated use of a web-based application (m-Palliative Care Link) as compared with telephone contact for African Palliative care Outcome Scale assessment twice weekly for up to 4 months for patients with incurable cancer and found that symptom severity decreased over time in both groups but that those in the phone contact had significantly lower overall symptom severity.[38]

Training and Education Initiatives for the Health Care Workforce

Several investigators have described medical education and training initiatives in LMICs for breast and gynecologic cancers. Breast cancer detection and treatment services were able to be expanded in Democratic Republic of Congo through a joint effort among Zambian, United States, and Congolese care providers. Five-day training trips were carried out 5 times over a 2-year period to teach clinical breast examination, axillary and breast ultrasound, ultrasound-guided core needle biopsy and fine-needle aspiration, and breast surgery.[44] They report 183 lumpectomies, 58 modified radical mastectomies, and 45 axillary lymph node dissections during the course of the training program.

Rosen and colleagues[45] describe development of a gynecologic oncology training program in western Kenya at Moi University. Per their report, there was only one gynecologic oncologist in Kenya as of 2009. Canadian and Kenyan physicians collaborated to develop a clinical program and initiation of fellowship training in Kenya. At the time of their 2017 publication, 5 fellows had graduated from a 2-year fellowship training program over the prior 4 years.

Erem and colleagues describes a model for sustainable impact on gynecologic cancer care in sub-Saharan Africa, which includes subspecialty training in Ghana. They developed a 4-year training program at Komfo Anokye Teaching Hospital in 2013 as part of a multidecade partnership between the University of Michigan and academic medical centers in Ghana.[46]

The International Gynecologic Cancer Society (IGCS) launched the Gynecologic Oncology Global Curriculum and Mentorship Program in 2017 to help address the need for increased workforce of gynecologic cancer specialists in LMICs.[47] The Global Curriculum is a 2-year training program aimed at developing oncologic expertise designed for regions that do not currently have formal training in gynecologic oncology. The program is tailored to each locality to equip physicians to address specific women's cancer care needs in their region. To do so, the program pairs international mentors from HICs with local mentors and fellows at institutions in LMICs. There is a web-based curriculum and monthly Extension for Community Healthcare Outcomes (Project ECHO) multidisciplinary tumor boards. International mentors travel to the training site 2 to 3 times per year for hands-on surgical training, and the fellows travel to the high-resource institutions for 1 to 3 months. Fellow progress is monitored through evaluation reports completed by local and international mentors, surgical case log review, project ECHO participation, and periodic knowledge assessments with a final examination upon completion of the training program. By the end of 2021, there were 15 global training sites with 41 fellows actively enrolled and 17 fellows who successfully completed training. Training sites are located in Asia, Africa, Oceana, Central America, and the Caribbean.[48]

Several countries were able to scale up radiation therapy providers in the first decade of the twenty-first century. International partnerships in Cambodia facilitated oncology training. Their first oncologist was trained in Vietnam and France; subsequently a 2-year program was developed where general practitioner could obtain a degree in oncology at University of Phnom Penh with support from 2 French professors from Strasbourg University.[49]

In a scoping review, 25 articles were identified that described oncology medical education initiatives in LMICs, most of which were aimed at continuing medical education for physicians; the investigators point out that education and training of nonphysician providers is integral to the workforce crisis in LMICs.[50] Further, the investigators raise concern that partnerships between HICs and LMICs may be driven by the funding and interests of the HIC partner, which may fail to address needs of the LMIC institution and may have focus on short-term goals rather than long-term capacity building and sustainability.

SUMMARY

Breast, ovarian, uterine, vaginal, and vulvar cancers are increasingly diagnosed in LMICs in part due to successful public health efforts geared toward other communicable and noncommunicable diseases that contribute to increased life expectancy and in part due to improving capacity to screen and diagnose these malignancies. Unfortunately, cancer care has often been left behind when addressing noncommunicable diseases. Many women in LMICs have extremely limited access primary and secondary prevention as well as early diagnosis and treatment. This problem is multifactorial, with issues related to lack of diagnostic equipment, treatment (surgical services, chemotherapy, and radiation), and palliative care as well as insufficient trained health care workforce to meet the needs of the women with cancer. However, reports of ongoing training efforts and capacity building give hope for the future of women's cancer care in LMICs. Great efforts are needed to ramp up training programs, quality assurance, radiation equipment maintenance, chemotherapy drug availability, and overall access to care to address the needs of women in LMICs who are diagnosed with breast and gynecologic cancers.

CLINICS CARE POINTS

- Limitations in health care workforce and infrastructure pose challenges to delivery of care.
- There is an opportunity of providing evidence-based alternatives to HIC methods of screening, diagnosis, and care in most LMICs.
- Strategies such as telehealth offer promise for home-based palliative and supportive care.
- Over the past decade, there has been a significant increase in training programs geared toward building up the health care workforce for breast and gynecologic cancer care.

DISCLOSURE

The authors report no conflict of interest.

REFERENCES

1. Ferlay J, Colombet M, Soerjomataram I, et al. Estimating the global cancer incidence and mortality in 2018: GLOBOCAN sources and methods. Int J Cancer 2019;144(8):1941–53.
2. Sung H, Ferlay J, Siegel RL, et al. Global cancer statistics 2020: GLOBOCAN estimates of incidence and mortality worldwide for 36 cancers in 185 countries. CA Cancer J Clin 2021;71(3):209–49.
3. Parkin DM, Bray F, Ferlay J, et al. Estimating the world cancer burden: Globocan 2000. Int J Cancer 2001;94(2):153–6.
4. Ferlay J, Shin HR, Bray F, et al. Estimates of worldwide burden of cancer in 2008: GLOBOCAN 2008. Int J Cancer 2010;127(12):2893–917.
5. International Agency for Research on Cancer. Breast cancer screening. IARC handbooks of cancer prevention. Lyon: IARC; 2002.
6. Nogueira MC, Fayer VA, Corrêa CSL, et al. Inequities in access to mammographic screening in Brazil. Cadernos de saude publica 2019;35(6):e00099817.
7. Nuche-Berenguer B, Sakellariou D. Socioeconomic determinants of cancer screening utilisation in Latin America: a systematic review. PLoS One 2019; 14(11):e0225667.
8. Gutnik LA, Matanje-Mwagomba B, Msosa V, et al. Breast cancer screening in low- and middle-income countries: a perspective from Malawi. J Glob Oncol 2016; 2(1):4–8.
9. Corbex M, Burton R, Sancho-Garnier H. Breast cancer early detection methods for low and middle-income countries, a review of the evidence. Breast 2012; 21(4):428–34.
10. da Costa Vieira RA, Biller G, Uemura G, et al. Breast cancer screening in developing countries. Clinics (Sao Paulo) 2017;72(4):244–53.
11. Black E, Richmond R. Improving early detection of breast cancer in sub-Saharan Africa: why mammography may not be the way forward. Globalization and Health 2019;15(1). https://doi.org/10.1186/s12992-018-0446-6.
12. Sankaranarayanan R, Ramadas K, Thara S, et al. Clinical breast examination: preliminary results from a cluster randomized controlled trial in India. J Natl Cancer Inst 2011;103(19):1476–80.
13. Shetty MK, Longatto-Filho A. Early detection of breast, cervical, ovarian and endometrial cancers in low resource countries: an integrated approach. Indian J Surg Oncol 2011;2(3):165–71.
14. Shalu R, Ritu Y, Meenakshi BC, et al. Challenges in Screening and Early Diagnosis of Female Cancers. J Gynecol Oncol 2021;4(4):1067.
15. Hampl M, Sarajuuri H, Wentzensen N, et al. Effect of human papillomavirus vaccines on vulvar, vaginal, and anal intraepithelial lesions and vulvar cancer. Obstet Gynecol 2006;108(6):1361–8.
16. Grossman DC, Curry SJ, Owens DK, et al. Screening for ovarian cancer: US preventive services task force recommendation statement. JAMA 2018;319(6): 588–94.
17. Rosenblatt KA, Thomas DB. Reduced risk of ovarian cancer in women with a tubal ligation or hysterectomy. The World Health Organization Collaborative Study of Neoplasia and Steroid Contraceptives. Cancer Epidemiol Prev Biomarkers 1996;5(11):933–5.
18. Pegoraro RJ, Moodley M, Rom L, et al. P53 codon 72 polymorphism and BRCA 1 and 2 mutations in ovarian epithelial malignancies in black South Africans. Int J Gynecol Cancer 2003;13(4):444–9.

19. Manchana T, Phoolcharoen N, Tantbirojn P. BRCA mutation in high grade epithelial ovarian cancers. Gynecol Oncol Rep 2019;29:102–5.
20. Meara JG, Leather AJ, Hagander L, et al. Global Surgery 2030: evidence and solutions for achieving health, welfare, and economic development. Lancet 2015; 386(9993):569–624.
21. Sullivan R, Alatise OI, Anderson BO, et al. Global cancer surgery: delivering safe, affordable, and timely cancer surgery. Lancet Oncol 2015;16(11):1193–224.
22. Agarwal R, Rajanbabu A, Nitu PV, et al. A prospective study evaluating the impact of implementing the ERAS protocol on patients undergoing surgery for advanced ovarian cancer. Int J Gynecol Cancer 2019;29(3):605–12.
23. Bhandoria GP, Bhandarkar P, Ahuja V, et al. Enhanced Recovery After Surgery (ERAS) in gynecologic oncology: an international survey of peri-operative practice. Int J Gynecol Cancer 2020;30(10):1471–8.
24. Deo S, Ray M, Bansal B, et al. Feasibility and outcomes of cytoreductive surgery and HIPEC for peritoneal surface malignancies in low-and middle-income countries: a single-center experience of 232 cases. World J Surg Oncol 2021; 19(1):164.
25. Mulisya O, Sikakulya FK, Mastaki M, et al. The challenges of managing ovarian cancer in the developing world. Case Rep Oncological Med 2020;2020:8379628.
26. World Health Organization. Global action plan for the prevention and control of noncommunicable diseases 2013-2020. Geneva, Switzerland: World Health Organization; 2013.
27. World Health Organization. Model List of Essential Medicines - 22nd List, 20213. Geneva: World Health Organization; 2021. p. IGO.
28. von Grünigen S, Geissbühler A, Bonnabry P. The safe handling of chemotherapy drugs in low-and middle-income countries: An overview of practices. J Oncol Pharm Pract 2022;28(2):410–20.
29. Zubizarreta EH, Fidarova E, Healy B, et al. Need for radiotherapy in low and middle income countries – the silent crisis continues. Clin Oncol (R Coll Radiol) 2015; 27(2):107–14.
30. Grover S, Xu MJ, Yeager A, et al. A systematic review of radiotherapy capacity in low-and middle-income countries. Front Oncol 2015;4. https://doi.org/10.3389/fonc.2014.00380.
31. DIrectory of RAdiotherapy Centres (DIRAC). International Atomic Energy Agency. DIRAC v2.0.7 (40659). Available at: https://dirac.iaea.org. Accessed March 1, 2022.
32. Abdel-Wahab M, Gondhowiardjo SS, Rosa AA, et al. Global Radiotherapy: Current Status and Future Directions—White Paper. JCO Glob Oncol 2021;7:827–42.
33. Hui D, Bruera E. Integrating palliative care into the trajectory of cancer care. Nat Rev Clin Oncol 2016;13(3):159–71.
34. Cain JM, Denny L. Palliative care in women's cancer care: global challenges and advances. Int J Gynecol Obstet 2018;143(Suppl 2):153–8.
35. Yamaguchi T, Kuriya M, Morita T, et al. Palliative care development in the Asia-Pacific region: an international survey from the Asia Pacific Hospice Palliative Care Network (APHN). BMJ Support Palliat Care 2017;7(1):23–31.
36. Tapsfield JB, Jane Bates M. Hospital based palliative care in sub-Saharan Africa; a six month review from Malawi. BMC Palliative Care 2011;10. https://doi.org/10.1186/1472-684X-10-12.
37. Pastrana T, Eisenchlas J, Centeno C, et al. Status of palliative care in Latin America: looking through the Latin America Atlas of Palliative Care. Curr Opin Support Palliat Care 2013;7(4):411–6.

38. Harding R, Selman L, Agupio G, et al. The prevalence and burden of symptoms amongst cancer patients attending palliative care in two African countries. Eur J Cancer 2011;47(1):51–6.
39. Munday D, Kanth V, Khristi S, et al. Integrated management of non-communicable diseases in low-income settings: palliative care, primary care and community health synergies. BMJ Support Palliat Care 2019;9(4). https://doi.org/10.1136/bmjspcare-2018-001579.
40. Spence D, Merriman A, Binagwaho A. Palliative care in Africa and the Caribbean. PLoS Med 2004;1(1). https://doi.org/10.1371/journal.pmed.0010005.
41. Vallath N, Rahul RR, Mahanta T, et al. Oncology-based palliative care development: the approach, challenges, and solutions from north-east region of india, a model for low-and middle-income countries. JCO Glob Oncol 2021;7(1): 223–32.
42. Ngoma M, Mushi B, Morse RS, et al. mPalliative care link: examination of a mobile solution to palliative care coordination among tanzanian patients with cancer. JCO Glob Oncol 2021;7:1306–15.
43. Agboola SO, Ju W, Elfiky A, et al. The effect of technology-based interventions on pain, depression, and quality of life in patients with cancer: a systematic review of randomized controlled trials. J Med Internet Res 2015;17(3). https://doi.org/10.2196/jmir.4009.
44. Mathieu KM, YouYou TG, Hicks ML, et al. Building a breast cancer detection and treatment platform in the Democratic Republic of the Congo by integrating training, service and infrastructure development. Ecancermedicalscience 2021; 15. https://doi.org/10.3332/ecancer.2021.1233.
45. Rosen B, Itsura P, Tonui P, et al. Development of a comprehensive and sustainable gynecologic oncology training program in western Kenya, a low resource setting. Gynecol Oncol Rep 2017;21:122–7.
46. Erem AS, Appiah-Kubi A, Konney TO, et al. Gynecologic oncology sub-specialty training in Ghana: a model for sustainable impact on gynecologic cancer care in sub-Saharan Africa. Front Public Health 2020;8:603391. https://doi.org/10.3389/fpubh.2020.603391.
47. Randall TC, Somashekhar SP, Chuang L, et al. Reaching the women with the greatest needs: Two models for initiation and scale-up of gynecologic oncology fellowship trainings in low-resource settings. Int J Gynecol Obstet 2021; 155(Suppl 1):115–22.
48. Gynecologic oncology global curriculum and mentorship program 2021 progress report. International Gynecological Cancer Society; 2022. Available at: https://igcs.org/global-curriculum-progress-report/. Accessed March 4, 2022.
49. Eav S, Schraub S, Dufour P, et al. Oncology in Cambodia. Oncology 2012;82(5): 269–74.
50. Karim S, Sunderji Z, Jalink M, et al. Oncology training and education initiatives in low and middle-income countries: a scoping review. Ecancermedicalscience 2021;15. https://doi.org/10.3332/ecancer.2021.1296.

Surgical Burden of Disease in Women

John E. Varallo, MD, MPH[a],*, Daisy Ruto, MMED[b], Anmol Patted, MBBS[c]

KEYWORDS

- Cesarean section • Safe surgery • Surgical safety checklist • Nontechnical skills
- Enhanced recovery after surgery

KEY POINTS

- An inequitable surgical burden exists, where greater than 90% of people living in low- and middle-income countries (LMICs) lack access to safe and affordable surgical care.
- Patients in LMICs who do access surgical care are at much higher risk of perioperative complications and death compared with those in high-income countries, resulting in 96% of perioperative deaths globally occurring in LMICs.
- In many LMICs, countries face a double burden of inequitable access to and use of cesarean delivery (CS) (ie, underuse and overuse) coupled with CS being performed unsafely.
- Obstetric fistula (due to neglected obstructed labor or iatrogenic from unsafe CS) and women's cancers, for example, breast and cervical cancers, contribute to the surgical burden of women in LMICs.
- A multicomponent approach, tailored to the local context, is essential to optimize surgical outcomes in LMICs; 2 vital elements of such an approach include improved nontechnical skills of the surgical team (eg, teamwork and communication) and use of evidence-based tools such as the WHO Surgical Safety Checklist and an Enhanced Recovery after Surgery (ERAS) program.

INTRODUCTION

Globally, 5 billion people lack access to safe and affordable surgical and anesthesia care, resulting in nearly 17 million lives lost each year. The situation is worst in low-income and middle-income countries (LMICs), where greater than 90% of people cannot access basic surgical care. This lack of access translates into surgical conditions accounting for roughly one-third of the global burden of disease and results in 5 to 6 times more deaths annually than human immunodeficiency virus/AIDS, tuberculosis, and malaria combined.[1] Women are particularly impacted by the surgical burden

[a] Safe Surgery, Jhpiego, Washington, DC, USA; [b] MNH and Safe Surgery, Jhpiego Kenya, PO Box 66119-00800, Nairobi, Kenya; [c] Johns Hopkins Bloomberg School of Public Health, 615 North Wolfe Street, Baltimore, MD 21231, USA
* Corresponding author. Jhpiego, 1615 Thames Street, Baltimore, MD 21231.
E-mail address: John.Varallo@jhpiego.org

Obstet Gynecol Clin N Am 49 (2022) 795–808
https://doi.org/10.1016/j.ogc.2022.08.003
0889-8545/22/© 2022 Elsevier Inc. All rights reserved.

and inequitable access to safe and affordable surgical care (eg, cesarean delivery [CS], prevention and treatment of obstetric fistula, and as part of management of breast and cervical cancers). The Lancet Commission on Global Surgery considers the ability to provide CS, along with laparotomy and treatment of open fracture, as bellwethers of a health system functioning at a level capable of providing most other surgical procedures, and these are therefore referred to as Bellwether procedures.[1]

CS is one of the first surgeries performed and has thought to have been around since ancient times. However, it was not until the twentieth century, with improvements in surgical techniques, anesthesia, and infection prevention practices, that the benefits of CS began to outweigh the risks of the procedure. Although these improvements have made CS safer, when performed unsafely or without a valid medical indication, it can negatively impact maternal and perinatal outcomes, waste human and financial resources, and jeopardize progress toward the Sustainable Development Goals targets for maternal and newborn health.[2]

Cesarean Delivery: Global and Regional Trends and Disparities

Today, CS is one of the most common surgeries performed worldwide and accounts for nearly a third of operations in most resource-poor settings.[3] CS is a lifesaving intervention for women and newborns when conducted safely, timely, and for the right reason, potentially preventing nearly 100,000 maternal deaths and reducing neonatal deaths by 30% to 70%.[4]

Globally over the past 30 years, CS rates have continued to increase across all regions, now accounting for 21.1% of all births, but with significant disparities across the regions, ranging from 5% in sub-Saharan Africa, to 31.6% in Northern America, and to 42.8% in Latin America and the Caribbean (LAC).[5] National data reveal even starker disparities in CS use, from 0.6% in South Sudan to 58.1% in the Dominican Republic.[6] Although there is debate on the appropriate CS rate at the population level,[7] the global average CS rate is above the level considered optimal (generally considered 10%–15%, to no more than 20% of births) to improve maternal and perinatal outcomes in a population.[8–11]

The lower levels of CS use (eg, 5% in sub-Saharan Africa) indicates underuse ("too little, too late"), whereas the higher levels of CS use (eg, 42.8% in LAC) suggests overuse ("too much, too soon"). The pace of change in the increase in CS rates is also different across the regions, with the largest increase in percentage occurring in Eastern Asia and the lowest increase occurring in sub-Saharan Africa. Furthermore, recent estimates project that by 2030, global CS rates will be 28.5%, ranging from 7.1% in sub-Saharan Africa to 63.4% in Eastern Asia.[5]

These population-based estimates mask equity differences within countries and among population groups, such that the problem of underuse and overuse of CS often coexists in a country. Within countries, CS use tends to be especially high among wealthier women, more educated women, those living in urban areas, as well as women giving birth in private facilities.[6,12] Underuse and lack of access to CS, particularly among rural and disadvantaged communities, can result in unnecessary birth complications and lead to maternal and neonatal mortality and morbidity. Similarly, overuse (ie, use of CS without medically indicated reasons) is also associated with increased risk of harm for women and their babies, as well as wasting scarce human and financial resources.

Owing to the issue of underuse and overuse, optimization of CS use should be a global health priority with (1) greater efforts to overcome underuse and ensure universal access to safe, timely CS for all women and (2) gaining a better understanding of drivers of overuse of CS and using multipronged approaches (clinical and nonclinical) that reduce unnecessary CS use. Key drivers of access to and use of CS can be viewed as 3 broader, interconnected, and sometimes overlapping categories: organizational and system factors, health professional individuals/teams, and women and community factors (**Fig. 1**).[13,14]

The Double Burden of CS

In many LMICs there is a double burden of inequitable access to and use of CS (ie, underuse and overuse) coupled with CS being performed unsafely. Surgical site infections (SSIs) are an important postoperative complication cause, and a significant contributor to post-CS morbidity and mortality globally, although occurring at much higher rates in LMICs than in high-income countries (HICs). For example, in sub-Saharan Africa, SSI rates following CS are approximately 5 times more common than in HICs, 15.6%[15] when compared with 2.9%.[16]

Nearly a quarter (23.8%) of pregnant women who died in LMICs had undergone a CS, with the most common CS-related causes of maternal death being postpartum

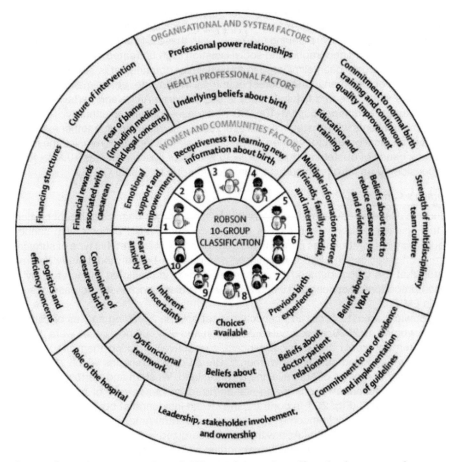

Fig. 1. Schematic representation of different factors that affect the frequency of cesarean section use. (Reprinted with permission from Elsevier. The Lancet, 2018, 392, 1358-1368. Betrán AP et al)

hemorrhage (32%), sepsis (22%), preeclampsia (19%), and anesthetic complications (14%).[17] Women giving birth in LMICs are 50 to 100 times more likely to die following CS than those in HICs, most often due to hemorrhage or infection, and CS maternal mortality risks have not improved in LMICs over the last 30 years.[17,18] Factors related to poor outcomes from hemorrhage at CS include system factors resulting in delay of surgical intervention (eg, dysfunctional referral systems, bottlenecks at facilities, lack of 24-hour CS services at some facilities), workforce numbers and capacity, not properly identifying mothers at risk (eg, preoperative anemia and previous CS), poor postoperative monitoring for complications, lack of quality medicines or blood, and lack of quality improvement systems in place.[19,20]

Such a staggering impact on women living in LMICs, along with the deep global inequities in the delivery of essential surgical care, are unacceptable, especially when we know how to prevent needless deaths.

Fistula

Women with obstetric fistula are evidence of the health system's failure to provide universally accessible, timely, and quality obstetric care, including safe CS. As noted in Saifuddin T. Mama and Mohan Chandra Regmi's article, "Pelvic Floor Disorders/ Obstetric Fistula," in this issue, obstetric fistula is a devastating injury sustained during childbirth resulting in severe lifelong morbidity, with these women often suffering from poverty, stigma, and geographic and social isolation if left untreated. Although obstetric fistula has largely been eliminated in the wealthier countries, it is still devastating the lives of many women in the poorest countries. Worldwide, an estimated 2 million women live with untreated fistula (mostly in sub-Saharan Africa and certain parts of Asia), with an additional 50,000–100,000 new cases occurring annually.[21,22] Yet, only 1 in 50 patients with obstetric fistula ever receive surgical repair, another example of unmet surgical burden for women.[22] Prolonged/obstructed labor remains the most common cause of obstetric fistula, at 80% to 90%[23] of cases, whereas 10% to 15% are considered an iatrogenic surgical complication due to unsafe CS.[22]

Women's Cancers

Cancer is a leading cause of death globally,[24,25] and women bear a significant portion of this disease burden with breast or cervical cancer.[26] Most patients with cancer require surgical treatment as part of their overall management, yet this type of surgical care is often lacking in LMICs. Alarmingly, a population-based model study has reported that the global demand for all cancer surgery is predicted to increase by 5 million procedures between 2018 and 2040, with a disproportionate increase occurring in LMICs.[27]

Worldwide, breast cancer and cervical cancer are the 2 leading causes of cancer among women. In 2020, an estimated 2.3 million and 604,000 new cases were attributed to female breast and cervical cancers, respectively, making them the 2 most commonly diagnosed cancers in women.[26] Breast cancer remains widely prevalent in HICs with the regions of Australia and New Zealand, Western and Northern Europe, and Northern America reporting age-standardized incidence rate of more than 80 cases per 100,000 (**Fig. 2**).[26] In contrast, the lowest incidence of breast cancer is reported in low- and middle-income regions such as Central America, Eastern and Middle Africa, and South-Central Asia with age-standardized incidence rates of less than 40 cases per 100,000.[26] Although underreporting and lack of screening for breast cancer remain a challenge in LMICs, the higher incidence of breast cancer in HICs has been explained by higher prevalence of reproductive, hormonal, and lifestyle risk factors[28]; higher penetrance of mutations in *BRCA-1* and *BRCA-2* genes among

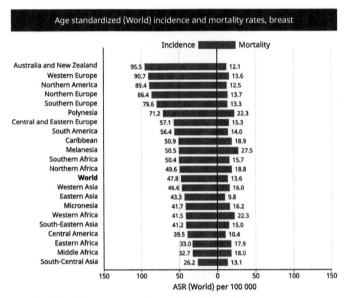

Fig. 2. Age-standardized incidence and mortality rates of breast cancer across world regions. (*From* World Health Organization International Agency for Research on Cancer (IARC). GLOBOCAN 2020: Breast fact sheet. Available at https://gco.iarc.fr/today/data/factsheets/cancers/20-Breast-fact-sheet.pdf.)

Ashkenazi Jewish population and certain populations of Europe[29]; and the presence of "organized and opportunistic mammographic screening."[28] However, despite their lower incidence, women in LMICs suffer higher breast cancer mortality rates than their counterparts in HICs (eg, sub-Saharan Africa); this likely reflects a weaker health infrastructure resulting in delay in timely diagnosis (ie, later stage at diagnosis) and limited access to treatment.[25,26]

The vast majority of new cervical cancer cases (84%) and deaths (90%) occur in LMICs, with age-standardized incidence and mortality rates in regions of Africa being 7 to 10 times higher than in some high-income regions, such as Northern America, Australia/New Zealand, and Western Asia (**Fig. 3**).[26] Persistent human papillomavirus (HPV) infection is the known cause of nearly all cases of cervical cancer. Yet, cervical cancer is nearly 100% preventable with effective primary prevention (eg, HPV vaccination) and secondary prevention (high-quality screening linked with effective treatment of precancerous lesions) strategies. The high cervical cancer incidence and mortality rates in LMICs, and other populations disproportionately affected by cervical cancer, represents a failure in the health system to prevent and to provide timely diagnosis and safe and effective treatment of both precancerous lesions and cervical cancer at its earliest stages.[27,28]

Improving Surgical Safety and Quality

Increasing access to surgical care for underserved populations is an important goal, but only if the surgical care provided is safe and of high quality. Expanding access to unsafe surgical care increases the risk of surgical complications and death, essentially trading the burden of untreated disease with the burden of preventable surgical complications and death. Patients who do access surgical care in LMICs are at much higher risk of perioperative complications and death

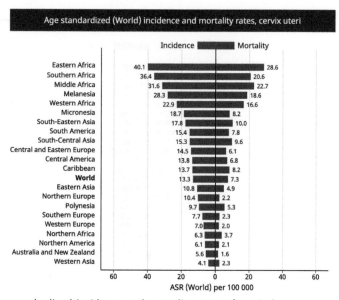

Fig. 3. Age-standardized incidence and mortality rates of cervical cancer across world regions. (*From* World Health Organization International Agency for Research on Cancer (IARC). GLOBOCAN 2020: Cervix uteri fact sheet. Available at https://gco.iarc.fr/today/data/factsheets/cancers/23-Cervix-uteri-fact-sheet.pdf.)

compared with HICs,[17,29] resulting in 96% of perioperative deaths globally occurring in LMICs.[1] A multicomponent approach, tailored to the local context, is essential to optimize surgical outcomes in LMICs. Two essential elements of such an approach include improved nontechnical skills of the surgical team (eg, teamwork and communication) and use of evidence-based tools such as the World Health Organization (WHO) Surgical Safety Checklist (SSC) and the Enhanced Recovery After Surgery (ERAS) program.

Importance of Nontechnical Skills

Providing safe, high-quality care requires effective teamwork and communication within and across health care teams and organizations.[30] The impact on poor surgical outcomes from ineffective teamwork and communication is exacerbated in the operating room (OR), where entrenched professional hierarchies can be potent barriers. Ineffective communication between surgical team members has been shown to be a cause of more than 50% of intraoperative surgical errors.[31] Strengthening nontechnical skills, defined as the social (leadership, communication, and teamwork) and cognitive (situational awareness and decision making) skills that support the technical skills (clinical knowledge and surgical skills) to perform safe surgery,[32] helps prevent perioperative complications and death.[33,34]

The Non-Technical Skills for Surgeons (NOTSS) framework was developed with surgical teams, educators, and researchers in mind to improve behaviors in the OR (ie, the social and cognitive skills) that improve performance and patient safety.[35] NOTSS emphasizes a multidisciplinary team-based approach to training and surgical care to increase surgical safety and quality. The NOTSS framework has been contextualized to be useful across diverse contexts (ie, language, culture, resources, level of the health system, and surgical epidemiology), and with the lessons learned from country implementation has the potential to improve the safety and quality and surgical care globally,[36] especially when coupled with evidence-based tools such as the SCC and ERAS.

Surgical Safety Checklist

In 2008 to 2009, WHO developed and introduced the SSC, a simple 19-item checklist designed to improve teamwork and communication and adherence to essential safety stops, with the goal to improve patient safety during surgery (**Fig. 4**).[37] The 3 pause points in the SSC (Sign In, Time Out, and Sign Out), prompt and foster discussion among team members and establishing a shared mental model of the surgical team members.[38] Correct use of the SSC improves surgical safety and quality by decreasing perioperative complications and deaths, globally and in resource-limited settings, by around 30% to 50%, with its impact likely greater in LMICs when adherence rates of SSC are high.[39,40]

However, successful implementation of the SSC in LMICs has been challenging, with adherence rates of around 30% in facilities from low Human Development Index (HDI) countries compared with nearly 90% in facilities from high-very high HDI,[41] and requires context-specific strategies to overcome specific barriers and achieve high adherence rates, for example, greater than 90% adherence.[41,42] The common barriers to successful SSC implementation include entrenched professional hierarchies that inhibit teamwork and communication, lack of team-based simulation training in the use of the SSC with ongoing support, and a general lack of a patient safety culture. Although evidence for the best SSC implementation strategies in LMICs is still limited, it seems that implementation success comes from a tailored approach that includes active leadership, adapting and tailoring to the local context, team-based simulation training, strengthening nontechnical skills (eg, teamwork and communication), ongoing real-time mentorship/support, audit, and feedback.[42–44]

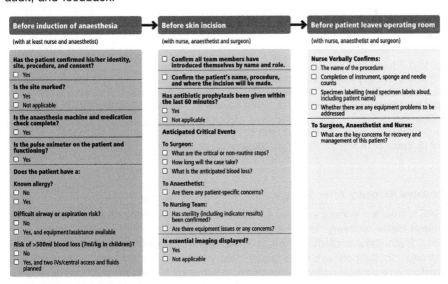

Fig. 4. WHO safe surgery checklist. (*From* Safe Surgery Checklist. 2019. World Health Organization (WHO). Available at: https://apps.who.int/iris/bitstream/handle/10665/44186/978924 1598590_eng_Checklist.pdf?sequence=2.)

Item	Recommendation	Evidence level	Recommendation grade
Antenatal pathway: OPTIMIZED			
Preadmission information, education and counselling (optimized element)	1. Although high-quality evidence is lacking, good clinical practice includes informing the patient about procedures before, during, and after cesarean delivery. The information should be adapted to whether cesarean delivery is an unscheduled or is a scheduled surgery.	Very Low-Low	Strong
	2. Cesarean delivery without medical indication should not be recommended without a solid preadmission evaluation of harms and benefits, both for the mother and her baby.	Very Low-Low	Strong
Preoperative pathway: FOCUSED			
Preanesthetic medications (focused elements)	1. Antacids and histamine H2 receptor antagonists should be administered as premedication to reduce the risk from aspiration pneumonitis.	Low	Strong
	2. Preoperative sedation should not be used for scheduled cesarean delivery because of the potential for detrimental effects on the mother and neonate.	Low	Strong
Preoperative bowel preparation (focused element)	1. Oral or mechanical bowel preparation should not be used before cesarean delivery.	High	Strong
Preoperative fasting (focused element)	1. Women should be encouraged to drink clear fluids (pulp-free juice, coffee, or tea without milk) until 2 hours before surgery.	High	Strong
	2. A light meal may be eaten up to 6 hours before surgery.	High	Strong
Preoperative carbohydrate supplementation (focused element)	1. Oral carbohydrate fluid supplementation, 2 hours before cesarean delivery, may be offered to nondiabetic women.	Low	Weak
Appendix: Preoperative maternal comorbidity optimization (optimized elements)	1. Maternal obesity (body mass index, >40 kg/m^2) significantly increases risks of maternal and fetal complications. Optimal gestational weight gain management should be used to control their weight during pregnancy. Surgical complexity requires multidisciplinary planning.	High	Strong
	2. Maternal hypertension should be managed during pregnancy because maternal chronic hypertension has been found to increase significantly the incidence of maternal and fetal morbidity and cesarean delivery.	High	Strong
	3. Maternal gestational diabetes mellitus has been found to significantly increase the risk for maternal and fetal morbidity. Maternal diabetes should receive timely and effective management during preconception and pregnancy.	High	Strong
	4. Maternal anemia during pregnancy is associated with low birthweight, preterm birth, and increases perioperative morbidity and mortality rates. The cause of the anemia should be identified and corrected.	Moderate	Strong
	5. Maternal cigarette smoking is associated with adverse medical and reproductive morbidity and should be stopped before or in early pregnancy.	High	Strong

Caughey. ERAS for cesarean delivery. Am J Obstet Gynecol 2018.

Fig. 5. Guidelines for perioperative care in cesarean delivery: Enhanced Recovery After Surgery (ERAS) Society recommendations. Preoperative care (Part 1). (*From* Wilson RD, Caughey AB, Wood SL, Macones GA, Wrench IJ, Huang J, Norman M, Pettersson K, Fawcett WJ, Shalabi MM, Metcalfe A, Gramlich L, Nelson G. Guidelines for Antenatal and Preoperative care in Cesarean Delivery: Enhanced Recovery After Surgery Society Recommendations (Part 1). Am J Obstet Gynecol. 2018 Dec;219(6):523.e1-523.e15. https://doi.org/10.1016/j.ajog.2018.09.015. Epub 2018 Sep 18. PMID: 30240657; with permission.)

Enhanced Recovery After Surgery

ERAS is another evidence-based tool that aims to standardize perioperative care to achieve faster recovery, improve patient safety and surgical outcomes, and reduce costs. Successful implementation of ERAS requires a multidisciplinary team-based approach to support evidence-based best practices, quality data collection, and monitoring of surgical patient outcomes using an audit system with comprehensive review during regular multidisciplinary meetings.[45] In addition to reduced surgical complications (20%–30%) and length of stay (20%–40%), ERAS has also been shown to reduce costs, with a return-on-investment analysis showing that every $1 invested in ERAS brought $7.3 in return, indicating that ERAS provides value.[38,45,46] Although

Guidelines for intraoperative care in cesarean delivery: Enhanced Recovery After Surgery Society recommendations

Item	Recommendation	Evidence level	Recommendation grade
Intraoperative pathway focused: preoperative antimicrobial prophylaxis and skin preparation (focused elements)	1. Intravenous antibiotics should be administered routinely within 60 min before the cesarean delivery skin incision. In all women, a first-generation cephalosporin is recommended; in women in labor or with ruptured membranes, the addition of azithromycin confers additional reduction in postoperative infections.	High	Strong
	2. Chlorhexidine-alcohol is preferred to aqueous povidone-iodine solution for abdominal skin cleansing before cesarean delivery.	Low	Strong
	3. Vaginal preparation with povidone-iodine solution should be considered for the reduction of postcesarean infections.	Moderate	Weak
Intraoperative pathway focused			
Pre- and intraoperative anesthetic management (focused element)	1. Regional anesthesia is the preferred method of anesthesia for cesarean delivery as part of an enhanced recovery protocol.	Low	Strong
Prevention of intraoperative hypothermia (focused element)	1. Appropriate patient monitoring is needed to apply warming devices and avoid hypothermia.	Low	Strong
	2. Forced air warming, intravenous fluid warming, and increasing operating room temperature are all recommended to prevent hypothermia during cesarean delivery.	High	Strong
Cesarean delivery surgical techniques/ considerations (focused element)	1. Blunt expansion of a transverse uterine hysterotomy at time of cesarean delivery is recommended to reduce surgical blood loss.	Moderate	Weak
	2. Closure of the hysterotomy in 2 layers may be associated with a lower rate of uterine rupture.	Low	Weak
	3. The peritoneum does not need to be closed because closure is not associated with improved outcomes and increases operative times.	Low	Weak
	4. In women with ≥2 cm of subcutaneous tissue, reapproximation of that tissue layer should be performed.	Moderate	Weak
	5. The skin closure should be closed with subcuticular suture in most cases, because of evidence of reduced wound separation in those women whose staples were removed ≤4 days postoperatively.	Moderate	Weak
Perioperative fluid management (focused element)	1. Perioperative and intraoperative euvolemia are important factors in patient perioperative care and appear to lead to improved maternal and neonatal outcomes after cesarean delivery.	Low-moderate	Strong
Neonate pathway focused: Immediate care of the newborn infant at delivery (focused element)	1. Delayed cord clamping for at least 1 minute at a term delivery is recommended.	Moderate	Strong
	2. Delayed cord clamping for at least 30 seconds at a preterm delivery is recommended.	Low-moderate	Strong
	3. Body temperature should be measured and maintained between 36.5°C and 37.5°C after birth through admission and stabilization.	Low-moderate	Strong
	4. Routine suctioning of the airway or gastric aspiration should be avoided and used only for symptoms of an obstructive airway (by secretions or meconium).	Low	Strong
	5. Routine neonatal supplementation with room air is recommended because the use of inspired air with oxygen may be associated with harm.	Low-moderate	Strong
	6. In all settings that perform cesarean delivery, a capacity for immediate neonatal resuscitation is mandatory.	High	Strong

Caughey. Guidelines for intraoperative care in cesarean delivery. Am J Obstet Gynecol 2018.

Fig. 6. Guidelines for perioperative care in cesarean delivery: Enhanced Recovery After Surgery (ERAS) Society recommendations. Intraoperative care (Part 2). (*From* Caughey AB, Wood SL, Macones GA, Wrench IJ, Huang J, Norman M, Pettersson K, Fawcett WJ, Shalabi MM, Metcalfe A, Gramlich L, Nelson G, Wilson RD. Guidelines for intraoperative care in cesarean delivery: Enhanced Recovery After Surgery Society Recommendations (Part 2). Am J Obstet Gynecol. 2018 Dec;219(6):533-544. https://doi.org/10.1016/j.ajog.2018.08.006. Epub 2018 Aug 15. PMID: 30118692; with permission.)

Guidelines for postoperative care in cesarean delivery: Enhanced Recovery After Surgery Society recommendations			
		Recommendation	
Variable	Item	Evidence level	Recommendation grade
Postoperative pathway			
Chewing gum after cesarean section (focused element)	Gum chewing appears to be effective and is low risk. It may be a redundant treatment if a policy for early oral intake is being used. However, it should be considered if delayed oral intake is planned.	Low	Weak
Nausea and vomiting prevention (focused element)	(1) Fluid preloading, the intravenous administration of ephedrine or phenylephrine, and lower limb compression are effective ways to reduce hypotension and the incidence of intraoperative and postoperative nausea and vomiting.	Moderate (multiple interventions)	Strong
	(2) Antiemetic agents are effective for the prevention of postoperative nausea and vomiting during cesarean delivery. Multimodal approach should be applied to treat postoperative nausea and vomiting.	Moderate	Strong
Postoperative analgesia (focused element)	Multimodal analgesia that include regular nonsteroidal antiinflammatory drugs and paracetamol is recommended for enhanced recovery for cesarean delivery.	Moderate	Strong
Perioperative nutritional care (focused element)	A regular diet within the 2 hours after cesarean delivery is recommended.	High	Strong
Perioperative glucose control (focused element)	Tight control of capillary blood glucose is recommended.	Low	Strong
Prophylaxis against thromboembolism (focused element)	(1) Pneumatic compression stockings should be used to prevent thromboembolic disease in patients who undergo cesarean delivery.	Low	Strong
	(2) Heparin should not be used routinely for venous thromboembolism prophylaxis in patients after cesarean delivery.	Low	Weak
Early post—cesarean delivery mobilization (focused element)	Early mobilization after cesarean delivery is recommended.	Very low	Weak
Post—cesarean delivery urinary drainage (focused element)	Urinary catheter should be removed immediately after cesarean delivery, if placed during surgery.	Low	Strong
Postoperative/ postpartum mother pathway			
Discharge counselling (focused element)	Standardized written discharge instructions should be used to facilitate discharge counselling.	Low	Weak

Macones et al. ERAS cesarean: part 3. Am J Obstet Gynecol 2019.

Fig. 7. Guidelines for perioperative care in cesarean delivery: Enhanced Recovery After Surgery (ERAS) Society recommendations. Postoperative care (Part 3). (*From* Macones GA, Caughey AB, Wood SL, Wrench IJ, Huang J, Norman M, Pettersson K, Fawcett WJ, Shalabi MM, Metcalfe A, Gramlich L, Nelson G, Wilson RD. Guidelines for postoperative care in cesarean delivery: Enhanced Recovery After Surgery (ERAS) Society recommendations (part 3). Am J Obstet Gynecol. 2019 Sep;221(3):247.e1-247.e9. https://doi.org/10.1016/j.ajog.2019.04. 012. Epub 2019 Apr 14. PMID: 30995461; with permission.)

most of these data come from HICs, the few established ERAS programs in LMICs are showing similar benefits as seen in HICs.[38]

Medical organizations around the world have embraced the principles of ERAS, following and promoting the guidelines that the ERAS Society has published in more than 20 specialties (including Obstetrics and Gynecology).[45] The ERAS Cesarean Delivery (ERAS CD) guideline was developed in 2018 and has the goal of enhancing the quality and safety of the cesarean delivery for improved maternal and fetal/neonatal outcomes.[46–48] The ERAS CD Guideline is organized into 3 sections: preoperative (Part 1, **Fig. 5**), intraoperative (Part 2, **Fig. 6**), and postoperative (Part

3, **Fig. 7**), and includes a "focused" pathway that starts 30 to 60 minutes before skin incision for cesarean deliveries until hospital discharge, along with a longer "optimized" pathway that includes antenatal education, maternal comorbidities, and immediate neonatal needs after delivery.[46]

SUMMARY

An inequitable, unmet global surgical need exists, as exemplified by greater than 90% of people living in LMICs lacking access to safe and affordable surgical care, with women particularly impacted (eg, CS, prevention and treatment of obstetric fistula, and as part of management of breast and cervical cancers). Although increasing access to surgical care for underserved populations is an important goal, it is essential that the surgical care provided is safe and of high quality. A multicomponent approach that is tailored to the local context will help optimize surgical outcomes in LMICs. Two essential components of this approach include (1) improved nontechnical skills of the surgical team (eg, teamwork and communication) and (2) use of evidence-based tools such as the WHO SSC and the ERAS program. Working in close collaboration with ministries of health and professional associations, combining this tailored approach with national surgical, obstetric, and anesthesia plans has the potential to improve the safety and quality of surgical care in LMICs, resulting in improved surgical outcomes for women and service efficiencies, which can be rapidly scaled and sustained, and can make a significant contribution to addressing the unmet surgical and anesthetic need of women, and the entire population, in LMICs.[38]

CLINICS CARE POINTS

- In many LMICs, countries face a double burden of inequitable access to and use of CS, that is, both underuse and overuse coexisting coupled with CS being performed unsafely. It is essential, therefore, to optimize CSs rates while simultaneously improving the safety and quality of the surgical procedure.

- A multicomponent approach, tailored to the local context, is essential to optimize surgical outcomes in LMICs. Two vital elements of such an approach include improved nontechnical skills of the surgical team (eg, teamwork and communication) and use of evidence-based tools such as the WHO SSC and the ERAS program.

- Correct use of the SSC, which includes adherence to the 3 pause points in the SSC (Sign In, Time Out, and Sign Out), prompting and fostering discussion among team members, and helping establish a shared mental model of the surgical team members, has been shown to reduce perioperative complications and deaths by approximately 30% to 50%, with its impact likely higher.

- ERAS is a multidisciplinary team-based approach that has been shown to reduce perioperative complications, speed recovery and reduce length of hospital stays, and save costs.

- Successful implementation of safe surgery practices comes from a customized approach that includes active leadership, adapting and tailoring to the local context, team-based simulation training, strengthening nontechnical skills (eg, teamwork and communication), ongoing real-time mentorship/support, audit, and feedback.

DISCLOSURE

The authors have nothing to disclose.

REFERENCES

1. Meara JG, Dr Leather, Andrew JM, et al. Global surgery 2030: Evidence and solutions for achieving health, welfare, and economic development. The Lancet (British edition) 2015;386(9993):569–624. Available at: https://www.clinicalkey.es/playcontent/1-s2.0-S014067361560160X.
2. United Nations. Transforming our world: The 2030 agenda for sustainable development. . 2015.
3. Weiser TG, Haynes AB, Molina G, et al. Size and distribution of the global volume of surgery in 2012. Bull World Health Organ 2016;94(3):201–209F. Available at: https://www.ncbi.nlm.nih.gov/pubmed/26966331.
4. Molina G MD, Esquivel MM, Uribe-Leitz T, et al. Avoidable maternal and neonatal deaths associated with improving access to caesarean delivery in countries with low caesarean delivery rates: An ecological modelling analysis. The Lancet 2015; 385:S33. Available at: https://www.clinicalkey.es/playcontent/1-s2.0-S014067361 5608285.
5. Betran AP, Ye J, Moller A, et al. Trends and projections of caesarean section rates: Global and regional estimates. BMJ Glob Health 2021;6(6):e005671.
6. Boerma T, Ronsmans C, Melesse DY, et al. Global epidemiology of use of and disparities in caesarean sections. The Lancet 2018;392(10155):1341–8.
7. Cavallaro FL, Cresswell JA, Ronsmans C. Obstetricians' opinions of the optimal caesarean rate: A global survey. PloS one 2016;11(3):e0152779. Available at: https://www.ncbi.nlm.nih.gov/pubmed/27031516.
8. Betran AP, Torloni MR, Zhang J, et al. What is the optimal rate of caesarean section at population level? A systematic review of ecologic studies. Reprod Health 2015;12(1):57. Available at: https://www.ncbi.nlm.nih.gov/pubmed/26093498.
9. Ye J, Betrán AP, Guerrero Vela M, et al. Searching for the optimal rate of medically necessary cesarean delivery. Birth (Berkeley, Calif.) 2014;41(3):237–44. Available at: https://api.istex.fr/ark:/67375/WNG-JRN7JMZP-M/fulltext.pdf.
10. Betran A, Torloni M, Zhang J, et al. WHO statement on caesarean section rates. BJOG 2016;123(5):667–70. Available at: https://onlinelibrary.wiley.com/doi/abs/10.1111/1471-0528.13526.
11. Molina G, Weiser TG, Lipsitz SR, et al. Relationship between cesarean delivery rate and maternal and neonatal mortality. JAMA 2015;314(21):2263–70.
12. Khan MN, Kabir MA, Shariff AA, et al. Too many yet too few caesarean section deliveries in bangladesh: Evidence from bangladesh demographic and health surveys data. PLOS Glob Public Health 2022;2(2).
13. Betrán AP, Temmerman M, Kingdon C, et al. Interventions to reduce unnecessary caesarean sections in healthy women and babies. The Lancet 2018;392(10155):1358–68.
14. Opiyo N, Kingdon C, Oladapo OT, et al. Non-clinical interventions to reduce unnecessary caesarean sections: WHO recommendations. Bull World Health Organ 2020;98(1):66–8. Available at: https://www.ncbi.nlm.nih.gov/pubmed/31902964.
15. Sway A, Nthumba P, Solomkin J, et al. Burden of surgical site infection following cesarean section in sub-saharan africa: A narrative review. Int J Women's Health 2019;11:309–18. Available at: https://www.ncbi.nlm.nih.gov/pubmed/31191039.
16. World Health Organization, Global Guidelines for the Prevention of Surgical Site Infection, Second Edition. patent CC BY-NC-SA 3.0 IGO. 2018. Available at: https://www.who.int/publications/i/item/global-guidelines-for-the-prevention-of-surgical-site-infection-2nd-ed. Accessed March 2022

17. Sobhy S, Arroyo-Manzano D, Murugesu N, et al. Maternal and perinatal mortality and complications associated with caesarean section in low-income and middle-income countries: A systematic review and meta-analysis. The Lancet 2019; 393(10184):1973–82.
18. Ndonga AKN, Samateh AL, Esterhuizen TM, et al. Maternal and neonatal outcomes after caesarean delivery in the african surgical outcomes study: A 7-day prospective observational cohort study. Lancet Glob Health 2019;7(4):e513–22.
19. Maswime S, Buchmann EJ. Why women bleed and how they are saved: A cross-sectional study of caesarean section near-miss morbidity. BMC Pregnancy and Childbirth 2017;17(1):15. Available at: https://www.ncbi.nlm.nih.gov/pubmed/28068945.
20. Buchmann E, Maswime TS. Near-miss maternal morbidity from severe haemorrhage at caesarean section : A process and structure audit of system deficiencies in south africa. SAMJ: South Afr Med J 2017;107(11):1005–9. Available at: http://hdl.handle.net/10520/EJC-abaaccfc4.
21. World Health Organization. Obstetric fistula. 2018. Available at: https://www.who.int/news-room/facts-in-pictures/detail/10-facts-on-obstetric-fistula. Accessed March 22, 2022.
22. Fistula Care Plus. Iatrogenic fistula. Available at: https://fistulacare.org/what-is-fistula/iatrogenic-fistula/. Accessed March 22, 2022.
23. Fistula Care Plus. Obstetric fistula. Available at: https://fistulacare.org/what-is-fistula/obstetric-fistula/. Accessed March 22, 2022.
24. Bray F, Laversanne M, Weiderpass E, et al. The ever-increasing importance of cancer as a leading cause of premature death worldwide. Cancer 2021;127(16): 3029–30. Available at: https://onlinelibrary.wiley.com/doi/abs/10.1002/cncr.33587.
25. Gelband H, Jha P, Sankaranarayanan R, et al. 3rd edition. Disease control priorities, vol. 3. Washington: World Bank Publications; 2015. Available at: http://portal.igpublish.com/iglibrary/search/WBB0000389.html. 10.1596/978-1-4648-0349-9.
26. Joko-Fru WY, Jedy-Agba E, Korir A, et al. The evolving epidemic of breast cancer in sub-Saharan africa: Results from the african cancer registry network. Int J Cancer 2020;147(8):2131–41. Available at: https://onlinelibrary.wiley.com/doi/abs/10.1002/ijc.33014.
27. Bray F, McCarron P, Parkin DM. The changing global patterns of female breast cancer incidence and mortality. Breast Cancer Res 2004;6(6):229–39. Available at: https://www.ncbi.nlm.nih.gov/pubmed/15535852.
28. Heer E, Harper A, Escandor N, et al. Global burden and trends in premenopausal and postmenopausal breast cancer: A population-based study. Lancet Glob Health 2020; 8(8):e1027–37. Available at: https://search.proquest.com/docview/2427294010.
29. Gordon CS, Samateh AL, Tumukunde JT, et al. Perioperative patient outcomes in the african surgical outcomes study: A 7-day prospective observational cohort study. The Lancet 2018;391(10130):1589–98.
30. Rosen MA, DiazGranados D, Dietz AS, et al. Teamwork in healthcare: Key discoveries enabling safer, high-quality care. Am Psychol 2018;73(4):433–50. Available at: http://psycnet.apa.org/journals/amp/73/4/433.
31. Gawande AA, Zinner MJ, Studdert DM, et al. Analysis of errors reported by surgeons at three teaching hospitals. Surgery 2003;133(6):614–21.
32. Yule S, Flin R, Paterson-Brown S, et al. Development of a rating system for surgeons' non-technical skills. Med Educ 2006;40(11):1098–104. Available at: https://api.istex.fr/ark:/67375/WNG-G93LF0SV-J/fulltext.pdf.
33. Christian CK, Gustafson ML, Roth EM, et al. A prospective study of patient safety in the operating room. Surgery 2006;139(2):159–73.

34. Catchpole KR, Giddings Anthony EB, Wilkinson M, et al. Improving patient safety by identifying latent failures in successful operations. Surgery 2007;142(1):102–10. Available at: https://www.clinicalkey.es/playcontent/1-s2.0-S0039606007001249.

35. The non-technical skills for surgeons (NOTSS) structuring observation, feedback and rating of surgeons' behaviours in the operating theatre system handbook v2.0. Available at: https://www.rcsed.ac.uk/media/682516/notss-system-handbook-v20.pdf. Accessed March 2022

36. Lindegger DJ, Abahuje E, Ruzindana K, et al. Strategies for improving quality and safety in global health: Lessons from nontechnical skills for surgery implementation in rwanda. Glob Health Sci Pract 2021;9(3):481–6. Available at: https://search.proquest.com/docview/2578778280.

37. WHO Patient Safety & World Health Organization, (2009). *WHO guidelines for safe surgery 2009: safe surgery saves lives*, World Health Organization https://apps.who.int/iris/handle/10665/44185.

38. Oodit R, Biccard B, Nelson G, et al. ERAS society recommendations for improving perioperative care in low- and middle-income countries through implementation of existing tools and programs: An urgent need for the surgical safety checklist and enhanced recovery after surgery. World J Surg 2021;45(11):3246–8. Available at: https://link.springer.com/article/10.1007/s00268-021-06279-x.

39. Haynes AB, Weiser TG, Berry WR, et al. A surgical safety checklist to reduce morbidity and mortality in a global population. New Engl J Med 2009;360(5):491–9. Available at: http://content.nejm.org/cgi/content/abstract/360/5/491.

40. Ademuyiwa AO, Medina AR, Nawara C, et al. Pooled analysis of WHO surgical safety checklist use and mortality after emergency laparotomy. Br J Surg 2019;106(2):e103–12. Available at: https://onlinelibrary.wiley.com/doi/abs/10.1002/bjs.11051.

41. Delisle M, Pradarelli JC, Panda N, et al. Variation in global uptake of the surgical safety checklist. Br J Surg 2020;107(2):e151–60. Available at: https://onlinelibrary.wiley.com/doi/abs/10.1002/bjs.11321.

42. Hellar A, Tibyehabwa L, Ernest E, et al. A team-based approach to introduce and sustain the use of the WHO surgical safety checklist in tanzania. World J Surg 2019;44(3):689–95. Available at: https://link.springer.com/article/10.1007/s00268-019-05292-5.

43. Conley DM, Singer Sara J, Edmondson L, et al. Effective surgical safety checklist implementation. J Am Coll Surg 2011;212(5):873–9. Available at: https://www.clinicalkey.es/playcontent/1-s2.0-S1072751511000858.

44. White MC, Peven K, Clancy O, et al. Implementation strategies and the uptake of the world health organization surgical safety checklist in low and middle income countries: A systematic review and meta-analysis. Ann Surg 2021;273(6):e196–205. Available at: https://www.ncbi.nlm.nih.gov/pubmed/33064387.

45. Ljungqvist O, de Boer HD, Balfour A, et al. Opportunities and challenges for the next phase of enhanced recovery after surgery: A review. JAMA Surg 2021;156(8):775–84.

46. Wilson RD, Caughey AB, Wood SL, et al. Guidelines for antenatal and preoperative care in Cesarean delivery: Enhanced recovery after Surgery Society recommendations (Part 1). Am J Obstet Gynecol 2018;219(6):523.e1-15.

47. Caughey AB, Wood SL, Macones GA, et al. Guidelines for intraoperative care in cesarean delivery: Enhanced recovery after surgery society recommendations (part 2). Am J Obstet Gynecol 2018;219(6):533–44.

48. Macones GA, Caughey AB, Wood SL, et al. Guidelines for postoperative care in cesarean delivery: Enhanced recovery after surgery (ERAS) society recommendations (part 3). Am J Obstet Gynecol 2019;221(3):247.e1-9.

Violence Against Women – A Global Perspective

Laura Keyser, PT, DPT, MPH[a],*, Raha Maroyi, MD[b,c], Denis Mukwege, MD, PhD[b,c]

KEYWORDS

- Violence against women • Intimate partner violence • Sexual violence
- Gender-based violence • Weaponized rape

KEY POINTS

- Violence against women affects approximately one-third of women and girls worldwide with an estimate 736 million women aged 15 years and older experiencing intimate partner and/or sexual violence during their lifetime. Prevalence varies by region with rates above the global average reported in many low- and middle-income regions.
- At a societal level, risk factors include gender inequality and social norms that promote harmful masculine behaviors, limit women's economic participation, and privilege men over women.
- Violence against women is known to increase during emergencies. During the COVID-19 pandemic, reports of domestic violence increased worldwide. Armed conflict is also characterized by a rise in sexual violence, whereby systematic rape by combatants is used as a weapon of war, often with the aim of physical, psychological, and economic destruction of individuals and communities.
- A holistic and integrated approach to care delivery that includes medical and psychosocial care, economic empowerment, and legal aid optimizes health outcomes and promotes rehabilitation and reintegration. Panzi Hospital's One Stop Center represents a comprehensive care model that has been replicated within and outside of the Democratic Republic of Congo and provides an example for other countries to develop similar health policies and programs.
- Justice plays an important role in the healing process; adjudication through the legal system not only holds perpetrators accountable for their crimes but serves to honor and empower survivors of physical and sexual violence.

[a] Department of Physical Therapy & Rehabilitation Science, University of California, San Francisco, 1500 Owens Street, Suite 400, San Francisco, CA 94158, USA; [b] Department of Uro-gynecology, Panzi General Referral Hospital, FV49+M53, Mushununu, Panzi, Bukavu, Dem Rep Congo; [c] Faculty of Medicine, Evangelical University in Africa (U.E.A), 10 Mushununu, Panzi, Bukavu, Dem Rep Congo
* Corresponding author:
E-mail address: lkeyser@mamallc.org

Obstet Gynecol Clin N Am 49 (2022) 809–821
https://doi.org/10.1016/j.ogc.2022.08.002
0889-8545/22/© 2022 Elsevier Inc. All rights reserved.

obgyn.theclinics.com

BACKGROUND AND DEFINITIONS

The term gender-based violence (GBV) distinguishes violent acts that target individuals or groups on the basis of their gender. This includes violence against women, defined in the UN Declaration on the Elimination of Violence Against Women as "any act of gender-based violence that results in, or is likely to result in physical, sexual, or mental harm or suffering to women, including threats of such acts, coercion or arbitrary deprivation of liberty, whether occurring in public or private life."[1] GBV occurs at the interpersonal level within families and communities and includes intimate partner violence (IPV) and sexual violence (SV). GBV is also perpetrated systematically and at a collective level and can include femicide, trafficking, and weaponized rape during conflict, among other forms.[2]

Table 1 provides definitions of the types of GBV that will be presented in this article. Though defined separately, there is a complex and mutually reinforcing dynamic between the micro and macro level determinants of interpersonal and collective violence.[3] Structural violence may be considered a form of collective violence that manifests in the political, economic, and social structures of societies. In the context of GBV, it includes restrictive policies that affect women's access to resources (eg, property, finances, health care). Structural violence reinforces gendered power dynamics that play out in daily life, creating an environment permissive to IPV and/or SV at individual and mass scale.[3] Consequently, SV, including rape occurs at both interpersonal and collective levels. Conflict-related SV or weaponized rape is noted explicitly in Table 1 because it is characterized by extreme violence not typically observed at the interpersonal level and is a special focus of the work at Panzi Hospital (PH) in the eastern Democratic Republic of Congo (DRC). This article will focus primarily on the clinical aspects of physical and sexual violence, including IPV and rape. A clinical profile of PH will highlight the ways in which interpersonal and collective

Table 1
Types and definitions of violence
Interpersonal violence: violence between family members and intimates, and violence between acquaintances and strangers that is not intended to further the aims of any formally defined group or cause[2] *Intimate partner violence*: physical, sexual, or psychological harm by a current or former intimate partner; includes physical aggression, sexual coercion, psychological abuse, and controlling behaviors[2]	*Collective Violence*: violence by people who identify as members of a group committed against another group or set of individuals, intended to achieve political, economic, or social aims[4] *Structural violence*: exploitative and unjust social, political, and economic systems that result in physical and psychological harm; examples: apartheid, slavery, institutional racism[2]

Sexual violence: nonconsensual sexual contact or noncontact of a sexual nature; includes rape, attempted rape, unwanted sexual touching, and other noncontact forms, such as sexual harassment, trafficking, and exploitation; occurs at interpersonal and collective levels[4]

Rape: physically forced or coerced penetration of the vulva or anus with a penis, other body part or object[4]

Conflict-related sexual violence and/or weaponized rape: systematic sexual torture carried out by combatants against civilians in the context of armed conflict or occupation; marked by severity of violence, high numbers of perpetrators and assaults, and the strategic use to terrorize and gain control over communities; considered a war crime and crime against humanity[5] violence intersect in the context of a complex humanitarian crisis, which has resulted in an epidemic of SV in the region. In this setting, PH has developed the One-Stop Center model to provide holistic care for survivors of IPV and SV. In addition to addressing individual health needs, PH works at the community, national, and international levels to educate and advocate for gender equity and an end to systemic violence and weaponized rape.

Epidemiology

The World Health Organization (WHO) estimates that 736 million women aged 15 years and older have experienced IPV and/or nonpartner SV during their lifetime.[6] Violence against women affects approximately 1 in 3 women worldwide and represents a significant global public health problem. IPV is the most common form of violence against women.[6] Prevalence estimates of IPV vary by region from 20% in high-income regions to 37% in low-income regions.[7] **Fig. 1** illustrates the global prevalence of IPV among women aged 15 to 49 years. Data includes lifetime and past year estimates from 2018 and is summarized by region.

Certain risk and protective factors at the individual, family, community, and societal levels are associated with IPV and SV. For example, greater socioeconomic status is associated with positive health outcomes.[3] Higher education, income, and access to employment are protective against IPV and SV. Social support and strong family linkages broadly are protective; however, the positive effect may be limited by gender roles and beliefs about a woman's place and duty.[3] Gender inequality and social norms that enable harmful masculine behaviors, limit women's economic empowerment, and privilege men above women are key contributors to IPV and SV.[8] Additional risk factors include low education, substance abuse, history of child abuse or exposure to family violence.[8] Moreover, it is known that violence against women increases during all types of emergencies. While data collection during the COVID-19 pandemic was limited, reports suggest a rise in violence against women globally.[9,10] Pandemic-related restrictions increased strain on families and communities and reduced access to health and social services. These effects were more pronounced among women experiencing unemployment and food insecurity, those living in rural areas, and for younger women living with children.[9,10]

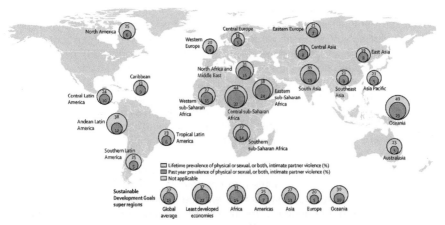

Fig. 1. Global prevalence estimates of intimate partner violence. (*Reprinted with permission from Elsevier. The Lancet, 2022, 399, 2022, Lynnmarie Sardinha PhD et al.*)

Health Consequences

IPV and SV are associated with a myriad of physical, mental, sexual, and reproductive health consequences contributing to high social and economic burdens not only for women, but their children and families, and society at-large. Those who experience IPV may sustain soft-tissue injuries, fractures, and/or traumatic brain injuries. The most common injuries involve the head, face, and neck, followed by musculoskeletal and genital injuries.[8] Women who survive SV are more likely to have a sexually transmitted infection (STI) and/or unintended pregnancy.[8] Common STIs include HIV, as well as hepatitis B and C, human papilloma virus, gonorrhea, and chlamydia, which may lead to cervical and other cancers and/or infertility. Unintended pregnancy is associated with increased risk of induced abortion.[8] Women with a history of IPV are more than twice as likely to report having an induced abortion, which may have significant health consequences in settings whereby safe and legal abortion care is unavailable. Unintended pregnancy as a result of IPV is also associated with increased risk of miscarriage and 41% greater likelihood of preterm birth, as well as significant economic implications and psychosocial consequences.[8] Other gynecologic problems associated with SV may include pelvic pain, urinary incontinence, fecal incontinence, and sexual dysfunction.[8,11,12] In the context of conflict-related SV, increased prevalence of pelvic fistula has also been reported.[12] Long-term physical health concerns associated with IPV and SV include hypertension, cardiovascular disease, cancer, gastrointestinal, neurologic, and metabolic disorders, chronic pain, including abdominal and pelvic pain, and premature death.[8] Mental health effects include posttraumatic stress disorder, anxiety, depression, sleep disturbances, substance abuse, and suicide. Survivors of IPV are nearly twice as likely to experience depression and over four times more likely to die by suicide.[8]

Human Rights-Based Approach to Health Service Delivery

WHO recommends a rights-based and survivor-centered approach to health care provision.[13] It is important for clinicians to recognize that GBV and specifically violence against women and girls stems from unequal power dynamics that exist between women and men. Clinicians must be aware of the factors that influence a woman's ability to access and receive health care, including her access to resources, ability to make decisions and communicate openly about her situation or experiences, and the social stigma she may face.[13]

Research demonstrates widespread attitudes of acceptance of violence against women, including among health workers who may assume predominant social norms, values, and attitudes that condone violence.[14] Moreover, worldwide, there is limited availability of trained health workers who are sensitized to the physical and mental health needs of survivors of IPV and SV. Training programs for health care professionals do not systematically include curricula related to GBV and survivor-centered care. Globally, there is an imperative to strengthen health systems to better respond to the needs of IPV and SV survivors, including training and capacity building, protocol implementation, effective coordination between organizations, and streamlined referral networks.[14]

Whether various forms of SV or IPV are considered criminal acts varies across states. Unfortunately, many countries do not have laws explicitly against GBV, and whereby laws do exist, they may not be enforced consistently. Domestic violence laws do not exist in 49 countries, and marital rape is not criminalized in 112 countries.[15] Legal requirements also differ with regard to reporting requirements and who may provide care to survivors of SV and IPV. National and state policies may also dictate clinical management, particularly regarding emergency contraception, abortion, and HIV testing and prevention. Additionally, national or provincial-level health guidelines may exist for some aspects of care provision for survivors of IPV or SV. This includes STI treatment protocols, emergency contraception, and postexposure prophylaxis (PEP) protocols, and/or vaccination schedules.

The availability of certain diagnostic tests, medications, and vaccines may affect clinical care. It is important to be aware of the available resources and regional supply chains, to appropriately manage resources, and advocate for what is needed, particularly in low resource and/or emergency settings. This also includes the availability of mental health care, psychosocial support services, and legal aid. Ideally, all services are provided within the same facility. When this is not possible, an integrated and efficient referral system is important to minimize the burden on the survivor. Collaboration between health facilities and local and international nongovernmental organizations may be helpful to fill resource gaps.

GUIDELINES AND TOOLS FOR CLINICAL PRACTICE

Beyond emergency medical care, survivors of IPV and SV require urgent care specific to the type of violence they have experienced. First-line support is essential and entails listening and responding to the survivor's needs, both emotional and practical, such as childcare or shelter. It is equivalent to "psychological first aid," can be lifesaving, and is an important first step before a medical examination is conducted.[16] Preparing the survivor and obtaining informed consent is also critical to ensure her agency and autonomy in making decisions about her care, including her right to refuse any aspect of examination and treatment. All aspects of the exam must be described, including forensic evidence collection, mandated reporting, and other legal requirements.

Patient history includes general medical information, noting vaccinations and HIV status, account of the IPV and/or SV incident(s) – may be limited or detailed depending on the patient's mental and emotional state, gynecologic history, and mental health assessment. For the physical and gynecologic examination, it is recommended that a witness is present, preferably a trained support person. If the clinician conducting the exam is male, it is recommended that a female health worker is present. Physical injuries must be well-documented using standard terminology or classification. Each area of the body must be examined, and injuries described in detail. **Box 1** provides guidelines for the clinical examination of survivors of IPV and/or SV, including descriptive characteristics of physical injuries, body parts involved, and types of injuries.[13]

A genital examination is indicated for survivors of SV and may include the collection of vaginal secretions to determine the presence of sperm.

For physical injuries, appropriate wound care should be provided, antibiotics if infection is suspected, analgesics for pain relief, and Tetanus prophylaxis if skin or mucosa have been disrupted.[13] For cases of SV, the most effective preventive care is delivered within 72 hours of the incident. This includes prophylactic STI treatment for Gonorrhea, Chlamydia, and Syphilis, Hepatitis B vaccination (if incomplete), postexposure prophylaxis (PEP) for HIV prevention (if survivor is not already living with HIV), and emergency contraception. Patient counseling is imperative to ensure adherence to all medications and vaccination schedules, and follow-up is recommended for repeat testing and patient monitoring at least once within 3 months and ideally more frequently at 2 weeks, 1, 3, and 6 months. Survivors of SV presenting for care beyond 72 hours are not eligible for PEP or emergency contraception. For these patients, diagnostic testing includes STI tests for HIV, Hepatitis B and C, Syphilis, Gonorrhea, and Chlamydia, and a pregnancy test. Care should be provided based on clinical

> **Box 1**
> **Clinical examination of physical and genital lesions**
>
> Description of Physical Injuries
> - Classification: Use accepted terminology (abrasion, contusion, laceration, gunshot wound, and so forth)
> - Site: Record anatomic position of each wound
> - Size: Measure dimensions of each wound
> - Shape: Describe shape of each wound (linear, curved, irregular, and so forth)
> - Surrounds: Note the condition of surrounding tissues (bruised, swollen, and so forth)
> - Color: Important when describing bruises
> - Course: Note the apparent direction of force applied
> - Contents: Note the presence of foreign material (dirt, glass, and so forth)
> - Age: Note evidence of healing
> - Borders: Characteristics of edges of wound may suggest the type of weapon used
> - Depth: Measure or estimate the depth of each wound
>
> Body parts to be examined
> - General appearance
> - Hands and wrists, forearms, inner surfaces of upper arms, armpits
> - Face, including the inside of mouth
> - Ears, including inside and behind ears
> - Head
> - Neck
> - Chest, including breasts
> - Abdomen
> - Buttocks, thighs, legs, feet
> - External genitals
> - Internal genitals, with speculum
> - Anal region
>
> Characteristics of injuries
> - Active bleeding or fresh wounds
> - Bruising
> - Redness or swelling
> - Cuts or abrasions
> - Evidence that hair has been recently pulled out
> - Evidence of recent loss of teeth
> - Injuries such as bite marks, scratches, stabbing, gunshot wounds
> - Evidence of internal, traumatic injuries to the abdomen
> - Ruptured ear drum
> - Foreign body presence
>
> *Adapted from* World Health Organization (WHO), United Nations Population Fund (UNFPA), United Nations High Commissioner for Refugees (UNHCR). Clinical Management of Rape and Intimate Partner Violence Survivors: Developing Protocols for Use in Humanitarian Settings. Geneva; 2020.

presentation and laboratory testing, including STI treatment, HIV counseling and treatment, and management of unintended pregnancy.[13]

Surgical intervention may be indicated for survivors who have sustained severe pelvic or abdominal injury, including traumatic or childbirth-related pelvic fistula or other internal injuries. Such intervention should be carried out only by specialty-trained surgeons and at facilities with adequate resources to provide perioperative care and postoperative convalescence. For those waiting for surgery and/or referral to a reference hospital, continence management solutions should be offered to those experiencing urinary or fecal incontinence, along with health education about hydration, bladder and bowel management, and personal hygiene.

In addition to caring for physical injuries and gynecologic conditions, basic psychological support should be offered to all survivors, and referral to appropriate mental health treatment, if available. In most cases, survivors require some level of psychosocial support and assistance with economic and/or legal resources. The acronym LIVES (Listening, Inquiring about needs and concerns, Validating, Enhancing safety, Supporting) may be used to guide clinicians in providing first-line support.[16] This includes expressing empathy and understanding, responding to immediate physical and emotional needs and practical concerns, ensuring safety, and providing access to information and social support. Each interaction presents an opportunity to provide this type of psychosocial support. Clinicians may also provide instruction on breathing and relaxation exercises and assist patients in identifying positive coping strategies.[16]

It is also important to monitor for more severe mental health concerns. While many trauma-informed psychotherapeutic strategies demonstrate effectiveness in reducing symptoms of posttraumatic stress disorder, anxiety, and depression, access to skilled providers is severely limited in resource-poor settings.[17] A recent review of mental health service delivery for GBV survivors in low- and middle-income countries indicates that most interventions are delivered by community health workers, in an effort to address access barriers. The authors cite challenges in integrating psychological treatment into health systems and report limited effectiveness and poor long-term follow-up.[18] Clinical advocacy may be focused on scaling mental health services through training and research efforts and promoting acceptance and integration of these services into existing health networks.

Clinical Profile: Panzi General Reference Hospital, Bukavu, Democratic Republic of Congo

For decades, armed conflict involving the national military and foreign and local militia groups has been persistent in DRC. This conflict has disproportionately affected eastern DRC and has contributed to crises of malnutrition, fractured health care and social systems, internally displaced persons, and insecurity. Additionally, SV including the use of rape as a weapon of war, has been a hallmark of the conflict.[19,20] In more recent years, it has been noted that civilian-perpetrated sexual violence is also a significant problem in DRC. Several factors contribute to this, including an environment of impunity surrounding sexual violence, the "normalization" of rape in society, and deeply rooted gender inequities.[21]

PH was established in 1999 in Bukavu, DRC, and is a full-service tertiary care referral hospital providing for the vast health needs of the region. PH is also a center of excellence and training for gynecologic surgery and the treatment of female pelvic floor disorders and is a pioneer in multidisciplinary care for women with fistula and survivors of SV. PH also supports several rural health centers and conducts regular mobile outreach programs to regions whereby there is no established specialty gynecologic care.[22] Such support focuses primarily on the identification and treatment of women and girls with fistula and individuals who have experienced SV.

Timely postrape care is challenging in eastern DRC, particularly in rural areas. It is ideal for women to present for medical evaluation within 72-h of sexual assault to document physical findings and receive postrape medications aimed at the prevention of pregnancy and STIs. However, many barriers exist to both accessing care and to maintaining a constant inventory of postrape care medications, particularly in rural health clinics, where individuals first present for care. In response to this challenge, PH partnered with the nongovernmental organization, Global Strategies to develop and implement the Prevention Pack program.[23] The program combines community sensitization, provision of prepackaged postrape medical kits, and a cloud-based, GPS-enabled inventory management system. Between 2013 and 2017, 2081 postrape medical kits were provided to survivors of SV at 13 sites in the South Kivu Province of DRC. Care was delivered continuously and without a single stockout. The Prevention Pack Program has improved the delivery of immediate postrape medical care in unstable and remote areas by addressing inventory challenges and creating a map of demand for postrape care across wide geographies.[23]

After years of caring for women and girls who had experienced rape, other sexual assault, and severe bodily harm, PH developed a holistic model of care, called "The One Stop Center" (OSC). This innovative, holistic, person-centered care model embodies the human rights-based approach to health. Its fundamental tenet is that women's empowerment is at the core of a functional and flourishing society, and these principles guide work at the individual, community, and national levels. The model comprises 4 pillars, covering medical care, psychosocial support, legal aid, and socio-economic needs. The goal is for the woman or girl to restore her health and reintegrate into society.

The OSC was first established by PH and the Panzi Foundation and has provided care for more than 70,000 survivors of SV. The success of this model has led to expansion to other regions of high need. An adapted OSC model has been established in some rural areas in DRC to bring services closer to communities most in need. In these areas, PH staff partner with health clinics to deliver medical care, train local providers, and provide community education. Implementation of the OSC model has also expanded across the region and beyond to Rwanda, Burundi, Kenya, Central African Republic, Guinea-Conakry, and Iraq.

Entry into the OSC model begins with the medical pillar, from which other services may be accessed. Each patient is assigned a personal nurse/social worker, who serves as a point of contact and coordinates her individual care plan across all four pillars. This system reduces the need for the patient to repeat her narrative to each provider or service. Medical care is provided according to the physical examination and treatment guidelines outlined above in the section, Guidelines and Tools for Clinical Practice. Forensic evidence collection is used to produce a medical certificate, which may be used for judicial proceedings, if/when the patient decides to pursue legal action. For survivors of SV, those arriving within 72 hours are offered STI prophylaxis, including PEP, emergency contraception, and appropriate vaccinations. As a result of the Prevention Pack Program and outreach efforts, most women present to PH-affiliated rural health clinics within the 72-h window. However, more than 80% arrive at PH in Bukavu beyond the 72-h window, and often require more complex medical and psychological treatment.[23]. Reasons for these delays may be due to transportation and other access barriers, including ongoing, active conflict in some regions.

Among adult survivors of SV, pelvic injuries may result from sudden, forceful, and/or repeated penile penetration or from the introduction of a foreign object (eg, firearm) into the vagina that causes tissue injury. These lesions may be treated surgically, similar to childbirth injuries, such as perineal tears or pelvic fistula. Traumatic pelvic fistula is less common, comprising about 4% of fistula cases.[24] Childbirth-related pelvic fistula is more frequent among survivors of SV and may be attributed to poor access to emergency obstetric care in the context of obstructed labor. Surgical outcomes of traumatic fistula are often superior to that of childbirth-related fistula because fibrosis is typically minimal. A more detailed discussion of fistula management is outside the scope of this article and may be found in Saifuddin T. Mama and Mohan Chandra Regmi's article, "Pelvic Floor Disorders/Obstetric Fistula," in this issue.

Classification of gender-based genitourinary and rectovaginal trauma in girls under 5 years of age

Type I

Bruising and superficial abrasions, and cutaneous and subcutaneous lesions without muscle or sphincter damage.

Type II

Cutaneous and musculoskeletal damage of the perineal body without fecal or urinary incontinence.

Type III

Cutaneous, musculoskeletal, and sphincter damage with fecal incontinence.

Type IV

Stellate cutaneous and musculoskeletal trauma with bladder and anal sphincter damage resulting in fecal and urinary incontinence.

Type V

Rupture of the posterior vagina into the posterior cul-de-sac (pouch of Douglas) with protrusion of abdominal contents.

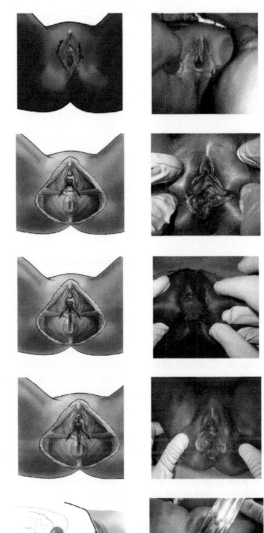

Fig. 2. Classification of rape-induced perineal lesions in girls under 5 years. (*From* Mukwege D. Classification of gender-based genitourinary and rectovaginal trauma in girls under 5 years of age. Int J Gynaecol Obstet. 2014;124(2):97-98. https://doi.org/10.1016/j.ijgo.2013.11.002; with permission.)

Due to a high volume of pediatric SV cases, PH has developed a classification system and treatment algorithm for child survivors of SV who have sustained genitourinary and/or rectovaginal trauma.[25] For children more than age 5, pelvic injuries appear similar to those seen in adult patients and may be treated as such. For children

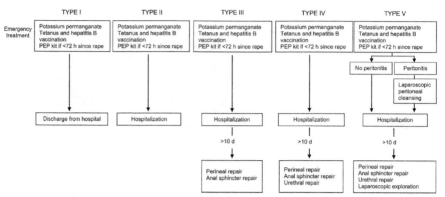

Fig. 3. Treatment algorithm for rape-induced perineal lesions in girls under 5 years. (*From* Mukwege D, Alumeti D, Himpens J, Cadière GB. Treatment of rape-induced urogenital and lower gastrointestinal lesions among girls aged 5 years or younger. Int J Gynaecol Obstet. 2016;132(3):292-296. https://doi.org/10.1016/j.ijgo.2015.07.034; with permission.)

under age 5, a specific classification scheme was developed (**Fig. 2**). Perineal lesions are described by the depth of the injury, extent of damage to the pelvic viscera, including sphincter involvement, and the presence or absence of urinary and/or fecal incontinence. Initial treatment of all cases includes a sitz bath in potassium permanganate solution and tetanus and hepatitis B vaccinations. Approximately 70% of cases under age 5 present within 72 hours of the incident, and thus, may be treated with PEP.[26] Following acute management, treatment diverges according to the type of lesions (**Fig. 3**). Children with mucocutaneous lesions only are discharged after a thorough evaluation. Those with muscular involvement, but no incontinence are admitted for observation and discharged once the lesion shows signs of healing. For those with muscular lesions and urinary and/or fecal incontinence, operative repair is indicated. This comprises approximately 10% of pediatric cases ranging in age from 18 to 60 months.[26] Surgery is typically delayed for a period of days or weeks due to the risk of infection following an acute assault.[26] Surgical procedures are performed by those with specialty training in pediatric gynecology. Medico-surgical care for most of these young survivors yields satisfactory outcomes. As with adult patients, psychosocial support and legal assistance are also provided to patients and their families. Unfortunately, long-term follow-up remains challenging. Understanding the developmental trajectories of these girls remains an area of interest and future research for PH.

Adjunctive interventions include individual and group-based physical therapy, which is provided to women with musculoskeletal and pelvic floor deficits and includes pre and postoperative rehabilitation for women with pelvic fistula. Psychosocial care involves individual and group mental health counseling, as well as music therapy and occupational therapy activities. Counseling may also be provided to close relatives, to aid family reintegration. Socioeconomic support and reintegration are also provided for those who have been displaced or lost property in the context of war. Legal aid includes educating survivors about their rights and the legal processes involved in pursuing a case against their perpetrator(s). Full legal assistance is provided for those who wish to prosecute. Lastly, socioeconomic needs are met through a number of life skills training programs that may include literacy programs, microfinance activities, and leadership training, among others. Beyond individual-level care, community sensitization and advocacy efforts are another key feature of the OSC model. Educational events are organized in community settings, such as schools, churches, or markets to raise awareness about human rights, GBV, and SV, as well as the free services offered at PH and the need for urgent medical care within 72 hours of an SV incident. In addition to local prevention and advocacy work, PH is engaged in national and international efforts to support holistic, survivor-centered care globally and to champion gender equitable policies to end violence against women.

SUMMARY

GBV is a pervasive public health threat that affects communities across the globe. Physical and sexual violence directed at women and girls occurs at the interpersonal and collective levels, and is exacerbated during crisis situations, such as financial hardships (eg, loss of income or employment) or political conflict (eg, war, occupation). Exposure to such violence is associated with significant long-term health consequences, and effective management of acute and chronic physical and mental health needs is paramount. Survivors of physical and sexual violence benefit from comprehensive, interdisciplinary care that includes medical treatment, psychosocial support, legal aid, and economic resources. Clinicians providing women's health care, particularly those working in humanitarian settings must understand the specific care needs of this population, as well as the resources available to meet these needs. Given the prevalence of GBV, prevention strategies are equally important, including community education and group training, economic development, and broad policies that promote gender equity.

CLINICS CARE POINTS

- Exposure to physical and sexual violence leads to significant short- and long-term physical and mental health consequences. Acute conditions include soft tissue injuries, fractures, concussions, and in cases of sexual assault, STIs, and unintended pregnancy. Pregnancies resulting from sexual violence are high risk and associated with miscarriage, preterm birth, and childbirth-related pelvic fistula, in areas whereby emergency obstetric care is not accessible.

- Survivors of physical and sexual violence require urgent physical and psychological care that includes acute management of physical injuries, mental health counseling, and appropriate social services. Postrape medications to prevent pregnancy and STIs may be administered within 72 hours of the assault. For those presenting after the 72-h window, care consists of STI treatment, referral for HIV counseling, and obstetric care, as appropriate.

- Medical treatment within 72 hours of a sexual assault can effectively prevent STIs, including HIV, as well as unintended pregnancy. Sensitizing patients and communities about the urgency of timely medical care and maintaining the supply of postrape medication kits in rural/community health clinics may help women access preventive care more readily.

- The One-Stop Center model integrates medical and psychosocial care, legal aid, and socioeconomic assistance and represents the optimal care model for survivors of sexual violence, particularly in humanitarian settings. When integrated care is not available, an efficient, streamlined referral system between agencies is essential.

ACKNOWLEDGMENTS

Jessica McKinney, PT, DScPT, MS.

DISCLOSURE

L. Keyser is the co-founder of Mama LLC, a consulting firm providing expertise in women's health and development. Mama LLC partners with Panzi Hospital and

Foundation on program development and research initiatives. All services provided are completely pro bono. No funding was provided to Mama LLC or any of the authors for this work. R. Maroyi and D. Mukwege have no disclosures.

REFERENCES

1. United Nations. Convention on the elimination of all forms of discrimination against women. General recommendation no. 19. Available at: https://www.un. org/womenwatch/daw/cedaw/recommendations/recomm.htm. Accessed May 19, 2022.
2. Rutherford A, Zwi AB, Grove NJ, et al. Violence: A glossary. J Epidemiol Community Health 2007;61(8):676–80.
3. Montesanti SR, Thurston WE. Mapping the role of structural and interpersonal violence in the lives of women: Implications for public health interventions and policy. BMC Women's Health 2015;15(1):1–13.
4. Krug EG, Dahlberg LL, Mercy JA, Zwi AB, Lozano R, eds. World report on violence and health. Geneva: World Health Organization, 2002.
5. Ba I, Bhopal RS. Physical, mental and social consequences in civilians who have experienced war-related sexual violence: a systematic review (1981–2014). Public Health 2017;142:121–35.
6. World Health Organization. Violence against Women Prevalence Estimates, 2018. 2018. https://www.who.int/publications/i/item/9789240022256. [Accessed 26 June 2022].
7. Sardinha L, Maheu-Giroux M, Stöckl H, et al. Global, regional, and national prevalence estimates of physical or sexual, or both, intimate partner violence against women in 2018. Lancet 2022;399(10327):803–13.
8. World Health Organization. Global and Regional Estimates of Violence against Women: Prevalence and Health Effects of Intimate Partner Violence and Non-Partner Sexual Violence. 2013. https://apps.who.int/iris/handle/10665/85239. [Accessed 26 June 2022].
9. Emandi R., Encarnacion J., Seck P., et al. Measuring the Shadow Pandemic: Violence Against Women During COVID-19. UN Women. 2021. https://data.unwomen.org/publications/vaw-rga (Accessed June 26, 2022).
10. World Health Organization. COVID-19 and violence against women what the health sector/system can do. Hum Reproctive Programme/WHO 2020;1(2):1–3. https://www.who.int/reproductivehealth/publications/emergencies/COVID-19-VAW-full-text.pdf?ua=1.
11. Andersson G, Kaboru BB, Adolfsson A, et al. Health Workers' Assessment of the Frequency of and Caring for Urinary and Fecal Incontinence among Female Victims of Sexual Violence in the Eastern Congo: An Exploratory Study. Open J Nurs 2015;05(04):354–60.
12. Dossa NI, Zunzunegui MV, Hatem M, et al. Fistula and Other Adverse Reproductive Health Outcomes among Women Victims of Conflict-Related Sexual Violence: A Population-Based Cross-Sectional Study. Birth 2014;41(1):5–13.
13. World Health Organization, United Nations Population Fund (UNFPA), United Nations High Commissioner for Refugees (UNHCR). Clinical Management of Rape and Intimate Partner Violence Survivors: Developing Protocols for Use in Humanitarian Settings. 2020. https://apps.who.int/iris/handle/10665/331535. [Accessed 26 June 2022].
14. García-Moreno C, Hegarty K, D'Oliveira AFL, et al. The health-systems response to violence against women. The Lancet 2015;385(9977):1567–79.

15. World Bank. Development Data Group. Atlas of sustainable development goals 2017 : From World Development Indicators. https://openknowledge.worldbank.org/handle/10986/26306. [Accessed 26 June 2022].

16. WHO. Health care for women subjected to intimate partner violence or sexual violence: a clinical handbook. World Health Organization. 2014. www.who.int/reproductivehealth. [Accessed 26 June 2022].

17. Coventry PA, Meader N, Melton H, et al. Psychological and Pharmacological Interventions for Posttraumatic Stress Disorder and Comorbid Mental Health Problems Following Complex Traumatic Events: Systematic Review and Component Network Meta-Analysis. Plos Med 2020;17(8):e1003262.

18. st. John L, Walmsley R. The Latest Treatment Interventions Improving Mental Health Outcomes for Women, Following Gender-Based Violence in Low-and-Middle-Income Countries: A Mini Review. Front Glob Women's Health 2021;2:1–7.

19. Mukwege DM, Mohamed-Ahmed O, Fitchett JR. Rape as a strategy of war in the Democratic Republic of the Congo. Int Health 2010;2(3):163–4.

20. Bartels S, Kelly J, Scott J, et al. Militarized Sexual Violence in South Kivu, Democratic Republic of Congo. J Interpersonal Violence 2013;28(2):340–58.

21. Lussy JP, Dube A, Lusi JKM, et al. Trends in sexual violence patterns and case management: a sex disaggregated analysis in Goma, Democratic Republic of Congo. Conflict and Health 2021;15(1):1–9.

22. Maroyi R, Keyser L, Hosterman L, et al. The mobile surgical outreach program for management of patients with genital fistula in the Democratic Republic of Congo. Int J Gynaecol Obstet 2020;148(Suppl 1):27–32.

23. Bress J, Kashemwa G, Amisi C, et al. Delivering integrated care after sexual violence in the Democratic Republic of the Congo. BMJ Glob Health 2019; 4(1):1–7.

24. Onsrud M, Sjøveian S, Luhiriri R, et al. Sexual violence-related fistulas in the Democratic Republic of Congo. Int J Gynecol Obstet 2008;103(3):265–9.

25. Mukwege D. Classification of gender-based genitourinary and rectovaginal trauma in girls under 5 years of age. Int J Gynecol Obstet 2014;124(2):97–8.

26. Mukwege D, Alumeti D, Himpens J, et al. Treatment of rape-induced urogenital and lower gastrointestinal lesions among girls aged 5 years or younger. Int J Gynecol Obstet 2016;132(3):292–6.

Quality Improvement Models and Methods for Maternal Health in Lower-Resource Settings

Victor Mivumbi Ndicunguye, MD, MMed, MSc[a],*,
Alison M. El Ayadi, ScD, MPH[b]

KEYWORDS

- Maternal health • Quality of care • Quality improvement • Implementation science

KEY POINTS

- Optimizing maternal health in lower-resource settings to prevent morbidity and mortality requires a joint focus to simultaneously increase skilled delivery care access and improve the quality of preventive and emergency maternal health care provided.
- Translation of evidence-based practices for optimizing maternal health is challenging in many settings; implementation science–guided approaches are needed to increase the adoption and sustainment of evidence-based practices.
- Quality improvement (QI) activities should be continuous and standardized and incorporate maternal morbidity and mortality surveillance and review as well as assessment of key processes to identify health systems gaps and implement remedial actions.
- Development of contextually specific valid core indicators for QI assessment and focus on identifying optimal implementation strategies for sustainable maternal health care improvement are key areas for future work.

INTRODUCTION

Despite global improvements in maternal mortality and morbidity over recent decades, rates remain substantial in lower-resource settings. Over the period 1990 to 2017, the global maternal mortality ratio (MMR) dropped from 385 maternal deaths per 100,000 live births to 211, representing a 45% reduction,[1,2] However, large disparities in maternal mortality persist globally, with the latest maternal mortality ratios

[a] Department of Reproductive, Maternal, Newborn, and Child Health, Jhpiego, Kigali, Rwanda; [b] Department of Obstetrics, Gynecology and Reproductive Sciences, University of California, San Francisco, 550 16th Street, Third Floor, UCSF Box 1224, San Francisco, CA 94158, USA
* Corresponding author. Remera, Gisimenti, KN 5 Road, UMUYENZI PLAZA, 2nd Floor, PO Box 1680, Kigali, Rwanda.
E-mail address: vndicunguye@jhpiego.org

Obstet Gynecol Clin N Am 49 (2022) 823–839
https://doi.org/10.1016/j.ogc.2022.08.009
0889-8545/22/© 2022 Elsevier Inc. All rights reserved.

obgyn.theclinics.com

(2017) among high-income countries 11 per 100,000 live births compared with 254 and 462 per 100,000 live births in World Bank–defined lower-middle-income and low-income countries, respectively.[2] Most maternal deaths occur in sub-Saharan Africa (~66%) and South Asia (~20%). Sustainable Development Goal 3.1 targets a reduction of the maternal mortality ratio to less than 70 per 100,000 live births, with no country having an MMR of more than 140 per 100,000 live births.[3] By 2015, 61.2% of 188 countries had already achieved this ratio, with national maternal mortality ratios ranging from 0.7 to 1073.9 per 100,000 live births.[4] However, projections using country-level trajectories from 1990 to 2015 suggest that without substantially accelerating global efforts, very few countries that have not yet met this level by 2015 are likely to achieve the rate of change required in order to achieve this target,[5] even before acknowledging the substantial impacts that the ongoing COVID-19 pandemic will exert on this trend.

Expanding attention to maternal near-miss, or severe maternal morbidity, serious complications during labor and childbirth that can have both short- and long-term effects on health, is an important transition given estimates that severe maternal morbidity occurs 50 to 100 times more frequently than maternal mortality.[6] It includes conditions such as hemorrhage, eclampsia, cardiovascular events, and sepsis, among others, which place birthing individuals at high risk of death. Severe maternal morbidity is a more sensitive focus for understanding maternal health and quality of obstetric care and an important proxy for maternal mortality whose infrequency makes it less feasible to study. In higher-resource settings, a minimum of 60% of maternal deaths and severe complications are considered preventable.[7,8]

Optimizing maternal health in lower-resource settings to prevent morbidity and mortality requires a joint focus to simultaneously increase skilled delivery care access and improve the quality of preventive and emergency maternal health care provided. Facility delivery rates have dramatically increased over time, with a recent analysis of 63 low- and middle-income countries identifying substantial increases in facility delivery in 60 countries (ranging from 13.7%–18.3% annually) from 1990 through 2018.[9] Gains in facility delivery rates were noted to decrease over time, with the highest annual increases observed from 1990 to 1999.[9] Disparities in both facility delivery levels and trend increases were observed by household wealth, rural versus urban residence, maternal education, and age, suggesting that concentrated efforts to improve equitable access are still warranted in most places.[9]

Evidence-based interventions to protect maternal health are well established by international and national obstetrics and gynecology professional societies and affiliated organizations and regularly updated for integration of newly identified best practices.[2,10–17] Core guidelines are relatively consistent across sources, and variations are related to health systems resources and complexities, facility levels, and outcomes targeted. The latest World Health Organization recommendations on intrapartum care for a positive childbirth experience (updated May 2017; summarized in **Fig. 1**) present a global evidence-based care package for optimizing women-centered quality of care and extend further to evidence-based management of childbirth complications in other guideline documents.[10–13] However, translation of evidence-based guidelines into practice remains challenging, and individual studies suggest that despite increasing access, poor quality is limiting health gains. Findings from the WHO Multicountry Survey on Maternal and Newborn Health reported that high coverage of essential interventions was not associated with reduced maternal mortality in facilities,[18] concluding that the coverage of interventions must co-occur with overall improvements in quality of care. Other recent studies from India, Malawi,

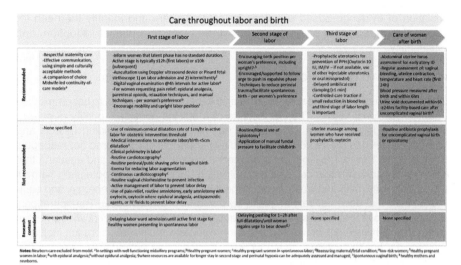

Fig. 1. Summary on World Health Organization recommendations: on intrapartum care for a positive childbirth experience.

and Rwanda showed that the higher rates of institutional deliveries and better access to antenatal care were not accompanied by reductions in maternal and newborn mortality.[19] These findings emphasize the imperative of assessing quality, identifying the determinants of quality performance, and implementing quality improvement (QI) approaches across varied health systems levels to address new health priorities in the United Nation's Sustainable Development Goals.

Modeling exercises have evaluated the potential impact of improving care access and quality across the intrapartum period using overlapping combinations of evidence-based interventions. One study identified that increasing both care coverage and quality of care for a core set of 16 preconception, antenatal, intrapartum, and postnatal interventions associated with reductions in stillbirth and neonatal mortality globally could avert 54% of maternal deaths globally.[20] Even where utilization is not increased beyond current levels, another study modeling the impact of 19 evidence-based maternal and neonatal interventions identified that QI alone, defined through the consistent implementation in 81 high-burden countries, would prevent 86,000 (95% confidence interval [CI] 77,800–92,400) maternal and 0.67 million (95% CI 0.59–0.75 million) neonatal deaths and up to 0.52 million (95% CI 0.48–0.55 million) stillbirths.[21] Integration and scaling up of some evidence-based interventions remains challenging, particularly in lower-resource settings. Quality of care remains key for continuous health systems improvement even in higher-resource settings where quality remains a serious concern, particularly with regard to health equity.

In this paper the authors review QI of maternal health in lower-resource settings through introducing prevalent frameworks used in health care quality and their application to maternal health and common monitoring approaches for maternal health quality including key indicator and adverse maternal event review. The authors then describe tools to support implementation of evidence-based maternity care such as checklists and the application of QI project approaches to improve maternal care. However, they are unable to delve into the extensive literature defining evidence-based maternal care. They describe the literature on facilitators and barriers to the translation of evidence-based practices in maternity care and identify the need for implementation science orientations in future work to optimize adoption and sustainability.

ORIENTATIONS TO QUALITY OF CARE

Quality of care has been conceptualized using a variety of frameworks to accommodate its multidimensional nature. The US Institute of Medicine considers quality of care to encompass 6 domains: safe (ie, avoiding harm), effective (ie, avoiding misuse and underuse of services, based on scientific knowledge), patient-centered (ie, respectful and responsive to individual patient preferences, needs, and values and ensuring that patient values guide clinical decisions), timely (ie, reducing wait and potentially harmful delay), efficient (ie, avoiding waste of equipment, supplies, ideas, and energy), and equitable (ie, care that does not vary in quality by personal characteristics). The operational definition used by the WHO also specifies that care be integrated, in acknowledgment of the fact that achievement of high-quality care requires a multilevel approach including governments, health systems, health workers, citizens, and patients.[9] In applying this model to implementation of quality maternal and newborn care in the facility setting, the WHO framework incorporates 8 domains focused on both provision and experience of care, which influence each other (**Fig. 2**).[16] These domains include both provision of care domains (evidence-based practices for routine care and management of complications, actionable information systems, and functional referral systems) and experience of care domains (effective communication, respect and preservation of dignity, and emotional support). Cross-cutting domains include competent, motivated human resources and essential physical resources available. The WHO has defined the relationship between the health system structure, these 8 qualities-of-care process

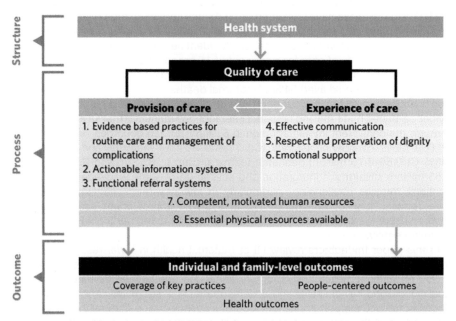

Fig. 2. World Health Organization framework for quality of maternal and neonatal health. (*From* WHO recommendations: intrapartum care for a positive childbirth experience. Geneva: World Health Organization; 2018. Licence: CC BY-NC-SA 3.0 IGO.)

domains, and individual and family level outcomes, which are coverage of key practices, people-centered outcomes, and health outcomes.

QUALITY-OF-CARE MONITORING

Approaches for monitoring the quality of maternal health care include tracking of key clinical practice and process indicators and review of adverse events, usually at the level of the health facility, with statistics aggregated to higher levels. These activities should be implemented continuously, integrated within care documentation, and accompanied by data review and strategic attention to remedy any deficiencies in care identified.

Key Clinical Practice and Process Indicators

Key indicators, or key performance indicators, are metrics designed to observe, analyze, or optimize a health care process to increase quality and/or patient satisfaction. Various key indicator sets have been developed by diverse international stakeholders including the WHO, international nongovernmental organizations (NGOs), and other implementation partners for use at population and facility levels.[22] Such indicators or indicator sets vary based on target outcome (eg, maternal vs neonatal health or focus on reducing a particular complication such as hemorrhage) and facility context (eg, facility location, level, or specific QI priorities).

Establishment of key indicators for monitoring maternal health care quality has occurred within a broader context of rapid expansion in health care performance metrics overall.[23] Although it is broadly recognized that high-quality indicators are needed for performance assessment, indicator development processes have been critiqued for both lack of coordination across various players as well as the lack of indicator validation. Two recent reviews have systematically assessed the literature on maternal health indicators. A systematic review of indicators for monitoring maternal, newborn, and child health care identified a large number of indicators (1445 in total, 297 for pregnancy, 299 for childbirth, and 119 for puerperium).[24] However, most were appraised as generally poor quality, lacking empirical testing or support, and inadequately distributed across the full continuum of care.[24] A scoping review of maternal and newborn indicators classified most of 140 indicators identified as addressing inputs and processes (39%), followed by outputs (21%), including service quality and safety.[25] The results of both reviews, and others, demonstrate a substantial international commitment to measurement yet confirm the need for indicator improvement and empirical testing as an important target for improving assessment of the quality of maternal health care.[24–26] Establishing a core set of high-quality standard indicators can improve impact assessment of various QI strategies as well as facilitate comparisons.

Maternal Adverse Event Review: Maternal Death and Near-Miss

Maternal death and near-miss (or severe morbidity) are considered sentinel events and serve as key indicators of health care quality, which are continuously reviewed. Maternal death and near-miss audit and feedback, ongoing systematic investigation into the occurrence of maternal deaths and near-miss events followed by concerted efforts to alter contributing factors, are a cornerstone of facility-based QI efforts and recommended by the WHO and others for reduction of preventable adverse events through collective action.[27]

The WHO's maternal near-miss assessment approach (2011) included implementation guidance and a standard definition and uniform identification criteria to facilitate facility, regional, and country-level comparisons.[28] The maternal near-miss audit and feedback cycle is designed to identify all facility maternal near-misses and deaths; examine morbidity patterns to identify support needs; and review underlying and contributory causes of near-miss in order to process indicators (eg, evidence-based care implementation), underlying causes of death or near-miss, and contributory or associated conditions.[28] Key to the implementation of near-miss assessment is a standardized definition, which WHO has specified as survival of a life-threatening complication during pregnancy, childbirth, or within 42 days after the termination of pregnancy. This definition has been operationalized as severe maternal complications (ie, severe postpartum hemorrhage, severe preeclampsia, eclampsia, sepsis/severe systemic infection, and ruptured uterus), receipt of critical interventions or intensive care unit use (ie, admission to intensive care unit, interventional radiology, laparotomy including hysterectomy but excluding cesarean section, or use of blood products), or cardiovascular, respiratory, renal, coagulation/hematological, hepatic, neurologic, or uterine dysfunction.[28]

The WHO, United Nations Population Fund (UNFPA), United Nations Children's Fund (UNICEF), and other international maternal and neonatal health partners have contributed to engaging countries to policy guidance and institutionalization, including the development and dissemination of national policy documents establishing maternal and perinatal death surveillance and response systems.[27,29] Maternal death reviews were initiated in the early 2000s in many sub-Saharan African countries, compared with European countries in the 1950s.[30–32] Countries have applied this approach to quantify the magnitude of maternal morbidity and its determinants, although consistent implementation has been a challenge in certain settings.[33,34] The maternal death audit approach consists of a multidisciplinary group that reviews the evidence surrounding a maternal death to determine the cause of death and what factors may have contributed to it.[35] The group makes recommendations for changes in clinical practice and identifies targets for social and behavior change communication.[29] In both higher- and lower-resource settings, maternal death review has resulted in improvement in quality of care and reduced maternal deaths through the identification and correction of poor care quality.[31,36] For example, a study conducted in Ghana showed a 15% reduction in odds of maternal mortality (odds ratio [OR] 0.85, 95% CI 0.73–0.98) and 26% reduction in odds of neonatal mortality (OR 0.74, 95% CI 0.61–0.90) with the implementation of maternal death review.[37] In Ethiopia, this strategy has been used to identify factors associated with maternal near-miss including multigravidity, lack of antenatal care, delay in reaching the hospital, and labor induction.[30] In Nigeria, it has been used to classify the distribution of maternal morbidity, identifying postpartum hemorrhage as the most common maternal morbidity in this setting.[30] Maternal death and near-miss review is a promising way to identify and review the quality of service provision, and its implementation across different settings has identified key human errors, systems weaknesses, and contributing factors, leading to strategic intervention for improvement. A systematic review and meta-analysis of 39 studies across sub-Saharan Africa and South Asia (n = 6205 audited deaths) identified 42 different avoidable factors across 4 key categories: health worker–oriented factors, patient-oriented factors, transport/referral factors, and administrative/supply factors.[38] The top 3 attributable factors for maternal deaths were substandard care by a health worker, patient delay, and deficiencies in blood transfusion.[38]

Evaluations of maternal near-miss review cycle implementation have identified positive outcomes in terms of quality of maternal care improvement and reductions in maternal mortality in high-burden countries, with low heterogeneity of results identified in a pooled analysis of 8 studies from sub-Saharan Africa and South Asia.[39] Despite its increasing institutionalization within maternal death audit structures in low- and middle-income countries as well as high-income countries, and the acknowledgment of near-miss review as an effective strategy for improving the quality of maternal care, evaluations of facility-based maternal near-miss review suggest that important opportunities for process improvement and expansion exist.[39] A recent systematic review identified ongoing deficits in this literature related to quality of scientific evidence in this area, the lack of attention paid to identification of strategies for successful implementation, lack of inclusion of patient experience, and challenges associated with effective translation of recommendations into practice.[39]

Maternal mortality or near-miss assessment is traditionally facility based; however, community-based death review through social or verbal autopsy can also help to identify factors contributing to these deaths, including social determinants of health.[40] For example, one study in Sri Lanka identified poverty, gender inequity, lack of relationship stability, and domestic violence contributed to inequities in maternal death risk, denoting the need for a socially sensitive health system.[41]

Other aids intended for monitoring and evaluation of quality of maternal care at the systems level include the maternal-newborn bottleneck analysis tool that evaluates skilled birthing attendance, basic emergency obstetric care, and comprehensive emergency obstetric care. This tool guides users to unpack critical bottlenecks by health system component to enable comparison between countries, regions, and higher and lower mortality contexts and identify critical focal targets for QI efforts.[42]

TOOLS TO SUPPORT IMPLEMENTATION OF EVIDENCE-BASED MATERNITY CARE

Ensuring the translation of evidence-based clinical practices for high-quality essential maternity care into practice in lower-resource settings remains a significant challenge due to multilevel barriers ranging across leadership and management, resources, and end-user–related factors.[43] A variety of innovations and systems target ensuring the provision of high-quality maternal health care, including tools to support implementation of evidence-based care such as care checklists and other job aids and formal QI approaches.

Care Checklists

Studies to improve patient safety have identified that care checklists improve adherence to care protocols, team communication, and reduce complications through facilitating teamwork and ensuring that critical tasks are completed to evidence-based standards.[44,45] Checklists are common as cognitive aids used across various industries to reduce variability and improve performance, particularly for complex processes and emergency situations.[46] Checklists common to the maternal health care setting include the WHO Safe Childbirth Checklist, the WHO Safe Surgery Checklist, and adaptations of these tools.[47,48]

The World Health Organization's Safe Childbirth Checklist (SCC) was publicly released in 2015 as a job aid for frontline health care providers to ensure the implementation of 28 essential birth practices addressing major childbirth-related morbidity and mortality.[47] The SCC was designed for implementation within a supportive environment incorporating key stakeholder buy-in; understanding and ownership; local adaptation for alignment with existing guidelines and protocols; technical training to overcome practice gaps; and support through ongoing coaching, monitoring, and evaluation.[47] Implementation of the checklist and associated mentorship plus continuous data feedback was found to increase adherence to evidence-based practices at primary level facilities in the northern India BetterBirth study; however, maternal or perinatal morbidity and mortality were not reduced.[49] Subanalysis of trial data identi-fied variation in adherence to the full set of evidence-based practices and found that each additional practice performed was associated with an 18% to 22% decrease in neonatal mortality, confirming a minimum required level of bundle adherence required for impact.[20] Overall implementation of the WHO SCC in Namibia found improvement in the average number of evidence-based practices implemented from 68% to 95% and associated reductions in perinatal mortality from 22 deaths per 1000 deliveries to 13.8, largely due to declines in fresh stillbirths.[50] A study among global SCC imple-menters identified key content and implementation adaptations.[51] Facilitators of suc-cessful SCC implementation included leadership commitment, QI capacity, organizational culture of accountability, staff appreciation, and openness to change.[51] Varied other trials assessing care bundles incorporating the SCC in combination with other components have found improvements in evidence-based practice implemen-tation,[50] reductions in stillbirth,[52] and severe complications.[53] Barriers to SCC imple-mentation include facility resources including supplies and utilities.[51,54]

Adaptations of the WHO Surgical Safety Checklist to maternity care in the context of cesarean section have been implemented in various settings and have resulted in reduced incidence of postoperative sepsis, higher-level care referral, and reopera-tion[55]; lower rates of maternal sepsis[56]; and improved team communication.[36] Users have emphasized the need for contextual adaptation to ensure implementation success.[57]

Quality Improvement Project Approaches

QI broadly refers to continuous systems change in clinical processes, with constant reassessment of changes in patient outcomes as iterative adjustments are made. QI is designed to operate within a supportive environment that can support systems changes within a robust, no blame educational program. Effective QI programs should be transparent; both administration and clinical staff should understand the goals and methods of a QI project.[58] Commonly used QI frameworks include (1) Plan-Do-Study-Act (PDSA) cycles; (2) define measure, analyze, improve, and control (DMAIC) problem-solving; and (3) results, approaches, deploy, assess, and refine (RADAR) ma-trix cycles, all of which have been adopted from other industries and applied to the health care setting.[59,60]

The PDSA cycle is a 4-step ongoing quality-of-care process approach (**Fig. 3**). It in-cludes (1) Plan: developing a plan and which outcomes are clearly stated and a clear plan is put into place (ie, recruit a team, draft an aim statement, describe current context, brainstorming, describe the problems as well as identification of causes and alternatives); (2) Do: implement the action plan; (3) Study: assess the impact of the action plan, as well as unintended side effects; and (4) Act: change practice based on plan and the target outcomes.[61,62] PDSA cycles have been found to be more effec-tive than adopting "the right-first-time" approaches[59] and enable 2 types of corrective action—temporary and permanent. Temporary actions are aimed at results by practi-cally tackling problems, whereas permanent corrective actions target improved pro-cess sustainability, including investigation and elimination of root causes.[37] PDSA cycles seem to be the most prevalent QI framework used in maternal health. Evalua-tions of maternal care quality improvement processes using PDSA cycles to improve early breastfeeding initiation in an Indian facility identified an increase from 72% to 98%.[63] Another Indian study at a tertiary care facility reported PDSA cycle use increased early maternal-neonatal skin-to-skin contact, delayed cord clamping, and early breastfeeding initiation compliance from minimal to a median of 54%, 59%, and 61%, respectively, over a 36-month period.[64]

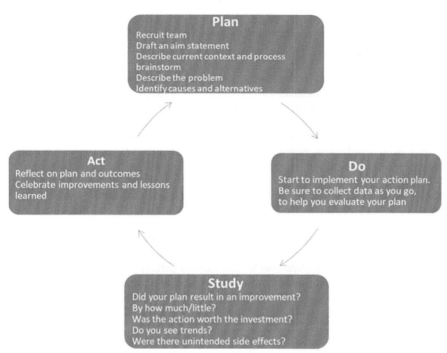

Fig. 3. Depiction of iterative Plan-Do-Study-Act cycle. (*Adapted from* Plan-do-study-act (PDSA) worksheet: IHI. Institute for Healthcare Improvement. https://www.ihi.org/resources/Pages/Tools/PlanDoStudyActWorksheet.aspx; with permission)

DMAIC is a quality improvement or problem-solving process, which stands for define measure, analyze, improve, and control.[62,65] DMAIC comes from a data-driven life-cycle approach to Six Sigma projects for process improvement and differs from the PDSA cycle approach through its incorporation of a more detailed planning phase and the use of more advanced tools, including statistical resources; thus it may be more complicated to implement within certain contexts. DMAIC is a popular and robust methodology for identifying areas of improvement and determining the appropriate actions to remedy them through structured organization or systems performance inquiry with targeted objectives. However, relatively fewer maternal health QI projects are oriented by DMAIC,[66] and its relative utility compared with other QI frameworks is therefore not well established.

RADAR matrix cycles are another option for structured assessment of organization or systems performance, and RADAR matrix cycles are oriented by a specific intended result. This cycle first defines the results that it is aiming to achieve, followed by development of an integrated set of approaches that are anticipated to achieve those results. Those approaches are then deployed in a systematic way ensuring full implementation and assessed. Approaches are refined based on ongoing monitoring and analysis as well as other ongoing learning activities. Similar to DMAIC, this framework is relatively less used in the context of maternal health care.

Although QI processes have successfully changed practice in many settings, contextual factors important for successful implementation are needed and may vary across sites, including capacity building and supervision, governance and regulation, multilevel orientation, and infrastructural support, in addition to a combination of interventions deployed simultaneously.[67–69] Further research should evaluate comparative QI frameworks, by facility level and context, in order to guide advances, and use implementation science frameworks, as described later, to support robust assessment.[58,70,71]

Intervention facilitators and challenges and implementation science priorities

Evidence-based care standards for improving the quality of maternal and newborn care at the health facility level have been established by the WHO and international, regional, and national professional societies, among others.[72] However, where standards are adopted to lower-resources settings from higher-resource settings, concerns around contextual adaptation exist including around appropriateness and feasibility for context both for the evidence-based practices being focused on and their targets and the data collection process itself.[73–75] Challenges in data collection for informing achievement of standards include variability in reliability and validity of survey versus registry data, as compared with observation, in terms of implementation of maternal and newborn care interventions.[76]

The increasing popularity of implementation science models and frameworks for understanding the translation of evidence-based practice is rapidly expanding our understanding of the key multilevel factors across settings.[77] A recent scoping review of the literature identified implementation facilitators and barriers for maternal health interventions in lower-resource settings (n = 58).[78] Facilitators include knowledge, training, service provider motivation, effective coordination, leadership, and effective communication. Barriers included cultural divides, differences between western and traditional health care, change capacity, and infrastructure, particularly workforce capacity and resources.[78] The review identified limited application of implementation science theory within the identified literature, highlighting an important opportunity for improving the evidence base. Indeed, implementation research priorities were heavily featured within an expert prioritization exercise defining key maternal health issues that have received inadequate attention from donors and researchers across the following domains: optimizing health worker distribution and retention, task shifting, hands-on skills development, promoting evidence-based practice, encouraging attitudinal and behavioral changes, and transforming managerial capacity across health system levels.[79] Research focused on optimizing the Consolidated Framework for Implementation Research for low- and middle-income settings confirms the utility of this framework for implementation research on a variety of health topics and suggests particular adaptations for greater attention to external implementation determinants that may hold greater importance in resource-limited settings.[71]

Provider educational strategies

Provider education strategies range from supporting health care workers in obtaining and retaining knowledge and skills to task shifting or sharing approaches, expanding the range of cadres who are trained to provide certain levels of care. Formal task shifting is a deliberate strategy to overcome shortages in the health workforce that limit a health system's ability to provide needed care. Task shifting strategies provide lower-level cadres with specific skills to implement specific clinical tasks normally reserved for higher-level cadres through formal training and certification processes. In the context of maternal health, this strategy allows for midwives and obstetricians to focus on meeting more complex care needs without sacrificing the quality of care provided. However, this strategy is not without controversy.[80,81] A systematic review of task shifting and sharing for maternal and reproductive health in low- to upper-middle-income country contexts including 20 papers reported obstetric surgery outcomes of nonphysician clinicians with physicians identified little difference in patient outcomes between cadres in postoperative maternal outcomes, cesarean case fatality rate, fetal deaths, and length of hospital stay.[82] Furthermore, task shifting has largely been reported to be acceptable to providers and perceived to be essential.[83] However, increased training and continuing education are called for to optimize health outcomes.[82]

Beyond well-structured preservice and in-service training, opportunities for implementation support of evidence-based interventions include shifts from traditional supervisory models to mentorship models. Mentorship models lead to improvements in quality of clinical care, leadership and accountability, and staff satisfaction, particularly where they are contextually adapted.[84] Mentoring-based models are considered more flexible than supervision-based models, and their relationship-oriented approach empowers both mentor and mentee through emphasis on an ongoing developmental orientation where honest appraisal, feedback, and skills building can take place.[49] Furthermore, mentorship models have been found to result in greater skilled personnel retention, a significant challenge in lower-resource settings both domestically and internationally.[85] Innovative approaches to overcome such challenges through expanding beyond on-job training supported through both onsite and virtual platforms are critical.

SUMMARY

Tremendous improvements in maternal health care have been achieved over the past 3 decades[1,2]; however, evidence-based care practices including those prioritizing patient-centered strategies are inconsistently implemented, limiting gains in maternal health and well-being. Expanding evidence-based maternity care implementation through various contextually adapted quality improvement strategies is an imperative for improving maternal health and well-being in lower-resource settings.

Quality assessment and improvement activities such as the implementation of maternal death and near-miss review and efforts to increase evidence-based care practices have been successful in increasing services and quality provision through providing feedback to the entire health system as well as informing the development and implementation of guidelines for clinical performance, service utilization, and patient satisfaction.[86] Strategies for enhancing ongoing QI programming are broad and must be contextually adapted given the range of internal and external influences. Incorporating implementation science–framed approaches is an important next step for implementers and researchers to facilitate an understanding of best practices to consistently achieve evidence-based care across varied settings. The availability of WHO maternal and newborn quality-of-care standards allows health systems to set up quality-of-care strategies and standards to overcome issues related to the improvement of quality of care in maternal and newborn health and integrate these standards into policy and guidance documents.

Factors critical to successful QI implementation include clarity of intervention concept, availability of providers, intervention design, and approaches. Key stakeholders need to be clear about the QI concepts, tools, and methods used to execute the intervention and the principles and philosophy behind those. Furthermore, environmental factors need to be supportive, including leadership.

This review reflects the need for enhancing standardized and valid monitoring strategies and varied options for QI approach implementation, based on the selection of any QI intervention, considering the varied needs of stakeholders within a particular geographic context, leading to appropriate implementation and knowledge management strategies to meet the needs of maternal health program planners and managers in lower-resource settings.

CLINICS CARE POINTS

- Assessment of key indicators for monitoring maternal health care quality in lower-resource settings were largely appraised as poor quality, lacking empirical testing or support, and inadequately distributed across the full continuum of care. Establishing a core set of high-quality standard indicators through harmonization and validation can improve impact assessment of various quality improvement strategies and facilitate comparisons.

- Systematic review of maternal deaths across sub-Saharan Africa and South Asia identified the top 3 attributable factors as substandard care by a health worker, patient delay, and deficiencies in blood transfusion.

- Consistent implementation of the WHO Safe Childbirth Checklist and adaptations of the WHO Safe Surgery Checklist are associated with improved adherence to evidence-based practices and reductions in mortality and morbidity.

- PDSA cycles are the most commonly used quality improvement framework in maternal care in lower-resource settings and have been found to effectively enable temporary and permanent corrective action.

- Key facilitators of maternal health intervention implementation include knowledge, training, service provider motivation, effective coordination, leadership, and effective communication. Key barriers included cultural divides, differences between western and traditional health care, change capacity, and infrastructure, particularly workforce capacity and resources.

- Overcoming external barriers to quality improvement such as limited human resources, commodities, and equipment require leadership commitments across multiple levels and creative approaches. Intermediate strategies such as task shifting and sharing may be considered. A systematic review of nonphysician clinicians' performance identified little difference in obstetric surgery patient outcomes, and this approach has been reported to be acceptable to providers.

DISCLOSURE

The authors have no conflicts of interest to disclose.

REFERENCES

1. Maternal mortality in 1990-2015 WHO, UNICEF, UNFPA, World Bank Group, and United Nations Population Division Maternal Mortality Estimation Inter-Agency Group.
2. World Health Organization. Trends in maternal mortality 2000 to 2017: estimates by WHO, UNICEF, UNFPA, World Bank group and the united Nations population Division: executive summary. World Health Organization; 2019. Available at: https://apps.who.int/iris/handle/10665/327596. Accessed April 15, 2022.
3. Koblinsky M, Moyer CA, Calvert C, et al. Quality maternity care for every woman, everywhere: a call to action. Lancet 2016;388:2307–20.
4. Lim SS, Allen K, Bhutta ZA, et al. Measuring the health-related Sustainable Development Goals in 188 countries: a baseline analysis from the Global Burden of Disease Study 2015. Lancet 2016;388:1813–50.

5. GBD 2017 SDG Collaborators. Measuring progress from 1990 to 2017 and projecting attainment to 2030 of the health-related Sustainable Development Goals for 195 countries and territories: a systematic analysis for the Global Burden of Disease Study 2017. Lancet Lond Engl 2018;392:2091–138.
6. Geller SE, Koch AR, Garland CE, et al. A global view of severe maternal morbidity: moving beyond maternal mortality. Reprod Health 2018;15:98.
7. Severe Maternal Morbidity: Screening and Review. Available at: https://www. acog.org/en/clinical/clinical-guidance/obstetric-care-consensus/articles/2016/ 09/severe-maternal-morbidity-screening-and-review. Accessed June 26, 2022.
8. Petersen EE. Racial/Ethnic Disparities in Pregnancy-Related Deaths — United States, 2007–2016. MMWR Morb Mortal Wkly Rep 2019;68. https://doi.org/10. 15585/mmwr.mm6835a3.
9. World Health Organization, OECD, The World Bank. Delivering quality health services: a global imperative for universal health coverage. Geneva (Switzerland): World Health Organzation, Organisation for Economic Co-operation and Development, and The WOrld Bank. Available at: https://www.who.int/publications-detail-redirect/9789241513906. Accessed April 17, 2022.
10. FIGO Statements. Figo. Available at: https://www.figo.org/resources/figo-statements. Accessed July 16, 2022.
11. American College of Obstetricians and Gynecologists. ACOG Clinical Topics. Available at: https://www.acog.org/en/topics. Accessed July 16, 2022.
12. Published guidance, NICE advice and quality standards | Guidance. NICE. Available at: https://www.nice.org.uk/guidance/published. Accessed July 16, 2022.
13. Sakala C, Corry MP, Milbank Memorial Fund (USA). Evidence-based maternity care: what it is and what it can achieve. New York: Milbank Memorial Fund; 2008.
14. World Health Organization. WHO recommendations on antenatal care for a positive pregnancy experience. Geneva, Switzerland: World Health Organization; 2016.
15. World Health Organization. WHO recommendations on maternal health: guidelines Approved by the WHO GUidelines review Committee. Geneva, Switzerland: World Health Organization; 2017.
16. World Health Organization. WHO Recommendations: Intrapartum care for a positive childbirth experience. 2018.
17. World Health Organization. WHO recommendations on newborn health: guidelines Approved by the WHO guidelines review Committee. Geneva, Switzerland: World Health Organization; 2017.
18. Akachi Y, Tarp F, Kelley E, et al. Measuring quality-of-care in the context of sustainable development goal 3: a call for papers. Bull World Health Organ 2016;94: 160-160A.
19. Okeke EN, Chari AV. Can Institutional Deliveries Reduce Newborn Mortality?: Evidence from Rwanda. RAND Corporation. 2015. Available at: https://www.rand. org/pubs/working_papers/WR1072.html. Accessed April 21, 2022.
20. Bhutta ZA, Das JK, Bahl R, et al. Can available interventions end preventable deaths in mothers, newborn babies, and stillbirths, and at what cost? Lancet Lond Engl 2014;384:347-70.
21. Chou VB, Walker N, Kanyangarara M. Estimating the global impact of poor quality of care on maternal and neonatal outcomes in 81 low- and middle-income countries: A modeling study. Plos Med 2019;16:e1002990.
22. Moran AC, Jolivet RR, Chou D, et al. A common monitoring framework for ending preventable maternal mortality, 2015–2030: phase I of a multi-step process. BMC Pregnancy Childbirth 2016;16:250.

23. Institute of Medicine. Vital signs: core metrics for health and health care progress. Washington, DC: The National Academies Press; 2015.

24. Saturno-Hernández PJ, Martínez-Nicolás I, Moreno-Zegbe E, et al. Indicators for monitoring maternal and neonatal quality care: a systematic review. BMC Pregnancy Childbirth 2019;19:25.

25. Moller A-B, Newby H, Hanson C, et al. Measures matter: A scoping review of maternal and newborn indicators. PLoS ONE 2018;13:e0204763.

26. Madaj B, Smith H, Mathai M, et al. Developing global indicators for quality of maternal and newborn care: a feasibility assessment. Bull World Health Organ 2017;95:445–452l.

27. UN agencies(WHO, UNICEF. Maternal and perinatal death surveillance and response: materials to support implementation. 2021. Available at: https://www.who.int/publications/i/item/9789240036666. Accessed March 15, 2022.

28. World Health Organization. Evaluating the quality of care for severe pregnancy complications: the WHO near-miss approach for maternal health. Geneva (Switzerland): World Health Organization; 2011. Available at: http://apps.who.int/iris/bitstream/10665/44692/1/9789241502221_eng.pdf.

29. Sayinzoga F, Bijlmakers L, van Dillen J, et al. Maternal death audit in Rwanda 2009-2013: a nationwide facility-based retrospective cohort study. BMJ Open 2016;6:e009734.

30. Kumela L, Tilahun T, Kifle D. Determinants of maternal near miss in Western Ethiopia. Ethiop J Health Sci 2020;30:161–8.

31. Tayebwa E, Sayinzoga F, Umunyana J, et al. Assessing Implementation of Maternal and Perinatal Death Surveillance and Response in Rwanda. Int J Environ Res Public Health 2020;17:4376.

32. Kurinczuk JJ, Draper ES, Field DJ, et al. Experiences with maternal and perinatal death reviews in the UK–the MBRRACE-UK programme. BJOG Int J Obstet Gynaecol 2014;121(Suppl 4):41–6.

33. Kinney MV, Walugembe DR, Wanduru P, et al. Maternal and perinatal death surveillance and response in low- and middle-income countries: a scoping review of implementation factors. Health Policy Plan 2021;36:955–73.

34. Smith H, Ameh C, Roos N, et al. Implementing maternal death surveillance and response: a review of lessons from country case studies. BMC Pregnancy Childbirth 2017;17:233.

35. Scott H, Dairo A. Maternal Death Surveillance and Response in East and Southern Africa. J Obstet Gynaecol Can 2015;37:915–21.

36. Kearns RJ, Uppal V, Bonner J, et al. The introduction of a surgical safety checklist in a tertiary referral obstetric centre. BMJ Qual Saf 2011;20:818–22.

37. Willcox ML, Price J, Scott S, et al. Death audits and reviews for reducing maternal, perinatal and child mortality. Cochrane Database Syst Rev 2020;3: CD012982.

38. Merali HS, Lipsitz S, Hevelone N, et al. Audit-identified avoidable factors in maternal and perinatal deaths in low resource settings: a systematic review. BMC Pregnancy Childbirth 2014;14:280.

39. Sotunsa JO, Adeniyi AA, Imaralu JO, et al. Maternal near-miss and death among women with postpartum haemorrhage: a secondary analysis of the Nigeria Near-miss and Maternal Death Survey. BJOG Int J Obstet Gynaecol 2019;126:19–25.

40. Kalter HD, Salgado R, Babille M, et al. Social autopsy for maternal and child deaths: a comprehensive literature review to examine the concept and the development of the method. Popul Health Metr 2011;9:45.

41. Lasandha Irangani. Social determinants of health pave the path to maternal deaths in rural Sri Lanka: reections from social autopsies. 2022. Available at: https://doi.org/10.21203/rs.3.rs-1585439/v1. Accessed March 15, 2022.
42. Dickson KE, Kinney MV, Moxon SG, et al. Scaling up quality care for mothers and newborns around the time of birth: an overview of methods and analyses of intervention-specific bottlenecks and solutions. BMC Pregnancy Childbirth 2015;15(Suppl 2):S1.
43. Nyamtema AS, Urassa DP, van Roosmalen J. Maternal health interventions in resource limited countries: a systematic review of packages, impacts and factors for change. BMC Pregnancy Childbirth 2011;11:30.
44. Lingard L, Regehr G, Orser B, et al. Evaluation of a Preoperative Checklist and Team Briefing Among Surgeons, Nurses, and Anesthesiologists to Reduce Failures in Communication. Arch Surg 2008;143:12–7.
45. Sewell M, Adebibe M, Jayakumar P, et al. Use of the WHO surgical safety checklist in trauma and orthopaedic patients. Int Orthop 2011;35:897–901.
46. Winters BD, Gurses AP, Lehmann H, et al. Clinical review: Checklists - translating evidence into practice. Crit Care 2009;13:210.
47. World Health Organization. WHO safe childbirth checklist implementation guide: improving the quality of facility-based delivery for mothers and newborns. 2015.
48. World Health Organization. Implementation manual: WHO surgical safety checklist. 2008. Available at: https://apps.who.int/iris/handle/10665/70046. Accessed March 15, 2022.
49. Semrau KEA, Hirschhorn LR, Marx Delaney M, et al. Outcomes of a Coaching-Based WHO Safe Childbirth Checklist Program in India. N Engl J Med 2017; 377:2313–24.
50. Kabongo L, Gass J, Kivondo B, et al. Implementing the WHO Safe Childbirth Checklist: lessons learnt on a quality improvement initiative to improve mother and newborn care at Gobabis District Hospital, Namibia. BMJ Open Qual 2017;6:e000145.
51. Molina RL, Benski A-C, Bobanski L, et al. Adaptation and implementation of the WHO Safe Childbirth Checklist around the world. Implement Sci Commun 2021; 2:76.
52. Walker D, Otieno P, Butrick E, et al. Effect of a quality improvement package for intrapartum and immediate newborn care on fresh stillbirth and neonatal mortality among preterm and low-birthweight babies in Kenya and Uganda: a cluster-randomised facility-based trial. Lancet Glob Health 2020;8:e1061–70.
53. Sousa K de M, Saturno-Hernández PJ, Rosendo TMS de S, et al. Impact of the implementation of the WHO Safe Childbirth Checklist on essential birth practices and adverse events in two Brazilian hospitals: a before and after study. BMJ Open 2022;12:e056908.
54. Maisonneuve JJ, Semrau KEA, Maji P, et al. Effectiveness of a WHO Safe Childbirth Checklist Coaching-based intervention on the availability of Essential Birth Supplies in Uttar Pradesh, India. Int J Qual Health Care 2018;30:769–77.
55. Naidoo M, Moodley J, Gathiram P, et al. The impact of a modified World Health Organization surgical safety checklist on maternal outcomes in a South African setting: A stratified cluster-randomised controlled trial. S Afr Med J 2017;107: 248–57.
56. Wurdeman T, Staffa SJ, Barash D, et al. Surgical Safety Checklist Use and Post-Caesarean Sepsis in the Lake Zone of Tanzania: Results from Safe Surgery 2020. World J Surg 2022;46:303–9.

57. Verwey S, Gopalan PD. An investigation of barriers to the use of the World Health Organization Surgical Safety Checklist in theatres. S Afr Med J 2018;108:336–41.

58. Lincoln EW, Reed-Schrader E, Jarvis JL. EMS Quality Improvement Programs. In: StatPearls. Treasure Island (FL): StatPearls Publishing. 2022. Available at: http://www.ncbi.nlm.nih.gov/books/NBK536982/. Accessed April 15, 2022.

59. Ahmed ES, Ahmad MN, Othman SH. Business process improvement methods in healthcare: a comparative study. Int J Health Care Qual Assur 2019;32:887–908.

60. Plan-Do-Study-Act (PDSA) Worksheet | IHI - Institute for Healthcare Improvement. Available at: https://www.ihi.org/resources/Pages/Tools/PlanDoStudyActWorksheet.aspx. Accessed August 5, 2022.

61. Christoff P. Running PDSA cycles. Curr Probl Pediatr Adolesc Health Care 2018;48:198–201.

62. M. Sokovic a,*, D. Pavletic b KKP. Quality Improvement Methodologies – PDCA Cycle, RADAR Matrix, DMAIC and DFSS. Ind Manag Organ; Volume 43. Available at: https://www.researchgate.net/publication/49600834_Quality_improvement_methodologies_-_PDCA_cycle_RADAR_matrix_DMAIC_and_DFSS. Accessed March 15, 2022.

63. Sharma S, Sharma C, Kumar D. Improving the Breastfeeding Practices in Healthy Neonates During Hospital Stay Using Quality Improvement Methodology. Indian Pediatr 2018;55:757–60.

64. Sachan R, Srivastava H, Srivastava S, et al. Use of point of care quality improvement methodology to improve newborn care, immediately after birth, at a tertiary care teaching hospital, in a resource constraint setting. BMJ Open Qual 2021;10:e001445.

65. de Mast J, Lokkerbol J. An analysis of the Six Sigma DMAIC method from the perspective of problem solving. Int J Prod Econ 2012;139:604–14.

66. Tufail MMB, Shamim A, Ali A, et al. DMAIC methodology for achieving public satisfaction with health departments in various districts of Punjab and optimizing CT scan patient load in urban city hospitals. AIMS Public Health 2022;9:440–57.

67. Strom KL. Quality improvement interventions: what works. J Healthc Qual 2001;23:4–14 [quiz: 14, 24].

68. Goyet S, Broch-Alvarez V, Becker C. Quality improvement in maternal and newborn healthcare: lessons from programmes supported by the German development organisation in Africa and Asia. BMJ Glob Health 2019;4:e001562.

69. Teviu EAA. Contributing Factors to Implementation of Quality Improvement Methods for Maternal, Neonatal and Child Health Services in Lower-Middle Income Countries, Using Ghana as a Case Study. 2017. Available at: https://bibalex.org/baifa/Attachment/Documents/zJF1NjiP8E_20180404112310255.pdf.

70. Keith RE, Crosson JC, O'Malley AS, et al. Using the Consolidated Framework for Implementation Research (CFIR) to produce actionable findings: a rapid-cycle evaluation approach to improving implementation. Implement Sci 2017;12:15.

71. Means AR, Kemp CG, Gwayi-Chore M-C, et al. Evaluating and optimizing the consolidated framework for implementation research (CFIR) for use in low- and middle-income countries: a systematic review. Implement Sci IS 2020;15:17.

72. WHO. STANDARDS FOR IMPROVING QUALITY OF MATERNAL AND NEWBORN CARE IN HEALTH FACILITIES. Available at: https://cdn.who.int/media/docs/default-source/mca-documents/qoc/quality-of-care/standards-for-improving-quality-of-maternal-and-newborn-care-in-health-facilities.pdf?sfvrsn=3b364d8_4. Accessed March 15, 2022.

73. Proctor E, Silmere H, Raghavan R, et al. Outcomes for implementation research: conceptual distinctions, measurement challenges, and research agenda. Adm Policy Ment Health 2011;38:65–76.
74. Theobald S, Brandes N, Gyapong M, et al. Implementation research: new imperatives and opportunities in global health. Lancet Lond Engl 2018;392:2214–28.
75. Boatin AA, Ngonzi J, Ganyaglo G, et al. Cesarean delivery in low- and middle-income countries: A review of quality of care metrics and targets for improvement. Semin Fetal Neonatal Med 2021;26:101199.
76. Day LT, Sadeq-ur Rahman Q, Ehsanur Rahman A, et al. Assessment of the validity of the measurement of newborn and maternal health-care coverage in hospitals (EN-BIRTH): an observational study. Lancet Glob Health 2021;9:e267–79.
77. Emmanuel Akwoulo Agyigewe Teviu. Contributing Factors to Implementation of Quality Improvement Methods for Maternal, Neonatal and Child Health Services in LowerMiddle Income Countries, Using Ghana as a Case Study. 2012; Available at: chrome-extension://efaidnbmnnnibpcajpcglclefindmkaj/http://bibalex.org/baifa/Attachment/Documents/zJF1NjiP8E_20180404112310255.pdf. Accessed March 15, 2022
78. Dadich A, Piper A, Coates D. Implementation science in maternity care: a scoping review. Implement Sci 2021;16:16.
79. Kendall T, Langer A. Critical maternal health knowledge gaps in low- and middle-income countries for the post-2015 era. Reprod Health 2015;12:55.
80. McPake B, Mensah K. Task shifting in health care in resource-poor countries. Lancet Lond Engl 2008;372:870–1.
81. Lehmann U, Van Damme W, Barten F, et al. Task shifting: the answer to the human resources crisis in Africa? Hum Resour Health 2009;7:49.
82. Gajewski J, Cheelo M, Bijlmakers L, et al. The contribution of non-physician clinicians to the provision of surgery in rural Zambia—a randomised controlled trial. Hum Resour Health 2019;17:60.
83. Dawson AJ, Buchan J, Duffield C, et al. Task shifting and sharing in maternal and reproductive health in low-income countries: a narrative synthesis of current evidence. Health Policy Plan 2014;29:396–408.
84. Alidina S, Chatterjee P, Zanial N, et al. Improving surgical quality in low-income and middle-income countries: why do some health facilities perform better than others? BMJ Qual Saf 2021;30:937–49.
85. Schwerdtle P, Morphet J, Hall H. A scoping review of mentorship of health personnel to improve the quality of health care in low and middle-income countries. Glob Health 2017;13:77.
86. uddin MN, Alvi MA, Malik MZ, et al. Approaches towards improving the quality of maternal and newborn health services in South Asia: challenges and opportunities for healthcare systems. Glob Health 2018;14:17.

Interprofessional Care in Obstetrics and Gynecology

Neil Joseph Murphy, MD, Reinou Sybrecht Groen, MD, MIH, PhD*

KEYWORDS

- Interprofessional care • Task sharing • Task shifting • Availability • Acceptability
- Affordability • Accessibility • Accommodation

KEY POINTS

- Interprofessional care strengthens a health-care system on micro and macro levels.
- Task sharing increases access to care.
- Task shifting decreases health-care costs.
- Acceptability of care is an important aspect of why task shifting and sharing should not be undertaken without keeping local specifics in mind.
- Task shifting and sharing can increase the quality of care.

INTRODUCTION

This article describes interprofessional care in obstetrics and gynecology (OBGYN). Interprofessional care relates to providing care to an individual in an integrated system of professionals. These professionals (including doctors, nurses, midwives, pharmacists) relate to each other in their specific roles, making patient care collaborative and open for discussion, and sharing tasks and decision-making, rather than the traditional top–down approach. By enabling each cadre of HCWs to contribute and by strengthening lower cadres with standards, appropriate check-ins at predetermined times and providing checklists before procedures and care events, medicine has become safer and more comprehensive.[1] Checklists have made transition of specific care to lower cadres of HCWs possible, as each component of care is clearly outlined. Interprofessional care can also include telemedicine with remote consultations, curbsides, and sharing of guidelines, expertise, or possibly remote direction of certain procedures.

Task shifting and sharing (TS/S) is globally acknowledged as one of the best solutions for the HCW crisis. With clear guidelines, checklists, and referral indications, an appropriate standard of care can be achieved, and patients who were not able to access health care in a timely manner due to remote living conditions, lack of transportation, or other barriers can be eliminated. The first experience in TS/S came from countries

OBGYN at Alaska Native Medical Center, 4441 Diplomacy Drive, Anchorage, AK 99508, USA
* Corresponding author.
E-mail address: rgroen@southcentralfoundation.com

Obstet Gynecol Clin N Am 49 (2022) 841–868
https://doi.org/10.1016/j.ogc.2022.08.006
0889-8545/22/Published by Elsevier Inc.

hardest hit by the HIV epidemic. These countries found that when specific outlined tasks were moved from the most highly qualified health workers to HCWs with shorter training and/or fewer qualifications, there was more efficient and effective use of the available human resources for health. With decentralization of health-care tasks, shifting care made access to care in remote locations possible and helped address the shortage of health workers.[2]

Health-care worker shortage is real. Doctors and nurses have been difficult to train and retain in many countries and rural areas across the globe. In a 2009 study, South-central Somalia had just 11 doctors, 193 nurses, and 32 community health workers for a population of 600,000. In Malawi, there is a 60% vacancy rate for nurses in rural areas and only 2 doctors for every 100,000 people. Moreover, in Niger, besides having few HCWs and a severe health crisis due to food insecurity, 90% of HCWs are in the few cities leaving a vast rural area with limited and sparsely distributed staff.[3] However, rural areas in the United States and Australia and elsewhere are facing similar disparities, although on a different scale.[4,5] Globally about half of the world population resides in rural areas but those areas are served by one-fourth of all physicians and less than two-fifth of nurses.[6,7]

Health-care worker shortage in rural areas across the globe has been addressed by policy makers through a variety of strategies, including increasing the lure of relocation with attractive housing, financial incentives, and professional support. In addition, there has been increased recruitment for rural HCWs by rural medical schools and nursing programs and attractive school-loan forgiveness programs linked to a rural posting for several years. However, increased recruitment and training of HCWs may not necessarily lead to their retention, which may rather be addressed by attention to job satisfaction, access to continuing medical education, and availability of virtual consultation. Health policies that promote both recruitment and retention of HCWs are generally grouped into education, regulation, financial compensation, and personal and professional support programs.[8,9]

Lower resourced countries cannot compete with the financial benefits offered by high-income countries, leading to another reason for HCW maldistribution globally, often referred to as "brain-drain."[10] There may also be intangible reasons for the difficulty of recruitment of rural health personnel. Race, ethnicity, religious, or gender disparities in admissions for nursing and medical educational programs has led to a cadre of HCWs with possibly less affinity to populations living in rural and more remote areas.

Task shifting and sharing (TS/S) can break down some of the barriers of access to health care in a different way. In TS/S, HCWs are generally trained in a local context, they already have affinity with the community, and their certification is less translatable internationally, improving retention. Training through TS/S is also less extensive, reducing the cost for those providers. Countries have come up with their own strategies for TS/S, including shorter specialty training for medical doctors directed to specific rural needs, to allow work in remote settings including performance of surgery; giving nonphysician providers training and legal privileges to perform specified surgical procedures; nurses providing HIV medications; use of Physician-Assistants and Nurse-Practitioners to provide basic and more specialized patient care; and development of community health workers or health surveillance assistants, who enter a medical workforce with limited training and very task specific roles.[11-17] OBGYNs are not new to the field of TS/S; there has always been an opportunity to work with midwifes and family physicians who chose to include OBGYN in their practice have been instrumental in delivering care in rural areas. There have also always been birth companions, birth workers, or birth attendants who have supported women in childbirth with knowledge passed down through generations.

In this article, we discuss the opportunities of TS/S based on evidence of benefit and with considerations of training, quality assurance, as well as permissive laws and regulations.

DEFINITIONS
Interprofessional Care

Interprofessional care happens when multiple health workers from different professional backgrounds work together with patients, families, caretakers, and communities to deliver the highest quality of care. It allows health workers to engage any individual whose skills can help achieve health goals.[18] Interprofessional care and TS/S are different from multidisciplinary care. In the latter, each health-care team member has their own specific plan of care based on specific and distinct knowledge and skill sets (**Box 1**); in the interprofessional care model, a team of health-care workers will share their knowledge and treatment plans and determine which and how HCWs will interact with patients.[19] Frequently, in interprofessional care, the tasks in treatment plans are distributed on a local-regional level; for example, vaccine distribution may be shifted or shared by pharmacist, nurse supervisors, and rural HCWs. The nurses can take on traditional pharmacist responsibilities and the pharmacist may take nurse supervising responsibilities to smoothly role out the vaccination campaign.

Task Sharing

Task sharing indicates that a specific health-care task can be done by different health providers, even though those health providers may not have the same full scope of care. The term can be used for an entire procedure or parts of the procedure or can include medication prescriptions by providers other than physicians. Task sharing gives flexibility to a team of health workers to deliver timely care. Health-care needs vary in time and place; task sharing assists health-care teams to deliver care when

Box 1
Differences in interprofessional care and multidisciplinary care

	Multidisciplinary	Interprofessional Care
Attitude	Each person is focused on own discipline-specific plan of care. Some disciplines are thought to be more suitable for team leadership roles	A biopsychosocial model, which includes team discussions on group processes in addition to patient care. Team development is encouraged and supported, and there is shared leadership
Knowledge	Knows core patient care functions of other disciplines but only knows own discipline well. Recognizes team leader and others' responsibilities	Knows part of training and competencies of other disciplines and can perform/supervise these and is licensed to do so. Is able to articulate role overlap and unique contributions
Behaviors	Each member of the team has their own assessment and treatment plans. Evaluates progress on their own	Joint assessment and treatment plans. Identifies role overlaps in an attempt to avoid duplication and enhance coverage

Adapted from Steffen, Ann M., Antonette M. Zeiss, and Michele Karel, 'Interprofessional Geriatric Healthcare: Competencies and Resources for Teamwork', in Nancy A. Pachana, and Ken Laidlaw (eds), The Oxford Handbook of Clinical Geropsychology, Oxford Library of Psychology (2014; online edn, Oxford Academic, 6 Jan. 2015), https://doi.org/10.1093/oxfordhb/9780199663170.013.021; with permission.

and where it is needed. Tasks are not taken away from one cadre of workers and given to another cadre but rather midlevel health-care professionals are given expanded tasks, enabling safe provision of procedures or other care that would otherwise be delayed or not possible due to limitations in number or availability of higher level HCWs. It can also refer to task sharing across disciplines, as in surgeons trained to perform cesarean deliveries or OBGYNs performing vasectomy or providing primary or psychiatric care.[20]

Task Shifting

Task shifting refers to a redistribution of tasks to different health cadres. Some tasks are shifted from highly trained HCWs to health workers with shorter training and fewer qualifications to expand the reach of the care in the population and to use the distinct qualifications of the more highly trained HCW to achieve better coverage of more complicated services.[2]

Task Shifting and Sharing

When adopting health-care models to meet the health-care needs of a population, there is often a combination of task shifting and task sharing. The most beneficial use of TS/S involves a better balance of health-care tasks and responsibilities across health cadres.

CADRES OF CARE

A cadre of care refers to the types of HCWs in the health-care system, generally consisting of doctors, nurses, midwives, nurse practitioners, physician assistants, pharmacists, physical therapists, and mental health workers but also including community health workers, health educators, and peer navigators.

HEALTH-CARE WORKERS

A HCW is any person providing an aspect of health care to an individual, group, or population. HCWs encompass those directly at the bedside or in clinics as well as public HCWs, health educators, including auxiliary and complementary health-care services such as physical therapists and pharmacists (**Table 1**).

Community Health Workers

A frontline public health worker who is a trusted member of and/or has a close understanding of the community served and has been trained to attend to the most common or most urgent care needs of the community. Within community, health workers have a variety of tasks, such as peer navigation through health-care visits and in peer support groups, including youth health peers, for mental health education and prevention of depression and suicide, as well as for other areas of health care. Organized peer support groups have been shown to have positive effects on many chronic illnesses, including navigation of health care and better treatment adherence and have shown to reduce hospitalizations and health-care costs in general.[21–23]

FRAMEWORKS AND GENERAL GUIDANCE FOR INTERPROFESSIONAL CARE
Prerequisites for Interprofessional Care and Task shifting and sharing

Interprofessional care implies teamwork rather than a top–down hierarchy. Lower level cadres should be empowered to speak up and participate as active members of the team and a less hierarchical structure is associated with better outcomes.[24]

Table 1
Health-care workers for women's health

Health-Care Worker Type	Example
Specialist	Gynecologist/obstetrician
Doctor otherwise specialized	Family doctor/pediatrician/urologist/general surgeon
Basic medical doctor degree	Assistant medical officer/clinical officer
Advanced associate or associate clinician	Physician assistant/surgical technician/nurse practitioner
Midwife	Nurse-midwife, registered midwife, community midwife, direct entry midwife
Nurse	Registered nurse, clinical nurse specialist, nurse researcher
Complementary services	Osteopath, physical therapist, dietician/nutritionist, traditional healer, acupuncturist, mental health workers
Pharmacist	Doctorate pharmacist, pharmacist assistant
Lay health worker	Community health worker, village health worker, traditional birth attendant, female community health volunteer
Peer support	Patient to patient teaching, youth as health advocates
User/self	Woman, client

Adapted from: WHO, Recommendations for Optimizing Health Worker Roles to Improve Access to Key Maternal and Newborn Health Interventions through Task Shifting, 2012 Geneva World Health Organization.

Interprofessional care can only occur if all cadres and disciplines accept the importance of collaborative care and the necessity of task shifting and sharing. Task shifting and sharing can only be safe and successful with permissive legislation, clear regulations, and guidelines on the procedures or medication prescribing that is shifted from one health cadre to another. Appropriate training and Continuing Education for the cadres who participate in the TS/S is critical for successful interprofessional care systems. Finally, referral access for those clinical scenarios that are not covered in the guidelines or checklists needs to be available for those cadres involved in TS/S.

A quality assurance/quality improvement (QA/QI) process is also critical for a TS/S program or interprofessional care delivery. Rather than reacting to morbidity and mortality, a QA/QI program continuously and proactively reviews care plans and follow-up in health care to indicate the need for continued medical education, supervision, or redirection.

Health-care administrators need to give opportunities for QA/QI to HCWs to stimulate self-reflection, increase local solution finding and ensure durability of the program by ownership of the care given. With task shifted HCWs being the front-line workers of the rural health-care system support through consultants is essential for good quality of care. If consultants are respectful and willing to educate this will help strengthen the TS/S program. If consultants have the willingness to be educated about the local situation, including the standard of living, cultural considerations, and the background qualifications of their colleagues in the remote area, there is more likely to be mutual respect and appreciation.

Where to Start

Randomized controlled trials on TS/S may not be feasible in each instance but are possible.[25] Frequently, TS/S is a response to an urgent need and therefore a more pragmatic approach is preferred. A TS/S approach must include ability to adjust to the real-world situation. Unlike traditional trials in medicine, pragmatic clinical trials occur in real-world settings where care happens; they require extensive collaboration between researchers, implementors and health administrators, and other members of the health-care system.

TS/S can benefit from an improvement model referred to as Plan Do, Study, Act (PDSA; **Fig. 1**) or in some medical literature indicated as Design, Implement, Evaluate and Adjust.[26]

PLAN: Design the Task Shifting and Sharing in Detail

The PDSA cycle begins with the planning of the TS/S. Planning can be done with the FOCUS algorithm (**Box 2**). This will include finding or defining the problem and then looking into solutions that previously have worked or used elsewhere. Carefully defining the problem is important because this process may lead to ideas for a direction of the TS/S. The problem definition should include insights from all parties on both the supply side and demand side (**Table 2**), in which each team member clarifies their current tasks and responsibilities. There is a vast body of literature on TS/S regarding selection of solutions for the defined problem (see **Table 5**). The selection of the ideal candidates or cadres for the TS/S must be determined and consideration will include training, supervision needs, and regulatory approaches. This will include laws, rules, and regulations as well as policies and guidelines to enable cadres of health-care workers to practice according to an extended scope of practice.[18] Finally, but most importantly, the sustainability of the TS/S needs to be considered, including compensation for those willing to undertake more training and more responsibilities.

DO: IMPLEMENT THE CHANGES THAT ARE LIKELY IMPROVING THE PROGRAM

With the implementation of TS/S, it is important to start with a pilot program. This involves testing the day-to-day implementation of the program in a single clinic or area before it is regionally or nationally scaled up. This includes evaluation of the program

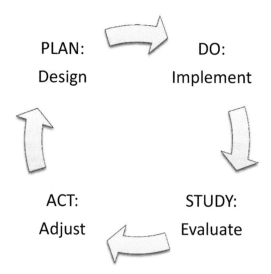

Fig. 1. PDSA.

Box 2	
FOCUS mentality of planning for TS/S	
F	Find the problem within health-care delivery
O	Organize a team to address this
C	Clarify current tasks and responsibilities
U	Understand the options of process variation
S	Select an ideal cadre for task sharing/shifting

and adjustment, a mini-PDSA cycle, before expanding the program. Ideally, there are several cycles leading to full implementation of the TS/S, which is the goal. Feedback from each cycle helps ensure greater likelihood of sustainability when the full program is implemented.

STUDY: EVALUATE THE CHANGES MADE TO THE PROGRAM

The evaluation of a TS/S program or proposal is best undertaken with a combined qualitative and quantitative approach. Predefined numerical targets can help evaluate if the TS/S had the expected effect in terms of uptake of care and number of patients seen. However, the qualitative aspect should not be overlooked. Qualitative data through focus group discussions or semistructured interviews with patients or providers can give insights into acceptability of the TS/S as well as perceived quality of the care.

ACT: Adjust the changes from what is leared in the evaluation process

The last component of the PDSA-cycle is the adjustment and actions based on the findings in the study phase. Both evaluation and adjustments will need to be ongoing

Table 2		
The 5A's and task shifting and sharing from a demand and supply side		
Demand Side		**Supply Side**
Cost of health care can be reduced by TS/S due to the lower cost of a midlevel provider instead of a doctor	Affordability	Health-care delivery can be less expensive due to less need for travel for HCWs and patients and less need for advanced training
The HCW is locally available and is not overbooked	Availability	More HCW can perform a task, therefore greater availability of the health service with more flexibility in scheduling for the HCWs
Because TS/S is oriented to being local there is less need for long transportation	Accessibility	The HCW is more likely to live in rural areas with no commute to work
TS/S can more likely accommodate care at convenient times, including walk-in clinics and remote care or telemedicine	Accommodation	TS/S can accommodate health-care coverage in a more life-friendly schedule for HCWs with possible flexible hours, or longer time off
TS/S can increase acceptability of the care due to the continuity of care provided by the local health-care team	Acceptability	HCW accepts the standards of the TS/S care because the local culture was considered in its design

to ensure high quality of care. In the initial pilot PDSA, adjustments may be needed in terms of number of people trained and depth of training, availability of supervision, and acceptability of TS/S for the population. Adjustments are also frequently required in population outreach and education around TS/S.

Increased Access to Care

Interprofessional care and TS/S are tools to be used with care and consideration of health-care deficiencies and for health-care strengthening. It is however not a fix for all problems encountered in health care, although it can address many barriers to health-care access.

A health-care access model described by Penchansky and Thomas suggests that access to health care is more than the road to a hospital but involves availability, affordability, accessibility, accommodation, and acceptability.[27] This structured approach has been adapted to include health-care demand and supply in relation to all aspects of access to care and TS/S (see **Table 2**).

Task Shifting and Sharing Examples in Women's Health

It is important to keep an individualized approach to TS/S programs and understand the prerequisite skills and qualifications of each health cadre, including literacy and numeracy for the more basic cadres and anatomy, physiology, and pharmacologic background knowledge for the more advanced cadres. **Table 3** indicates 4 different cadres of HCWs who can assist in OBGYN care.

Antenatal Care

Most of the components of antenatal care can be delivered safely by health-care workers with limited but focused health tasks than physicians and midwives if given the right education, tools, and guidelines. In an example from our own setting, the Alaska Native Tribal Health Consortium, the OBGYN department has established clear protocols for Midwives and General Practitioners in all Tribal affiliates on screening with a 2-hour glucose test, curb siding OBGYNs with glucose logs and issues of delivery timing, and inclusion of the pharmacist for those patients who are treated with insulin. To increase consistency in follow-up, women who are on insulin submit their glucose logs to the pharmacist who gives a summary to the OBGYN on call for direction on medication changes. This integration and task shifting and sharing has led to increased patient compliance and access to more regular follow-up for diabetes care in pregnancy.

Intrapartum Care

Intrapartum care is provided by many different cadres of HCWs, with the most basic assistance given by mothers, aunties, community health workers, or birth attendants (**Fig. 2**). Many generations have had traditional birth attendants with a variety of customs, training paths, and status in their respective cultures. The training required for attending the birthing process and for needed medical interventions by skilled birth attendants, midwives, general doctors, and obstetricians, as well as the terminology used for specific cadres, varies significantly around the globe. This can be confusing but is important to understand for individual settings.

The World Health Organization[28] has differentiated the basic care in obstetrics (basic emergent obstetric and neonatal care [BEmONC]) and a next level of care (comprehensive emergent obstetric and neonatal care [CEmONC]) see **Table 4**. This distinction is helpful when setting up health-care centers logistically and related to the training and human resources needed. In rural areas where access to an operating room may be limited,

Table 3
Cadres of care that can expand their health-care capabilities within Obstetrics and Gynecology

Lay health Workers	• Malaria prevention • Labor support • Prevention of postpartum hemorrhage • Neonatal resuscitation • Management of newborn sepsis • Initial dose of antibiotics for maternal sepsis • All short-acting contraceptives, plus injectables • HIV counseling and testing • Lactation services
Auxiliary nurse midwives	All above mentioned, plus: • Labor and birth • Initial antibiotic for premature rupture of membranes • BEmONC • Intrauterine devices
Midwives/nurses	All above mentioned, plus: • Manual vacuum aspiration • Prenatal corticosteroids for preterm labor • Antiretrovirals for treatment/prevention of HIV • Contraceptive implants • Blood transfusion
Nonspecialist physicians	All above mentioned, plus: • Cesarean deliveries • Tubal ligations

Adapted from Deller B, Tripathi V, Stender S, Otolorin E, Johnson P, Carr C. Task shifting in maternal and newborn health care: key components from policy to implementation. Int J Gynaecol Obstet. 2015 Jun;130 Suppl 2:S25-31. https://doi.org/10.1016/j.ijgo.2015.03.005. PMID: 26115853; with permission.

the services indicated in the BEmONC are to prevent death and provide initial care before transportation to a higher level of care. All of the interventions in BEmONC are medical/obstetric interventions, and HCW providing care in rural areas will need additional training and attention to an expanded scope of practice within the TS/S model. Approximately

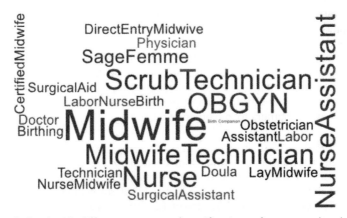

Fig. 2. Word cloud with different names and certifications of names and cadres of care involved in care around the birthing mother.

Table 4	
Basic and advanced/comprehensive obstetric care	
BEmONC	**CEmONC**
• Administration of injectable or intravenous infusions and medications, including antibiotics • Administration of uterotonic drugs • Administration of parenteral anticonvulsants for preeclampsia and eclampsia • Manual removal of the placenta • Manual vacuum extraction or dilatation and curettage • Assisted vaginal delivery with vacuum or forceps • Neonatal resuscitation (bag and mask)	• Perform all basic services • Perform surgeries including cesarean deliveries • Perform blood transfusions

Adapted from World Health Organization, United Nations Population Fund, Mailman School of Public Health. Averting Maternal Death and Disability & United Nations Children's Fund (UNICEF). (2009). Monitoring emergency obstetric care : a handbook. World Health Organization. https://apps.who.int/iris/handle/10665/44121.

5% to 10% of all neonates born need simple stimulation to help them breathe, 3% to 6% require basic resuscitation (bag-and-mask ventilation), and less than 1% require more advanced resuscitation. A meta-analysis of observational before-and-after studies reported a 30% reduction in intrapartum-related neonatal mortality after introduction of training in basic neonatal resuscitation, with a broad range of HCWs, including nonphysician clinicians, traditional birth attendants, and community health workers able to perform neonatal resuscitation.[29]

With CEmONC, TS/S is implemented in places where OBGYNs are scarce. Medical officers (MOs; physicians completing medical school, but without specialized training) and/or clinical officers (Cos; nonphysicians) have been trained to perform cesarean deliveries, tubal ligations, and cesarean hysterectomy in several countries. In India with MOs performing cesarean deliveries, sustainability was dependent on proper selection of facilities, trainees, and support for those trainees.[30] Nonphysician clinicians in Ethiopia often perform the bulk of emergency obstetric procedures including cesarean deliveries, manual removal of placenta, and uterine evacuations. Outcomes (maternal death, fetal death, and length of hospital stay) were comparable to those procedures performed by physicians.[31] In Tanzania, there were no significant differences in outcomes or quality of major obstetric surgeries performed by nonphysician clinicians who received an additional 2 years of training and MOs.[32] A recent review of 15 studies addressing task shifting of cesarean deliveries to nonphysician clinicians found comparable outcomes to procedures performed by physicians; enablers for task shifting included supportive policies, preexisting human resources for health shortage, well-resourced health facilities, and appropriate supervision. Weak health systems were major barriers to implementation.[33]

Family Planning

Family planning allows women to attain their desired number of children, and to determine the spacing of their pregnancies. The Sustainable Development Goals aim to meet 75% of the world's contraceptive needs by 2030; without TS/S, this will not be possible. The WHO has a detailed plan on task sharing to increase access to family planning, which includes the use of laypersons, nurses, midwives, general physicians, and specialists.[34] The information women use to decide on contraceptive use often comes from their own network; the main reason to use a certain type of contraceptive is based on local availability.[35]

The use of laypersons in family planning has been studied in several settings. A study in Madagascar used 61 nonmedically trained lay health workers in community-based distribution of injectable depomedroxyprogesterone acetate (DMPA).[36] The program maintained quality standards because they offered this new service and demonstrated sustained competency through knowledge scores measured 7 months after training and from qualitative reviews of supervisors and satisfied clients.

Abortion Care

Unsafe abortion is a major cause of morbidity and mortality in many low and middle income countries (LMICs). Abortion care was made more accessible in Bihar and Jharkhand where 10 physicians and 10 nurses were trained in performing manual vacuum aspirations (MVAs). More than 800 women with pregnancies less than 10 weeks gestation presented for abortion care; nurses were as skilled as physicians in assessing gestational age, counseling the women about her options and completing an abortion with an MVA. The overall failure and complication rates were low (Nurse 1.2% and 1.4% and physician 0.9% and 0.9%, respectively). Importantly, both provider types were equally acceptable to women who underwent the procedure.[37]

A holistic approach to women who seek abortion care includes birth control counseling and provision or preconception counseling, as well as addressing mental health and sexual health needs, and, when appropriate, safety concerns and social justice issues.[38] These issues should be addressed when the woman presents for her care. Interprofessional care is critical to making this happen.

Breast Cancer Screening

Remote or low resource settings may have limited capacity to follow clinical guidelines for early detection, diagnosis, and treatment of breast cancer.[39] Although mammography is the current standard screening method for breast cancer in high-income countries, population-based screening with this modality is not feasible in many LMICs due to high costs of the required equipment and personnel to do the screening and read the images[40]; population education and clinical breast examination (CBE) by CHW offers a feasible alternative (**Table 5**). This alternative was studied extensively in a cluster-randomized controlled screening-trial for cervix and breast cancer in Mumbai, India,[41] and found that CBE (with a 2-year interval and 8-year follow-up) was associated with good compliance in seeking treatment of screen-positive women.[42]

Cervical Cancer Screening

From health workers providing self-collection kits for human papillomavirus (HPV) testing to specially trained nurses performing visual inspection with acetic acid (VIA), cryotherapy and thermal ablation, cervical cancer screening and prevention is representative of the breadth and depth of TS/S,[43] which is critical, considering the large burden of cervical cancer globally and the disparities in cancer incidence, survival and treatment resources among socioeconomically disadvantaged women, especially in LMICs.[44,45]

In Ibadan, Nigeria, a total of 51 HCWs including doctors, nurses, community health extension workers (CHEWs), and community health officers (CHOs) were trained to screen for cervical cancer using VIA. In the subsequent 12 months, a total of 950 women were screened, close to 90% by the trained CHEWs and CHOs. A total of 63 women were rescreened for quality control and 88.1% of the women screened

Table 5
Examples of Task shifting and sharing in Obstetrics and Gynecology

Topic	Author (Year of Publication)	Study Type/Methodology/Control Group	Country	Cadre Shift from -> to	Health-Care Aspect	Impact Goal
Antenatal care	Deller,[55] 2015	Observational study	Mozambique	Nurses/Midwives -> CHW	HIV counseling and rapid diagnostic testing	Increased screening
	Deller[55] 2015	Observational study	Mozambique	Physicians -> maternal health nurses	Initiation and management of antiretroviral therapy	Increased access to care
	Deller[55] 2015	Observational study	Nigeria	Midwives and CHEWs -> Volunteer community distributors	Malaria prevention, medication, and bednet promotion	Increased prevention of malaria
	Deller[55] (2015)[55]	Observational study	South Africa	Physicians -> Nurses and midwives	Initiation and management of antiretroviral therapy	Increased access to care
	Deller[55] (2015)[55]	Observational study	Zambia	Nurses/midwives/laboratory personnel -> CHWs	HIV counseling and rapid diagnostic testing	Increased access to screening
	Jennings[56] (2011)[56]	Noninferiority study with direct observation and patient exit interviews	Benin	Midwives -> Nurse Aids	Birth counseling and birth preparedness was as effective and perceived well either done by midwife or well instructed nurse aids	Increased access to counseling

Ruizendaal[57] 2017	Observational study	Burkina Faso	Nurses/midwives -> CHW	Malaria screening and treatment in pregnancy	Increased access to screening and treatment of malaria
Ivers[58] 2011	Mixed qualitative/quantitative study	Haiti	Physicians -> Nurses and CHW	HIV counseling, screening and treatment initiation	Increased access to HIV care and less loss to follow up.
Deller[55] 2015	Mixed qualitative/quantitative study	Malawi	Community health nurses -> CHW	Antenatal care and newborn assessment.	Increased access to screening
Intrapartum care					
Deller[55] 2015	Observational	Malawi	Nurse Midwives -> Midwive technicians	Education in BEmONC	Increased access
Deller[55] 2015	Observational	Rwanda	Physicians (OBGYNs) -> Nurses and midwives	BEmONC including management of breech births	Increased competencies
Deller[55] 2015	Observational	Nigeria	Physicians and nurse midwives -> CHEWs	Clean and safe delivery BEmONC and FP counseling and services	Increased access

(continued on next page)

Table 5
(continued)

Topic	Author (Year of Publication)	Study Type/ Methodology/ Control Group	Country	Cadre Shift from —> to	Health-Care Aspect	Impact Goal
	Chilopora[59] 2007	Noninferiority outcome	Malawi	Medical Officers —> clinical officers (nonphysicians)	90% obstetric surgeries performed by nonphysicians with no major differences in postop outcomes compared with physicians	Increased access to CD
	Hounton[60] (2009)[60]	Descriptive study	Burkina Faso	OBGYNS —> clinical officers, surgical aids	Descriptive survey of records, qualitative interviews and cost-effectiveness analysis to increase EmOC	Increased access to Obstetric care
	Evans[30] 2009/ JHPIEGO[61] 2009	Pilot study and expansion program	India	OBGYNs —> MBBS (general medical doctors)	CEmONC coverage given by general doctors rather than specialized trained OBGYNs.	Increased access to Obstetric care

Study	Study type	Country	Task shift	Description	Outcome
Mavalanka[53] 2009	Observational	India	Anesthesiologist –> Medical officers	Evaluating a training program for anesthetic skills	Increased access to safe anesthesia
Deller[55] 2015	Observational	Nepal	Skilled birth attendants –> Female CHW	Community distribution of misoprostol for PPH prevention	Increased availability
Deller[55] 2015	Observational	Rwanda	Physicians and nurses –> CHWs	Community based postpartum hemorrhage prevention and family planning	Increased knowledge
Deller[55] 2015	Pilot study and expansion program	Afghanistan	Midwifes –> CHW	Distribution of misoprostol for PPH prevention	More access to misoprostol
Smith[62] 2013	Intergrated review of 18 programs	Many	Heath center/ hospital –> Community distribution	Community distribution of misoprostol for PPH prevention	Increased access, less hemorrhage and safety established
Gessessew[31] 2011	Quality control study	Ethiopia	Medical doctors –> clinical officers (non-physicians)	CEmONC comparable for trained clinical officers and medical officers	Increased access to CEmONC
McCord,[32] 2009	Quality control study	Tanzania		Obstetric surgeries done by nonphysician clinicians	Increased access to CEmONC

(continued on next page)

Table 5
(continued)

Topic	Author (Year of Publication)	Study Type/ Methodology/ Control Group	Country	Cadre Shift from -> to	Health-Care Aspect	Impact Goal
Family planning	Hoke[36] 2012	Observational study	Madagascar	Health professionals -> lay health workers (LHW)	Acceptability and effectiveness of injectable birth control	Increased access to family planning
	Deller[55] 2015	Pilot study and expansion program	Afghanistan	Midwifes -> CHW	Increased access to postpartum family planning	Increased access to family planning
	Deller[55] 2015	Observational study	Bangladesh	Facility-based health providers -> CHW	Increased access to postpartum family planning	Increased access to family planning
	Deller[55] 2015	Observational study	Kenya	OBGYNs -> Midwives	Postpartum family planning including IUD placements postpartum	Increased access to IUD
	Stanback[63] 2007	Noninferiority study	Uganda	Nurse/midwife -> CHW	Comparison of safety and quality of injections; safety guaranteed; and similar continuation rates	Increased access to Depo injections
	Mhlanga,[64] 2019	Noninferiority study	Multiple countries	Physicians -> Nonphycisians	IUD placement: safe and and expulsion rate nonsignificant different	Increased access to IUD

Category	Author/Year	Study type	Country	Task shifting	Findings	Outcome
Abortion/ miscarriage care	Dickson-Tetteh,[65] 2002	Observation and review of records	South Africa	Doctors -> Midwives	Trained midwives provided comprehensive/ safe abortion care (MVA) to 85 women	Increased access to abortion care
	Jejeebhoy,[37] 2011	Case control study: Doctor vs Nurses	India	Doctor -> Nurses	Counseling and manual vacuum aspirations for abortion care satisfactory when done by trained nurses	Increased counseling and abortion care access
	Nielsen[66] 2009	Observational study	Tanzania	Doctors -> Midlevel providers	Manual vacuum aspiration training and FP counseling for incomplete miscarriages	Increased access to comprehensive reproductive care
	Patel[67] 2009	Quantitative study	India	Midlevel providers -> CHW	Identify interest and barriers to training in early medical abortion	Increased understanding of health-care workers perspectives
	Warriner,[68] 2006	Case control study: Doctor vs Midlevel	Vietnam and South Africa	Doctor -> Midlevel provider	Evaluation of safety of first trimester MVA by midlevel providers	Increased access to comprehensive reproductive care
	Warriner,[69] 2011	Case control study: Doctor vs Midlevel	Nepal	Doctor -> RN and nurse-midwifes	Midlevel providers can safely and effectively provide MVAs in the first trimester	Increased access to comprehensive reproductive care
	Deller[55] 2015	Proof of concept	Guinea	Physicians -> Nurses/ midwives	Increased access to postabortion care	Increased access to comprehensive reproductive care

(continued on next page)

Table 5
(continued)

Topic	Author (Year of Publication)	Study Type/ Methodology/ Control Group	Country	Cadre Shift from --> to	Health-Care Aspect	Impact Goal
Breast cancer	Gutnick,[70] 2016]	Pilot program	Malawi	Doctors/Nurses --> Laywomen	Clinical breast examinations	Increased screening
	Mittra,[41] 2009	Randomized controlled study	India	Doctors/Nurses --> Primary health workers	Clinical breast examinations	Increased screening
	Pace,[71] 2016	Opinion paper/ review of literature	India, Sudan, China, Tanzania	Doctors --> community or volunteers	Clinical breast examinations	Increase in screening and some studies indicate increased finding of early-stage breast cancer but impact of CBE on survival not yet clear
	Donovan,[72] 2020	Literature review	Multiple	Doctors/nurses --> CHW	16 study review on CHW inclusion in breast cancer screening and treatment	Increased screening

Cervical cancer	Arrossi,[73] 2015	Randomized case control study	Argentina	Health-care visit -> Self-collection kit (as advised by CHW)	Women were randomly assigned to self-collection kits vs advice for a health clinic visit, uptake of screening increased with self-collection kit distribution	Increased screening
	Lazcano-Ponce,[74] 2011	Randomized case control	Mexico	Health-care visit vs Self-collection kits (as advised by nurses)	More uptake in screening with self-collection kits	Increased screening
	Awolude,[46] 2018	Observational and quality control study	Nigeria	Doctors -> CHEW and CHO	Visual inspection with acetic acid and cryotherapy	Increased treatment
	Shastri,[47] 2014	Cluster randomized controlled study	India	Doctors -> Midlevel providers	VIA-based cervical cancer screening and treatment	Increased treatment
	White,[48] 2017	Observational study	Kenya, Nigeria, Tanzania, Uganda, Zambia, and Zimbabwe	Integration of services with efforts from CHW and providers	Integration of cervical cancer screening and treatment with family planning	Increased access to family planning
	Mwanahamuntu,[49] 2013	Observational study	Ethiopia, Kenya, Malawi, Tanzania, Zambia, Zimbabwe	Integration of services with efforts from CHW and providers	Integration of cervical cancer screening and treatment with HIV services	Increased access to screening

(continued on next page)

Table 5 (*continued*)

Topic	Author (Year of Publication)	Study Type/ Methodology/ Control Group	Country	Cadre Shift from –> to	Health-Care Aspect	Impact Goal
	Deller[55] 2015	Observational study	Ghana	Physicians –> Nurses/ midwives	Cervical cancer screening with VIA, guidelines and treatment with cryotherapy	Increased access to screening and treatment
	Deller[55] 2015	Observational study	Thailand	Physicians –> Nurses	Cervical cancer screening with VIA, guidelines and treatment with cryotherapy	Increased access to screening and treatment
	Stulac[75] 2015	Observational	Rwanda	Nobody (since no OBGYNs available) –> General doctors and nurses	100 Doctors and 130 nurses at district hospitals were trained in cervical cancer diagnosis and treatment with VIA, cryotherapy, the loop electrosurgical excision procedure, and colposcopy	Increased access to screening and treatment
	Strother[76] 2013	Observational	Kenya	Nobody (since no OBGYNs available) –> Nurses	Palliative care is a nurse-driven service, as are the breast and	Increased access to screening and treatment

cervical screening programs, in which nurses have been trained in clinical breast examination, cervical visual inspection under acetic acid (VIA), and cryotherapy

Abbreviations: CBD, Community based distribution; CHEW, Community Health Extension Workers (used in Nigeria); CHW, community health workers; CME, continuing medical education; CO, clinical officer (3 y health program followed by internship); HIV, human immunodeficiency virus; LHW, lay health workers; LMICs, low and middle income countries; MO, medical officers (education includes medical school and some form of internship); NP, nurse practitioner; NPC, Nonphysician clinician; PA, physician assistant; PSP, nonspecialist physician; WHO, World Health Organization.

by CHEWs/CHOs and 92.3% of the women screened by nurses, agreed with expert team review.[46]

A cluster-randomized controlled study in Mumbai, India, found that VIA performed by trained midlevel providers significantly reduced cervical cancer mortality. It was estimated that this strategy could prevent 22,000 cervical cancer deaths in India and 72,600 deaths in resource-poor countries annually.[47]

Cervical cancer services have been combined with existing family planning programs, as well as integrated into HIV/AIDS programming in several countries, which has resulted in increased cervical cancer screening and prevention in those programs.[48,49] This integration was possible due to the sustained efforts of providers and community health educators to educate women in the community.

Fistula Care

Fistula care overall is a multidisciplinary enterprise involving most cadres of HCWs, as well as community involvement. Although it is unusual to have nonsurgeons involved in fistula surgery, Mulu Atesbaha is a passionately committed exception (**Box 3**).

Mulu's story is exceptional but not unheard of; however, currently the largest component of task shifting and sharing revolves around fistula prevention and removal of barriers to care. Primary prevention includes health promotion, encouraging planned pregnancies and birth spacing through counseling, contraception provision, and community awareness. Secondary prevention includes basic obstetric care with antenatal care, use of a skilled health birth attendant who can catheterize the bladder during labor if indicated and who is trained in the use of partograph to diagnose obstructed labor in a timely fashion and refer. Tertiary prevention of fistulas primarily includes timely and safe cesarean delivery by a trained/competent surgeon/obstetrician when obstructed labor occurs. Within these prevention strategies, many tasks can be shifted or shared to expand reach and decrease barriers to fistula care. Barriers to care for women with fistula are plentiful, and Tripathi and coworkers developed a strategy, which included multiple communication channels to disseminate fistula information to the population, followed by a fistula screening algorithm by community partners and barrier screening to assist women in accessing care.[50]

Fistula treatment encompasses much more than the surgical repair[51]; it involves a long stay away from home; due to past trauma and stigmatization many women need mental health care and resocialization; financial aid and skills are needed to be economically self-sustainable while undergoing (sometimes staged) repair and

---

Box 3
Mulu's fistula care commitment

Mulu is a health officer working on his master's degree in public health. With the mentoring of Dr Melaku Abraha, a seasoned gynecologist at the Mekelle Hamlin Fistula Center in Addis Ababa, Ethiopia, Mulu is learning to repair obstetric fistulas. He first encountered obstetric fistulas as an employee of the Ethiopian government, serving in the eastern Tigray region. The first woman with fistula whom he referred had lived with her obstetric fistula for 7 years, and surgical repair at Mekelle was a success. Seeing the transformation made possible by fistula repair, Mulu eagerly applied when he heard that there was a position open at the Fistula Center. Mulu got the job and learned about how to diagnose women with urinary incontinence, a bit about anesthesiology, and he began to learn about surgery by watching Dr Abraha perform fistula repairs. Now, Mulu is skilled enough to perform simple repairs himself, with Dr Abraha's guidance. As Mulu hones his skills over time, he will increase the capacity of the Mekelle Hamlin Fistula Center to provide fistula repairs.

treatment. There are many opportunities for TS/S roles and optimal outcomes are seen when working with local resource specialists and community workers.

Challenges to Task shifting and sharing

There are several challenges encountered with the implementation of TS/S programs. Problems have occurred when there is insufficient training or exposure before being responsible for providing certain procedures, such as cesarean deliveries[30] or neonatal care.[52] A need for continuing medical education in anesthesia was noted for nonspecialist physicians working in obstetrics.[53]

There are concerns regarding inadequate financial compensation and/or incentives for medical personnel to remain in a rural area, and low salaries for nonphysician clinicians may result in illicit fees to supplement income.[53] Incentives could include salary increases or entry into postgraduate health programs with possibilities for career advancement.[54]

Supervision of TS/S cadres in health care is a prerequisite but there is a need for improvement in this area.[52,53] In addition to onsite supervision and remote support for clinical tasks, coordination of placement based on skillset is important. Medical posts with anesthesia specialists or anesthesia trained clinicians were better in retaining their HCWs (physicians and nonphysicians) than programs where no anesthesia was available, since the physicians felt better supported in their study.[53]

Training fatigue and lack of receptiveness was noted by 15 participants who felt forced into EmOC training in India and did not perform any cesarean delivery after the training during the study period.[30] Compensation for training was frequently noted as too limited and did not compensate for time away from family and travel expenses, decreasing morale and attentiveness to the courses provided.

SUMMARY

Interprofessional care has long been a part of women's health care. From the first birth attended by an experienced relative or friend in a remote rural setting to the use of thermal ablation for high-grade cervical lesions, women's health care has always been a collaborative effort. This article has emphasized that there are many ways to create interprofessional care systems and that most systems rely on some form of task sharing or task shifting. Today this includes telemedicine with remote consultations and sharing of guidelines, expertise, or remote direction of certain procedures. Interprofessional care is providing care to an individual in an integrated system of professionals who share and shift the care given, depending on the individual and community need. It is hoped that interprofessional care in OB/GYN continues to thrive, from the community level to the most advanced health facilities, with an emphasis on expanding data driven evidence to promote excellence in women's health.

DISCLOSURE

None of the authors of this article has any financial conflicts of interest. The article was written without financial compensation.

REFERENCES

1. Haynes AB, Weiser TG, Berry WR, et al. A Surgical Safety Checklist to Reduce Morbidity and Mortality in a Global Population. N Engl J Med 2009;360(5):491–9.

2. WHO, Recommendations for Optimizing Health Worker. Roles to improve access to key maternal and newborn health interventions through task shifting. Geneva World Health Organization; 2012.

3. The new Humanitarian 2010. Africa Ten countries desperately seeking doctors available via. Last checked 4/10/2022. Available at: https://www.thenewhumanitarian.org/report/89186/Africa-ten-countries-desperately-seeking-doctors.

4. Hart-Hester Susan, Thomas Charlotte. Access to Health Care Professionals in Rural Mississippi. South. Medical Journal (Birmingham, Ala 2003;96(2):149–54.

5. Chen FM, Fordyce MA, Andes S, Hart LG. U.S. Rural Physician Workforce: Analysis of Medical School Graduates from 198801997. WWAMI: the rural health working Paper Series 2008.

6. Zurn P, Dal Poz MR, Stilwell B, et al. Imbalance in the health workforce. Hum Resour Health 2004;2:13. https://doi.org/10.1186/1478-4491-2-13.

7. Dussault G, Franceschini MC. Not enough there, too many here: understanding geographical imbalances in the distribution of the health workforce. Hum Resour Health 2006;4:12. https://doi.org/10.1186/1478-4491-4-12.

8. Dolea Carmen, Stormont Laura, Braichet Jean-Marc. Evaluated Strategies to Increase Attraction and Retention of Health Workers in Remote and Rural Areas. Bull World Health Organ 2010;88(5):379–85.

9. Grobler L, Marais BJ, Mabunda SA, et al. Interventions for increasing the proportion of health professionals practising in rural and other underserved areas. Cochrane Database Syst Rev 2009;1:CD005314.

10. World Health Organization. International nurse mobility : trends and policy implications/by James Buchan, Tina Parkin, Julie Sochalski. World Health Organization. 2003. Available at: https://apps.who.int/iris/handle/10665/68061.

11. Msidi ED, Sinkala M, Bositis A, et al. The Zambian HIV nurse practitioner diploma program: preliminary outcomes from first cohort of zambian nurses. Int J Nurs Education Scholarship 2011;8:1–19.

12. Falk R. Surgical Task-Sharing to Non-Specialist Physicians in Low-Resource Settings Globally: A Systematic Review of the Literature. World J Surg 2020;44(5):1368–86.

13. Sani R, Nameoua B, Yahaya A, et al. The Impact of Launching Surgery at the District Level in Niger. World J Surg 2009;33(10):2063–8.

14. Wren Sherry M, Kushner AL. Task Shifting in Surgery—What US Health Care Can Learn From Ghana. JAMA Surg 2019;154(9):860.

15. Courtenay M. Nurse prescribing and community practitioners. J Fam Health Care 2010;20(3):78–80. PMID: 20695351.

16. Lack A, Saddik M, Engels P, et al. The emergence of the physician assistant role in a Canadian acute care surgery setting. Can J Surg 2020;63(5):E442–8.

17. Ishikawa M. Current state and future direction of task shifting in obstetric and gynecological care: A survey of obstetrician-gynecologists across Japan. Medicine (Baltimore) 2022;101(2):e28467. https://doi.org/10.1097/MD.0000000000028467.

18. WHO Framework for action on interprofessional education & collaborative practice. World Health Organization. 2010. Available at: http://www.who.int/hrh/nursing_midwifery/en/Last checked: 3/30/2022; https://hsc.unm.edu/ipe/resources/who-framework-.pdf.

19. Steffen Ann M. Antonette M. Zeiss, and Michele Karel, 'Interprofessional Geriatric Healthcare: Competencies and Resources for Teamwork. In: Pachana Nancy A, Laidlaw Ken, editors. The Oxford Handbook of clinical Geropsychology. online edn. Oxford Library of Psychology; 2014. https://doi.org/10.1093/oxfordhb/9780199663170.013.021. Oxford Academic.

20. Schaefer L. Task sharing implant insertion by community health workers: not just can it work, but how might it work practically and with impact in the real world. Glob Health Sci Pract 2015;3(3):327–9. https://doi.org/10.9745/GHSP-D-15-00230.

21. Fisher EB, Ballesteros J, Bhushan N, et al. Key Features Of Peer Support In Chronic Disease Prevention And Management. Health Aff (Millwood) 2015;34:1523–30.

22. Fisher EB, Boothroyd RI, Elstad EA, et al. Peer support of complex health behaviors in prevention and disease management with special reference to diabetes: systematic reviews. Clin Diabetes Endocrinol 2017;3:4.

23. Kaunonen M, Hannula L, Tarkka MT. A systematic review of peer support interventions for breastfeeding. J Clin Nurs 2012;21(13–14):1943–54.

24. Rosen MA, DiazGranados D, Dietz AS, et al. Teamwork in healthcare: Key discoveries enabling safer, high-quality care. Am Psychol 2018;73(4):433–50.

25. Beard JH, Ohene-Yeboah M, Tabiri S, et al. Outcomes After Inguinal Hernia Repair With Mesh Performed by Medical Doctors and Surgeons in Ghana. JAMA Surg 2019;154(9):853–9.

26. Taylor MJ, McNicholas C, Nicolay C, et al. Systematic review of the application of the plan–do–study–act method to improve quality in healthcare. BMJ Qual Saf 2014;23:290–8.

27. Penchansky R, Thomas JW. The concept of access: definition and relationship to consumer satisfaction. Med Care 1981;19(2):127–40.

28. World Health Organization, United Nations Population Fund, Mailman school of public health. Averting maternal death and Disability & United Nations Children's Fund (UNICEF) (2009). Monitoring emergency obstetric care : a handbook. World Health Organization. Available at: https://apps.who.int/iris/handle/10665/44121.

29. Wall SN, Lee AC, Carlo W, et al. Reducing intrapartum-related neonatal deaths in low- and middle-income countries–what works? Semin Perinatol 2010;34(6):395–407.

30. Evans CL, Maine D, McCloskey L, et al. Where there is no obstetrician—increasing capacity for emergency obstetric care in rural India: an evaluation of a pilot program to train general doctors. Int J Gynecol Obstet 2009;107:277–82.

31. Gessessew A, Barnabas GA, Prata N, et al. Task shifting and sharing in Tigray, Ethiopia, to achieve comprehensive emergency obstetric care. Int J Gynecol Obstet 2011;113(1):28–31.

32. McCord C, Mbaruku G, Pereira C, et al. The quality of emergency obstetrical surgery by assistant medical officers in Tanzanian district hospitals. Health Aff (Millwood) 2009;28(5):w876–85.

33. Matinhure S, Chimbari MJ. Barriers and enablers to task shifting for Caesarean sections in sub-Saharan Africa: A scoping review. Afr J Reprod Health 2019; 23:149–60. https://doi.org/10.29063/ajrh2019/v23i3.13.

34. WHO Task sharing to improve access to Family Planning/Contraception. World Health Organization; 2018. Available via: https://www.who.int/publications/i/item/WHO-RHR-17.20 last checked 4/10/2022.

35. Duvall S, Thurston S, Weinberger M, et al. Scaling up delivery of contraceptive implants in sub-Saharan Africa: operational experiences of Marie Stopes International. Glob Health Sci Pract 2014;2(1):72–92. https://doi.org/10.9745/GHSP-D-13-00116. PMID: 25276564; PMCID: PMC4168608.

36. Hoke TH, Wheeler SB, Lynd K, et al. Community-based provision of injectable contraceptives in Madagascar: 'task shifting' to expand access to injectable contraceptives. Health Policy Plan 2012;27:52–9.

37. Jejeebhoy SJ, Kalyanwala S, Zavier AJF, et al. Can nurses perform manual vacuum aspiration (MVA) as safely and effectively as physicians? Evidence from India. Contraception 2011;84:615–21.

38. Mehrtash H, Kim CR, Ganatra B, et al. What's needed to improve safety and quality of abortion care: reflections from WHO/HRP Multi-Country Study on Abortion across the sub-Saharan Africa and Latin America and Caribbean regions. BMJ Glob Health 2021;6:e007226. https://doi.org/10.1136/bmjgh-2021-007226.

39. Harford E Azavedo, Fischietto M. Guideline implementation for breast healthcare in low- and middle-income countries: breast healthcare program resource allocation. Cancer 2008;113(S8):2282–96.

40. Wadler BM, Judge CM, Prout M, et al. Improving Breast Cancer Control via the Use of Community Health Workers in South Africa: A Critical Review. J Oncol 2011;2011:1–82011.

41. Mittra I, Mishra GA, Singh S, et al. A cluster randomized, controlled trial of breast and cervix cancer screening in Mumbai, India: methodology and interim results after three rounds of screening. Int J Cancer 2010;126:976–84.

42. Dinshaw K, Mishra G, Shastri S, et al. Determinants of compliance in a cluster randomised controlled trial on screening of breast and cervix cancer in mumbai, India. 2. Compliance to referral and treatment. Oncology 2007;73(3–4):154–61. https://doi.org/10.1159/000126498.

43. Dawson AJ, Buchan J, Duffield C, et al. Task shifting and sharing in maternal and reproductive health in low-income countries: a narrative synthesis of current evidence. Health Policy Plan 2014;29(3):396–408.

44. Sung H, Ferlay J, Siegel RL, et al. Global Cancer Statistics 2020: GLOBOCAN Estimates of Incidence and Mortality Worldwide for 36 Cancers in 185 Countries. CA Cancer J Clin 2021;71(3):209–49.

45. Ginsburg O, Bray F, Coleman MP, et al. The global burden of women's cancers: a grand challenge in global health. Lancet 2017;389(10071):847–60.

46. Awolude OA, Oyerinde SO, Akinyemi JO. Screen and Triage by Community Extension Workers to Facilitate Screen and Treat: Task-Sharing Strategy to Achieve Universal Coverage for Cervical Cancer Screening in Nigeria. J Glob Oncol 2018;4:1–10.

47. Shastri Aditi, Srinivas Shastri Surenda. Cancer Screening and Prevention in Low-Resource Settings. Nat Rev Cancer 2014;14(12):822–9.

48. White HL, Meglioli A, Chowdhury R, et al. Integrating cervical cancer screening and preventive treatment with family planning and HIV-related services. Int J Gynaecol Obstet 2017;138(Suppl 1):41–6.

49. Mwanahamuntu MH, Sahasrabuddhe VV, Blevins M, et al. Utilization of cervical cancer screening services and trends in screening positivity rates in a 'screen-and-treat' program integrated with HIV/AIDS care in Zambia. PLoS One 2013;8(9):e74607.

50. Tripathi Vandana, Arnoff Elly, Sripad Pooja. Removing barriers to fistula care: Applying appreciative inquiry to improve access to screening and treatment in Nigeria and Uganda. Health Care Women Int 2020;41(5):584–99.

51. Watt MH, Mosha MV, Platt AC, et al. A nurse-delivered mental health intervention for obstetric fistula patients in Tanzania: results of a pilot randomized controlled trial. Pilot Feasibility Stud 2017;3:35.

52. Cumbi A, Pereira C, Malalane R, et al. Major surgery delegation to mid-level health practitioners in Mozambique: health professionals' perceptions. Hum Resour Health 2007;5:27.

53. Mavalankar D, Callahan K, Sriram V, et al. Where there is no anesthetist— increasing capacity for emergency obstetric care in rural India: an evaluation of a pilot program to train general doctors. Int J Gynecol Obstet 2009;107:283–8.

54. De Brouwere V, Dieng T, Diadhiou M, et al. Task shifting for emergency obstetric surgery in district hospitals in Senegal. Reprod Health Matters 2009;17:32–44.

55. Deller B, Tripathi V, Stender S, et al. Task shifting in maternal and newborn health care: key components from policy to implementation. Int J Gynaecol Obstet 2015; 130(Suppl 2):S25–31.

56. Jennings L, Yebadokpo AS, Affo J, et al. Task shifting in maternal and newborn care: a non-inferiority study examining delegation of antenatal counseling to lay nurse aides supported by job aids in Benin. Implementation Sci 2011;6. https://doi.org/10.1186/1748-5908-6-2.

57. Ruizendaal E, Schallig HDFH, Scott S, et al. Evaluation of Malaria Screening during Pregnancy with Rapid Diagnostic Tests Performed by Community Health Workers in Burkina Faso. Am J Trop Med Hyg 2017;97(4):1190–7.

58. Ivers LC, Jerome JG, Cullen KA, et al. Task-shifting in HIV care: a case study of nurse-centered community-based care in rural Haiti. PLoS One 2011;6:e19276.

59. Chilopora G, Pereira C, Kamwendo F, et al. Postoperative outcome of caesarean sections and other major emergency obstetric surgery by clinical officers and medical officers in Malawi. Hum Resour Health 2007;5:17.

60. Hounton S, Newlands D, Meda N, et al. A cost-effectiveness study of caesarean-section deliveries by clinical officers, general practitioners and obstetricians in Burkina Faso. Hum Resour Health 2009;7:34.

61. Jhpiego. Strengthening the provision of high-quality emergency obstetric and newborn care services in India in collaboration with the Federation of obstetric and Gynaecological Societies of India and the Indian College of obstetrics and Gynaecology Jhpiego annual Report March 2007–February 2009. 2009. Baltimore, (MD): Jhpiego; 2009.

62. Smith JM, Gubin R, Holston MM, et al. Misoprostol for postpartum hemorrhage prevention at home birth: an integrative review of global implementation experience to date. BMC Pregnancy Childbirth 2013;13:44.

63. Stanback J, Mbonye AK, Bekiita M. Contraceptive injections by community health workers in Uganda: a nonrandomized community trial. Bull World Health Organ 2007;85(10):768–73.

64. Mhlanga FG. Feasibility and Safety of IUD Insertion by Mid-Level Providers in Sub-Saharan Africa. Int Perspect Sex Reprod Health 2019;45(1):61–9.

65. Dickson-Tetteh K, Billings DL. Abortion care services provided by registered midwives in South Africa. Int Fam Plan Perspect 2002;28:144.

66. Nielsen K, Lusiola G, Kanama J, et al. Expanding comprehensive postabortion care to primary health facilities in Geita District, Tanzania. Afr J Reprod Health 2009;13:129–38.

67. Patel L, Bennett TA, Halpern CT, et al. Support for provision of early medical abortion by mid-level providers in Bihar and Jharkhand, India. Reprod Health Matters 2009;17:70–9.

68. Warriner IK, Meirik O, Hoffman M, et al. Rates of complication in first-trimester manual vacuum aspiration abortion done by doctors and mid-level providers in South Africa and Vietnam: a randomised controlled equivalence trial. Lancet 2006;368:1965–72.

69. Warriner IK, Wang D, Huong NT, et al. Can midlevel health-care providers administer early medical abortion as safely and effectively as doctors? A randomised controlled equivalence trial in Nepal. Lancet 2011;377:1155–61.

70. Gutnik L, Moses A, Stanley C, et al. From Community Laywomen to Breast Health Workers: A Pilot Training Model to Implement Clinical Breast Exam Screening in Malawi. PLOS ONE 2016;11(3):e0151389.

71. Pace EL, Shulman LN. Breast Cancer in Sub-Saharan Africa: Challenges and Opportunities to Reduce Mortality. Oncologist 2016;21(6):739–44.
72. O'Donovan J, Newcomb A, MacRae MC, et al. Community health workers and early detection of breast cancer in low-income and middle-income countries: a systematic scoping review of the literature. BMJ Glob Health 2020;5(5). e002466.
73. Arrossi S, Thouyaret L, Herrero R, et al. EMA Study team. Effect of self-collection of HPV DNA offered by community health workers at home visits on uptake of screening for cervical cancer (the EMA study): a population-based cluster-randomised trial. Lancet Glob Health 2015;3(2). e85–94.
74. Lazcano-Ponce E, Lorincz AT, Cruz-Valdez A, et al. Self-collection of vaginal specimens for human papillomavirus testing in cervical cancer prevention (MARCH): a community-based randomised controlled trial. Lancet 2011; 378(9806):1868–73. https://doi.org/10.1016/S0140-6736(11)61522-5.
75. Stulac S, Binagwaho A, Tapela NM, et al. Capacity building for oncology programmes in sub-Saharan Africa: The Rwanda experience. Lancet Oncol 2015; 16:e405–13.
76. Strother RM, Asirwa FC, Busakhala NB, et al. AMPATH-Oncology: A model for comprehensive cancer care in sub-Saharan Africa. J Cancer Policy 2013; 1(3–4):e42–8.

UNITED STATES POSTAL SERVICE®
Statement of Ownership, Management, and Circulation (All Periodicals Publications Except Requester Publications)

1. Publication Title	2. Publication Number	3. Filing Date
OBSTETRICS AND GYNECOLOGY CLINICS OF NORTH AMERICA	000 – 276	9/18/2022

4. Issue Frequency	5. Number of Issues Published Annually	6. Annual Subscription Price
MAR, JUN, SEP, DEC	4	$345.00

7. Complete Mailing Address of Known Office of Publication (Not printer) (Street, city, county, state, and ZIP+4®)

ELSEVIER INC.
230 Park Avenue, Suite 800
New York, NY 10169

Contact Person: Malathi Samayan
Telephone (Include area code): 91-44-4299-4507

8. Complete Mailing Address of Headquarters or General Business Office of Publisher (Not printer)

ELSEVIER INC.
230 Park Avenue, Suite 800
New York, NY 10169

9. Full Names and Complete Mailing Addresses of Publisher, Editor, and Managing Editor (Do not leave blank)

Publisher (Name and complete mailing address)

DOLORES MELONI, ELSEVIER INC.
1600 JOHN F KENNEDY BLVD. SUITE 1800
PHILADELPHIA, PA 19103-2899

Editor (Name and complete mailing address)

KERRY HOLLAND, ELSEVIER INC.
1600 JOHN F KENNEDY BLVD. SUITE 1800
PHILADELPHIA, PA 19103-2899

Managing Editor (Name and complete mailing address)

PATRICK MANLEY, ELSEVIER INC.
1600 JOHN F KENNEDY BLVD. SUITE 1800
PHILADELPHIA, PA 19103-2899

10. Owner (Do not leave blank. If the publication is owned by a corporation, give the name and address of the corporation immediately followed by the names and addresses of all stockholders owning or holding 1 percent or more of the total amount of stock. If not owned by a corporation, give the names and addresses of the individual owners. If owned by a partnership or other unincorporated firm, give its name and address as well as those of each individual owner. If the publication is published by a nonprofit organization, give its name and address.)

Full Name	Complete Mailing Address
WHOLLY OWNED SUBSIDIARY OF REED/ELSEVIER, US HOLDINGS	1600 JOHN F KENNEDY BLVD. SUITE 1800 PHILADELPHIA, PA 19103-2899

11. Known Bondholders, Mortgagees, and Other Security Holders Owning or Holding 1 Percent or More of Total Amount of Bonds, Mortgages, or Other Securities. If none, check box ▶ ☐ None

Full Name	Complete Mailing Address
N/A	

12. Tax Status (For completion by nonprofit organizations authorized to mail at nonprofit rates) (Check one)
The purpose, function, and nonprofit status of this organization and the exempt status for federal income tax purposes:
☒ Has Not Changed During Preceding 12 Months
☐ Has Changed During Preceding 12 Months (Publisher must submit explanation of change with this statement)

PS Form 3526, July 2014 [Page 1 of 4 (see instructions page 4)] PSN: 7530-01-000-9631   PRIVACY NOTICE: See our privacy policy on www.usps.com.

---

13. Publication Title	14. Issue Date for Circulation Data Below
OBSTETRICS AND GYNECOLOGY CLINICS OF NORTH AMERICA	JUNE 2022

15. Extent and Nature of Circulation			Average No. Copies Each Issue During Preceding 12 Months	No. Copies of Single Issue Published Nearest to Filing Date
a. Total Number of Copies (Net press run)			215	172
b. Paid Circulation (By Mail and Outside the Mail)	(1)	Mailed Outside-County Paid Subscriptions Stated on PS Form 3541 (Include paid distribution above nominal rate, advertiser's proof copies, and exchange copies)	54	45
	(2)	Mailed In-County Paid Subscriptions Stated on PS Form 3541 (Include paid distribution above nominal rate, advertiser's proof copies, and exchange copies)	0	0
	(3)	Paid Distribution Outside the Mails Including Sales Through Dealers and Carriers, Street Vendors, Counter Sales, and Other Paid Distribution Outside USPS®	109	91
	(4)	Paid Distribution by Other Classes of Mail Through the USPS (e.g., First-Class Mail®)	0	0
c. Total Paid Distribution (Sum of 15b (1), (2), (3), and (4))		▶	163	136
d. Free or Nominal Rate Distribution (By Mail and Outside the Mail)	(1)	Free or Nominal Rate Outside-County Copies included on PS Form 3541	34	17
	(2)	Free or Nominal Rate In-County Copies Included on PS Form 3541	0	0
	(3)	Free or Nominal Rate Copies Mailed at Other Classes Through the USPS (e.g., First-Class Mail)	0	0
	(4)	Free or Nominal Rate Distribution Outside the Mail (Carriers or other means)	34	17
e. Total Free or Nominal Rate Distribution (Sum of 15d (1), (2), (3) and (4))		▶	34	17
f. Total Distribution (Sum of 15c and 15e)		▶	197	153
g. Copies not Distributed (See Instructions to Publishers #4 (page #3))		▶	18	19
h. Total (Sum of 15f and g)		▶	215	172
i. Percent Paid (15c divided by 15f times 100)			82.74%	88.88%

* If you are claiming electronic copies, go to line 16 on page 3. If you are not claiming electronic copies, skip to line 17 on page 3.

PS Form 3526, July 2014 (Page 2 of 4)

16. Electronic Copy Circulation	Average No. Copies Each Issue During Preceding 12 Months	No. Copies of Single Issue Published Nearest to Filing Date
a. Paid Electronic Copies ▶		
b. Total Paid Print Copies (Line 15c) + Paid Electronic Copies (Line 16a) ▶		
c. Total Print Distribution (Line 15f) + Paid Electronic Copies (Line 16a) ▶		
d. Percent Paid (Both Print & Electronic Copies) (16b divided by 16c × 100) ▶		

☒ I certify that 50% of all my distributed copies (electronic and print) are paid above a nominal price.

17. Publication of Statement of Ownership

☒ If the publication is a general publication, publication of this statement is required. Will be printed   ☐ Publication not required.
in the DECEMBER 2022 issue of this publication.

18. Signature and Title of Editor, Publisher, Business Manager, or Owner

Malathi Samayan - Distribution Controller

Malathi Samayan   Date 9/18/2022

I certify that all information furnished on this form is true and complete. I understand that anyone who furnishes false or misleading information on this form or who omits material or information requested on the form may be subject to criminal sanctions (including fines and imprisonment) and/or civil sanctions (including civil penalties).

PS Form 3526, July 2014 (Page 3 of 4)   PRIVACY NOTICE: See our privacy policy on www.usps.com

Printed and bound by CPI Group (UK) Ltd, Croydon, CR0 4YY

08/05/2025

01864723-0004